W9-BLC-329

Prenatal care: effectiveness and implementation

This book evaluates the effectiveness of prenatal care interventions and provides a framework for prenatal care that looks beyond the limited perspective of immediate neonatal outcomes. Ultimately, this book seeks to improve the content and the implementation of prenatal care by shifting the focus away from short-term technocentric medical advances to concentrate on the broader public health issues. A unique aspect of this book is its focus on the effectiveness of prenatal care interventions on longer-term benefits for women's and children's health. Traditional medical interventions, as well as social support and behavioral interventions during prenatal care, are reviewed. Effectiveness is considered within the context of its implications for public policy and service delivery.

This book is an important resource for maternal and child health professionals, policy makers and health care managers because it provides a thorough discussion of the practice and potential of prenatal care services for improving the long-term health of women and children.

Prenatal care

Effectiveness and Implementation

Edited by

Marie C. McCormick

Harvard School of Public Health, Boston, Massachusetts
www.hsph.harvard.edu/children

and

Joanna E. Siegel

Arlington Health Foundation,
Arlington, Virginia

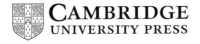

CAMBRIDGE
UNIVERSITY PRESS

PUBLISHED BY THE PRESS SYNDICATE OF THE UNIVERSITY OF CAMBRIDGE
The Pitt Building, Trumpington Street, Cambridge, United Kingdom

CAMBRIDGE UNIVERSITY PRESS
The Edinburgh Building, Cambridge CB2 2RU, UK www.cup.cam.ac.uk
40 West 20th Street, New York, NY 10011–4211, USA www.cup.org
10 Stamford Road, Oakleigh, Melbourne 3166, Australia
Ruiz de Alarcón 13, 28014 Madrid, Spain

© Cambridge University Press 1999

This book is in copyright. Subject to statutory exception
and to the provisions of relevant collective licensing agreements,
no reproduction of any part may take place without
the written permission of Cambridge University Press.

First published 1999

Printed in the United Kingdom at the University Press, Cambridge

Typeset in Minion 10.5/14pt [v n]

A catalogue record for this book is available from the British Library

ISBN 0 521 66196 X paperback

Every effort has been made in preparing this book to provide accurate and up-to-date information which
is in accord with accepted standards and practice at the time of publication. Nevertheless, the authors,
editors and publisher can make no warranties that the information contained herein is totally free from
error, not least because clinical standards are constantly changing through research and regulation. The
authors, editors and publisher therefore disclaim all liability for direct or consequential damages resulting
from the use of material contained in this book. Readers are strongly advised to pay careful attention to
information provided by the manufacturer of any drugs or equipment that they plan to use.

Contents

Contributors

Peter Bernstein, MD, MPH
Assistant Professor
Department of Obstetrics and Gynecology
and Women's Health
Albert Einstein College of Medicine
Bronx, New York

Marisa Brett, MD
Resident
Children's Hospital, Boston and
Boston Medical Center
Boston, Massachusetts

Wendy Chavkin, MD, MPH
Associate Professor of Public Health and
Obstetrics and Gynecology
Center for Population and Family Health
Columbia University School of Public
Health
New York, New York

James J. Crall, DDS, ScD
Department of Pediatric Dentistry
University of Connecticut Health Center
Farmington, Connecticut

Mark I. Evans, MD
Director, Division of Reproductive Genetics
Department of Obstetrics and Gynecology
Wayne State University
Detroit, Michigan

**Lisa M. Garceau, CNM, MSN, PhD
candidate**
Johns Hopkins School of Hygiene and
Public Health
Baltimore, Maryland

Robert L. Goldenberg, MD
Professor and Chair
Department of Obstetrics and Gynecology
University of Alabama at Birmingham
Birmingham, Alabama

Linda J. Heffner, MD, PhD
Associate Professor of Obstetrics and
Gynecology and Reproductive Biology
Harvard Medical School
Director of Maternal Fetal Medicine
Brigham and Women's Hospital
Boston, Massachusetts

Mark P. Johnson, MD
Associate Professor, Obstetrics, Gynecology,
Molecular Medicine and Genetics, and
Pathology
Wayne State University
Detroit, Michigan

Lorraine V. Klerman, DrPH
Professor and Chair
Department of Maternal and Child Health
University of Alabama at Birmingham
School of Public Health
Birmingham, Alabama

Ralph L. Kramer, MD
Fellow
Wayne State University
Detroit, Michigan

Marie C. McCormick, MD, ScD
Director, Harvard Center for Children's
Health
Chair, Department of Maternal and Child
Health
Harvard School of Public Health
Professor of Pediatrics
Harvard Medical School
Boston, Massachusetts

Jacques Milliez, MD
Professor
Service de Gynécologie-Obstétrique
Hôpital Saint-Antoine
Paris, France

Kathleen G. Nelson, MD
Professor of Pediatrics and Associate Dean
for Students
University of Alabama School of Medicine
Birmingham, Alabama

Lisa L. Paine, CNM, DrPH
Associate Professor of Obstetrics and
Gynecology
Boston University School of Medicine
Associate Professor of Public Health and
Chair, Department of Maternal and Child
Health
Boston University School of Public Health
Boston, Massachusetts

Richard B. Parad, MD, MPH
Instructor in Pediatrics
Harvard Medical School
Joint Program in Neonatology, Brigham and
Women's Hospital
Boston, Massachusetts

Lisa M. Pastore, PhD
Post Doctoral Fellow
Department of Epidemiology
University of North Carolina School of
Public Health
Chapel Hill, North Carolina

Kathleen Maher Rasmussen, ScD, RD
Professor, Division of Nutritional Sciences
Cornell University
Ithaca, New York

Dwight J. Rouse, MD
Assistant Professor
Department of Obstetrics and Gynecology
University of Alabama at Birmingham
Birmingham, Alabama

David A. Savitz, PhD
Professor and Chair
Department of Epidemiology
University of North Carolina School of
Public Health
Chapel Hill, North Carolina

Joanna E. Siegel, ScD
Director of Evaluation
Arlington Health Foundation
Arlington, Virginia

Joan M. Stoler, MD
Instructor in Pediatrics
Harvard Medical School
Assistant in Pediatrics, Genetics and
Teratology Unit
Massachusetts General Hospital
Boston, Massachusetts

Phillip G. Stubblefield, MD
Professor and Chair
Department of Obstetrics and Gynecology
Boston University School of Medicine
Chief of Obstetrics and Gynecology
Boston Medical Center
Boston, Massachusetts

Paul H. Wise, MD, MPH
Director of Social and Health Policy
Research
Department of Pediatrics
Boston Medical Center
Associate Professor
Boston University School of Medicine
Boston, Massachusetts

Yuval Yaron, MD
Fellow, Reproductive Genetics
Wayne State University
Detroit, Michigan

Foreword

Lisa A. Simpson, MB, BCH, MPH and Carolyn M. Clancy, MD

The Agency for Health Care Policy and Research (AHCPR) holds the main responsibility at the federal level for examining the relationship between how health care is organized, financed, and delivered and the care outcomes and health of those it is intended to serve. Since its inception, AHCPR has struggled to balance the need for rigorous research that addresses the question of what works with the impatience of all stakeholders in the health care system for solutions rather than ever more refined questions. Increased demands by public policy makers, health systems leaders, and even patients for better evidence to inform decisions at all levels of health care delivery is exciting – but also creates an unprecedented opportunity and challenge to the research community, and underscores the lacunae in the knowledge base supporting many areas of health care delivery. It was in recognition of this opportunity that AHCPR supported the conference that formed the basis for this book on the practice and the potential of prenatal care.

Research on effectiveness and cost-effectiveness can and does affect health policy. In 1985, the Institute of Medicine published *Preventing Low Birthweight*, a work often cited as the prime example of the impact research can have. The finding that every dollar spent on providing more adequate prenatal care for low-income, poorly educated women could reduce medical expenditures by $3.38 in the first year of the baby's life was a potent stimulus for subsequent policies that expanded Medicaid benefits for pregnant women and children. Providing early and adequate prenatal care has subsequently become a sentinel indicator for the success of public health and private care systems, whether at the local, state, or national level. The Healthy People initiatives and the HEDIS reporting requirements are two noteworthy examples. It is no wonder, then, that recent challenges to the evidence base underlying the premise – and the promise – of prenatal care have been presented cautiously. Many fear that asking hard questions, and finding too few hard answers, may reverse this Nation's incremental progress toward improving the health of women and children.

However, as the leaders of this conference recognized, failure to address the issues discussed here may obscure opportunities to understand which interventions are most effective in reducing preterm delivery as well as infant morbidity and mortality – and for which populations. In addition, a narrow focus on medical services included within standard definitions of prenatal care limits opportunities to consider how prenatal care fits within and complements women's health needs across the lifespan. Women's health care has historically been fragmented in the U.S., with reproductive needs juxtaposed with "all other" health care services. This book represents an important effort to challenge researchers and all others who have a stake in the health of families to reconsider both the questions and the possible solutions, and additionally, to motivate the research community to focus on areas where our knowledge base remains deficient.

We salute the conference organizers and participants for accepting these challenges. We are hopeful that readers of this book will assist AHCPR in its efforts to identify opportunities for translating research into practice and policy, and then to report on the impact of the changes that have been brought about. As John Eisenberg has said, it is not enough just to publish. It is our highest hope and expectation that this book represents a first of many steps to reconceptualize and redesign prenatal care within a broader context of women's health needs.

Acknowledgments

In June 1997, the Harvard Center for Children's Health and the Department of Maternal and Child Health at the Harvard School of Public Health hosted a conference examining prenatal care and its impact on the health of women and children. The conference, which was the genesis of this book, brought together researchers and practitioners in pediatrics and women's health to analyze the evidence linking prenatal interventions to improved health outcomes for women and children. For their contributions to the conference and ultimately to this book, we owe our sincere thanks to many individuals and organizations.

First and foremost, we would like to thank the Agency for Health Care Policy and Research (AHCPR) for their financial support of the conference. We are especially grateful to Heddy Hubbard and Denise Dougherty at AHCPR for their guidance and support. Additional financial support from the Massachusetts Chapter of the March of Dimes and Ross Laboratories made it possible for several health professionals from community-based organizations to attend the conference.

In planning the conference, we convened an Advisory Committee to help us refine the scope and content of the program. We are indebted to the members of this committee, Judyann Bigby, Jennifer Haas, Jody Heymann, Lorraine Klerman, Alan Leviton, Ellice Lieberman, and James Perrin, for their valuable insights and advice. We also thank Julie Henry who, as Chair of the Advisory Council for the Harvard Center for Children's Health, provided behind-the-scenes encouragement and practical advice throughout the process.

We wish to express our gratitude to the invited authors and their co-authors, who generously gave of their time and effort. These individuals are leaders in their fields, and we feel privileged to include their writing in this volume. Several other individuals served as discussants and invited speakers at the conference: Florence Haseltine, Claudia Holzman, Woodie Kessel, Mark Klebanoff, Deborah Klein Walker, Milton Kotelchuch, Evelyn Murphy, and Susan Pauker. Their stimulating presentations, comments and insights are also reflected in this book. For her role in preparing the reference sections of the manuscript, we also owe our thanks to Patricia Schmieg.

Finally, we wish to thank two individuals who were instrumental to the success of this project. Deborah DuFault Denhart served as project manager for the conference and the preparation of this book. In addition to managing countless details, she helped keep the book true to its vision. We are also deeply indebted to Anne Brown Rodgers for her careful, thoughtful, and professional editing of this manuscript. Her talents and good humor kept this book on track through its many revisions, and her contributions greatly influenced the quality of the final product. We have been very fortunate to work with such talented individuals.

Introduction

Over the past 30 years, the United States has experienced a major decrease in infant mortality, especially mortality in the neonatal period. Despite this dramatic change, the United States remains at a very disadvantaged position among industrialized countries when they are ranked by infant mortality rate. This situation reflects the conjunction of two trends. The first is the increasing technological sophistication and success of perinatal services in sustaining the survival of ever tinier infants (Richardson et al., 1998). The second trend, which offsets the first, is the persistence of high rates of low birth weight and prematurity, and even increases in rates of such births among African Americans. Another contributing factor is the persistence of a steady rate of major congenital malformations. Despite the fact that most industrialized countries experience similar malformation rates, they have been able to reduce the percentage of preterm deliveries while also incorporating technological interventions into the care of those who are born prematurely (Guyer et al., 1996).

The strategy that has been advocated to reduce the rate of preterm and low birth weight births in the U.S. reflects a short-term, clinical approach that consists of increasing access to early and regular prenatal care (IOM, 1985, 1988). Advocates for changing financial and other barriers to prenatal care base their arguments on conclusions of cost-effectiveness of prenatal care in changing birth weight or duration of gestation (Gorsky and Colby, 1989; IOM, 1985; Korenbrot, 1984). In response, national policy has been changed to expand the financing of access to prenatal care for low-income women. A variety of national and local demonstration programs to increase access to various types of enhanced prenatal services have also been launched (Gold et al., 1993; Howell et al., 1997).

The persistence of high rates of prematurity and low birth weight births and the modest outcomes from demonstration programs has led to a questioning of this strategy, however, and an erosion of support for these services. To what extent, then, does the evidence support either the advocates or the critics?

The premise of *Prenatal Care: Effectiveness and Implementation* is that the arguments for and the critiques of prenatal care are based on a very narrow conceptualization of both the definition of prenatal care and the relevant outcomes. The purpose of this book is to expand the range of our thinking about prenatal care. Both the problems addressed by prenatal care and the outcomes that need to be considered in addressing its effectiveness should reflect the true potential of these programs so that we may gain a more accurate understanding of the extent to which services meet this potential.

In overt recognition that at least two individuals participate in prenatal care, the first two chapters of the book (Part I) describe the role of prenatal care in women's health, taking into account both clinical and behavioral issues related to pregnancy. The next nine chapters (Part II, III and IV) consider the role of prenatal care in mitigating the major disruptions to fetal development: (1) premature delivery and/or intrauterine growth restriction, resulting from inadequate fetal growth, and (2) malformation, resulting from abnormal growth. Each chapter consists of a description of prevalence and risk factors, followed by information on what is known about prevention or intervention, and a discussion of long-term outcomes. The final five chapters (Part V) return to women's health to consider prenatal care as part of a continuum of health care for women over their entire lives. The book concludes with a brief epilogue summarizing some of the key themes articulated by the authors in light of a broad perspective on the effectiveness and cost-effectiveness of prenatal care.

Prenatal Care: Effectiveness and Implementation regards prenatal care as a flexible package of services and considers the extent to which this whole accomplishes a range of goals. We have deliberately not attempted to assess the evidence of efficacy or effectiveness of individual prenatal interventions. Substantial and systematic efforts to synthesize this information have been published recently and are ongoing (Enkin et al., 1996; Lindmark, 1992; Sinclair and Bracken, 1992). Instead, the contributors to this book provide an overview of a broad array of areas where the effect of prenatal care should be examined, including areas where prenatal care has been thought or is intended to have its effect, and areas of potential effect that have, as yet, rarely been assessed.

Part I: Prenatal care and complications of pregnancy

In Part I, we are reminded by Dr. Philip Stubblefield that the original focus of prenatal care was to improve the chances of the woman surviving pregnancy, and the schedule of visits was designed to detect the most common complication of pregnancy, pre-eclampsia. The notion of prenatal care to improve fetal well-being is of more recent origin. In one sense, prenatal care can be considered highly successful as the rates of maternal mortality in the U.S. are extraordinarily low (Sachs et al., 1987). Using the example of the management of the women with juvenile diabetes mellitus, Dr. Stubblefield illustrates the power of modern pre-natal care to sustain safe child-bearing in women with established chronic illness. He also discusses the management of other problems, but notes, however, that little attention has been given to assessing the utility of prenatal care on women's overall health.

Prenatal care also represents a "teachable moment," a time when women may be particularly willing to modify their health behaviors. Dr. Lisa Paine and colleague Lisa Garceau describe the results of a literature search on prenatal interventions in eight health-related behaviors: smoking cessation, substance avoidance, alcohol avoidance, nutrition, exercise, stress reduction and social support, sexual behavior, and violence. What they have discovered is that of the almost 300 articles on these behaviors, only about 50 reflect intervention studies. Most of these are related to smoking cessation, alcohol avoidance, and nutrition, and none addresses the issue of violence. They conclude by stating that interventions for many problematic health-related behaviors affecting women are lacking, and recommend that if we truly wish to influence women's health behaviors during the prenatal period, much more work is needed to develop appropriate interventions.

Part II: Preventing prematurity

The prevention of premature birth and the management of preterm infants constitute major clinical challenges. Drs. David Savitz and Lisa Pastore have provided a review of the association between prematurity and a broad array of risk factors and health behaviors. They conclude that the literature offers no clear examples of a risk factor amenable to modification that would reduce the rates of prematurity substantially. Thus, the reduction in prevalence of individual risk factors may produce only small improvements. Further, they conclude that we are very far from understanding how many of these factors act to influence premature delivery.

This lack of knowledge is further reflected in the review by Drs. Robert Goldenberg and Dwight Rouse on interventions to prevent or improve the outcomes of prematurity. As they note, preterm delivery results from spontaneous labor, spontaneous rupture of membranes, or iatrogenic intervention for the health of the mother, the latter most often a result of severe pre-eclampsia. They conclude that few interventions currently available will prevent preterm delivery, but that delaying delivery to provide an opportunity to give corticosteroids reduces neonatal morbidity. Finally, they review new information on the potential role of bacterial vaginosis in the risk of prematurity, but note that trials of antibiotic therapy have not reduced rates of preterm delivery.

The importance of reducing prematurity rates, especially extreme prematurity, is underscored by Dr. Marie McCormick's review of the longer-term outcomes of premature infants. This review reveals that premature infants are at increased risk for many subsequent health problems, not just the neurodevelopmental problems usually presented. However, the factors influencing or ameliorating the adverse outcomes among premature infants are still being elucidated, and the outcomes may not solely be attributable to preterm delivery.

Part III: New findings and long-term evidence on intrauterine growth restriction

Preterm delivery is not the sole complication of inadequate fetal development; a variety of factors result in intrauterine growth restriction (IUGR). Dr. Kathleen Rasmussen begins her chapter with a discussion of the challenges of defining IUGR, which makes estimates of its prevalence difficult. She then goes on to contrast the situation of developing countries, where undernutrition is a major risk factor, to that of developed countries, where cigarette smoking plays a significant role. In considering the role of nutrition, she indicates that much still needs to be learned about how nutritional programs affect birth weight, and about effective ways of intervening in IUGR that are not related to nutrition.

In discussing the management of IUGR, Dr. Linda Heffner stresses the importance of accurate detection and diagnosis of the condition and of careful monitoring. She identifies several conditions and behaviors that are associated with IUGR, but notes that not all are amenable to intervention, hence the importance of those that are, such as smoking and substance abuse. An important management strategy is early delivery in the context of the infant experiencing distress, but as stated above, that strategy incurs the risks associated with preterm delivery.

In her review of some of the outcomes among infants with IUGR, Dr. Kathleen Nelson concludes that IUGR is associated with higher infant mortality rates, lower physical growth attainment, and poorer neurodevelopmental outcomes. More controversial are the recent reports linking IUGR to adult conditions, such as cardiovascular disease, schizophrenia, and poor reproductive performance of women who experienced IUGR. However, if these longer-term outcomes are shown to be related to IUGR, the impact of reducing this complication of pregnancy could be substantially greater than currently appreciated.

Part IV: Preventing and treating birth defects

The use of vital statistics data tends to reduce the attention paid to congenital malformations, but these problems represent what will be a frontier between genetic research and clinical care. In her description of the origin and prevalence of birth defects, Dr. Joan Stoler underscores the heterogeneity of the conditions in this category. She also notes the difficulty of establishing the incidence of these conditions, as many anomalies result in spontaneous abortion or stillbirth. Risk factors for anomalies include low birth weight, twinning, gender, and consanguinity. However, the etiology of close to half of birth defects remains unknown, and thus primary prevention remains elusive.

In view of the heterogeneity among birth defects, no attempt is made to examine long-term outcomes in total. Instead the remainder of Part IV is devoted to the potential for detection and intervention.

Dr. Richard Parad's chapter describes the emerging imaging and cytogenetic technologies used to improve early diagnosis of birth defects. Such information could be used to aid parents in making a decision to terminate the pregnancy or to aid the medical team to enhance prenatal care. Dr. Parad describes these techniques, and while recognizing that much of the technology is still in the laboratory development stage, discusses their potential utility in clinical practice.

Dr. Mark Evans and his colleagues describe currently available approaches when a birth defect is detected. They note that the ability to detect birth defects reflects the recent dramatic improvement in the quality of prenatal ultrasound imaging, but that the knowledge of syndromes and correct approaches to counseling may not be as highly advanced as the technology available to detect the defects. They then carefully describe the steps and options in the diagnosis and management of birth defects. Finally, they review the utility of fetal surgical, medical, and gene therapies.

Part V: Linking prenatal care with women's health

In this section, we return to the notion that prenatal care should also focus on the health of the woman. Not only is prenatal care a necessary (although not sufficient) set of services to assure or improve pregnancy outcomes, it is also an opportunity to engage women in health care more generally.

Dr. James Crall argues the case for greater attention to women's oral health in pregnancy. He bases his argument on the types of oral health problems that emerge with the hormonal changes of pregnancy, the linkage between maternal oral health and infant health, and the potential relationship between maternal periodontal disease and preterm labor. Although substantially more research is needed to elucidate these relationships, Dr. Crall concludes that if current research is born out, pregnancy may represent an opportunity to reduce mother–infant transmission of the bacteria responsible for periodontal disease, and that greater collaboration between obstetric and dental health care providers may contribute to a reduction in prematurity.

As Dr. Lorraine Klerman suggests, one important component of a broader array of health care services for women is in regard to fertility. However, the lack of access to such services is indicated by the high proportion of pregnancies that are unintended in this country, as well as the proportion of subsequent births following short intervals. She argues that family planning should be part of preconceptional, prenatal, and interconceptional care, but studies reveal that few women get such counseling, and generalist physicians do not seem to consider it their role.

Dr. Wendy Chavkin suggests that part of the recent failure to be as concerned with women's health as with fetal health may be a false notion of conflict between the needs of the mother and those of the fetus. This concept emerges from a legal and ethical debate on abortion. She presents several illustrative situations to demonstrate that this notion presents a false dichotomy. She concludes that the best outcomes are achieved when the woman and fetus are seen as an inseparable whole.

Dr. Paul Wise summarizes the substantial changes that will be needed in research, clinical practice, and programs and policies to achieve this integration. Almost more important is changing the nature of public discourse, especially by child advocates. He notes that efforts to elevate the rights and needs of children often come at the expense of the rights and needs of their parents. Dr. Wise concludes that only when both are considered are the best outcomes achieved.

Finally, Dr. Jacques Milliez presents the proposition that the ultimate success of a system of care for women and young children is critically dependent on its comprehensiveness. He describes the French system of prenatal care, which strives to meet the goal of comprehensiveness by linking prenatal care to postpartum care and pediatric services for young children, and by participating in a universal social security system that provides health insurance, pensions, family support, and maternal and child support to more than 99% of France's 60 million citizens. Dr. Milliez credits these legal and social measures, along with technological breakthroughs and a general improvement in living standards, for the achievements in perinatal medicine that have occurred in France over the last three decades.

In the Epilogue of *Prenatal Care: Effectiveness and Implementation,* Drs. Joanna Siegel and Marie McCormick recap themes articulated by the authors of the book regarding the past and present contributions of prenatal care and its potential. In doing so, they aim to bring readers back to the broadened frame of reference that is the premise of this book. By looking beyond the narrow set of maternal and fetal outcomes that have traditionally been used to assess the effectiveness and cost-effectiveness of prenatal care, they seek to encourage a new consideration of the value of this care and stimulate discussion about the place of prenatal care in a continuum of ongoing care for women and their families.

REFERENCES

Enkin M, Keirse MJNC, Renfrew M, Neilson J, eds. A guide to effective care in pregnancy and childbirth. 2nd edition. New York: Oxford University Press, 1996.

Gold RB, Singh S, Frost J. The Medicaid eligibility expansions for pregnant women: evaluating the strength of state implementation efforts. Family Planning Perspectives 1993; **25**: 196–207.

Gorsky RD, Colby JP Jr. The cost-effectiveness of prenatal care in reducing low birth weight in New Hampshire. Health Services Research 1989; **24**: 583–9.

Guyer B, Strobino DM, Ventura SJ, MacDorman M, Marin JA. Annual summary of Vital Statistics–1995. Pediatrics 1996; **98**: 1007–19.

Howell EM, Devaney B, Foot B, et al. The implementation of Healthy Start. Lessons for the future. Washington (DC): Mathematica Policy Research, Inc., 1997.

Institute of Medicine, Committee to Study Outreach for Prenatal Care. Prenatal care: reaching mothers, reaching infants. Washington (DC): National Academy Press, 1988.

Institute of Medicine, Committee to Study the Prevention of Low Birthweight. Preventing low birthweight. Washington (DC): National Academy Press, 1985.

Korenbrot CC. Risk reduction in pregnancies of low income women: comprehensive prenatal care through the OB Access Project. Mobius 1984; **4**: 34–43.

Lindmark G, ed. The scientific basis of antenatal care routines. International Journal of Technology Assessment in Health Care 1992; **8**: Suppl.

Richardson DK, Gray JE, Gortmaker S, et al. Declining severity-adjusted mortality: evidence of improving neonatal intensive care. Pediatrics 1998; **102**: 893–9.

Sachs BP, Brown DA, Driscoll SG, et al. Maternal mortality in Massachusetts. Trends and prevention. New England Journal of Medicine 1987; **316**: 667–72.

Sinclair JC, Bracken MB. Effective care for the newborn infant. Oxford: Oxford University Press, 1992.

Part 1

Prenatal Care and Complications of Pregnancy

Effect of prenatal care upon medical conditions in pregnancy

Phillip G. Stubblefield

Introduction

The practice of prenatal health care (regular visits to a health professional throughout pregnancy) is well accepted as essential to the well-being of mother and fetus. This chapter examines in some detail this issue of prenatal care and its effect on maternal medical conditions. First, maternal juvenile diabetes mellitus is presented as an example of the superb benefits that prenatal care can bring to both mother and fetus. This paradigm is then considered with regard to a number of other conditions, including hypertensive disease, assessment of fetal growth, cardiovascular disease, maternal smoking, autoimmune diseases, hematologic disorders, disorders of coagulation, renal disease, neurologic disease, and liver disease. The chapter concludes by acknowledging the need to rigorously evaluate the effectiveness of new therapies and their outcomes in prenatal care.

Historical perspective on prenatal care

Organized prenatal care began in the United Kingdom early in the present century and the structure of visits defined by the British Ministry of Health in 1929 is still practiced (Banta et al., 1984). Prenatal care is comparatively recent in the United States. The first edition of the American classic, Williams' *Obstetrics*, published in 1903, had no section on prenatal care, and only a few pages on the diagnosis of pregnancy (Williams, 1903). By the 13th Edition, published in 1966, prenatal care still received only 12 pages, with the acknowledgment that "before the rise of present-day obstetrics, the physician usually had but one interview with the patient before he saw her in labor and often at that interview merely sought to compute the expected date of confinement" (Eastman et al., 1966). In contrast, a representative current obstetric text includes detailed sections on prenatal care totaling more than 200 pages and several hundred additional pages dealing with specific conditions affecting pregnancy (Gabbe et al., 1996).

Historically, the first focus of prenatal care was to improve maternal safety. The accepted plan of visits, consisting of monthly visits in early pregnancy, becoming more frequent in the mid trimester, then weekly in the last month, was an attempt to detect the most common serious illness of women in pregnancy – pre-eclampsia. Epidemiologic studies support the benefit of this approach, as they appear to demonstrate lower maternal and perinatal mortality for women who receive prenatal care (Greenberg, 1983).

However, the utility of prenatal care in reducing hazards to the pregnant woman has been little examined until relatively recently, and there are comparatively few randomized trials or other studies that demonstrate the global efficacy of prenatal care upon maternal health (Enkin, 1992; Villar et al., 1993). In fact, the authors of a recent systematic review concluded that because healthier women are more likely to receive care, selection bias could explain the apparent benefit (Fink et al., 1992).

The issue of prenatal care's utility was explored in a recent Norwegian study, which evaluated the effectiveness of care in terms of the detection rates for five conditions thought to represent the bulk of non-symptomatic disease in pregnancy and the main reasons for screening pregnant women (Backe and Nakling, 1993). The conditions were: twin pregnancy, placenta previa, breech presentation, small-for-gestational-age (SGA) infant (birth weight < 10th percentile), and pre-eclampsia. The study examined a sample of 1908 women giving birth in one Norwegian county in a 12–month period during 1988–1989. Sensitivity, specificity, predictive values, and prevalence are shown in Table 1.1. The low rate at which pre-eclampsia was detected is directly relevant to this discussion of maternal impact. It is not clear from the article whether the failure to diagnose this condition before hospitalization for labor reflected true failure or was because these women did not develop the signs of pre-eclampsia until labor began (Backe and Nakling, 1993). SGA is another case in point. The very poor ability of prenatal care in this study to detect this problem is disappointing in light of the fact that SGA may also reflect maternal health. However, screening was only carried out by measuring the height of the uterine fundus, not by the frequent use of ultrasound, as is current in the U.S. The effectiveness of screening upon outcome was not reported.

The utility of prenatal care in reducing morbidity from maternal illness in pregnancy depends upon the prevalence of the illness among childbearing women, our ability to detect the illness, and our application of effective therapy or preventive strategies. The economic evaluation of prenatal care is more complicated, and is discussed elsewhere (Bahaug, 1992). Theoretically, prenatal care as currently practiced in the U.S. should be of marked benefit to the pregnant woman. As listed in Table 1.2, screening women for a variety of illnesses is routine

Table 1.1 Effectiveness of prenatal screening for five conditions

Condition	Sensitivity	Specificity	Positive predictive value	Negative predictive value	Prevalence per 100
Twins	94.1	100.0	100.0	99.9	0.9
Placenta previa	57.1	100.0	100.0	99.8	0.4
Breech	69.4	100.0	100.0	99.2	2.5
SGA	13.6	99.5	75.0	91.1	10.1
Pre-eclampsia	74.6	99.5	84.7	99.1	3.5

Source: Backe and Nakling, 1993.

Table 1.2 Summary of pre-pregnancy and prenatal health intervention strategies

Before pregnancy
✓   Obtain general medical history, reproductive history.
✓   Conduct physical examination.
✓   Review outcome of previous pregnancies and assess pregnancy risk. Obtain previous records if any abnormal outcome.
✓   Detect previous pregnancy wastage that might have a remediable cause (uterine septum, uterine duplication, incompetent cervix).
✓   Perform genetic history, screening for inherited illness and malformations.
✓   Provide indicated genetic carrier testing, e.g., cystic fibrosis, Tay-Sachs Disease, hemoglobinopathies.
✓   Screen for STDs, including HIV, and counsel about prevention strategies.
✓   Determine rubella status. Consider immunization, if patient is using reliable contraception.
✓   Screen for hepatitis B; consider immunization.
✓   Perform cervical cytology; evaluate and treat abnormal findings.
✓   Encourage smoking cessation.
✓   Prescribe folate to prevent neural tube defects.
✓   Ensure control of blood sugar for women with diabetes mellitus.
✓   Counsel about avoiding environmental exposure to volatile household chemical (e.g., paints, oven cleaners, cleaning fluid, lead, other heavy metals).
✓   Counsel about avoiding eating raw meat and contact with cat litter (toxoplasmosis).
✓   Counsel about common teratogenic drugs (e.g., isotretinoin, valproate).
✓   Encourage weight gain for very slender women.
✓   Counsel about avoiding exposure to sick children who might have transmissible viral illness.
✓   Determine if woman is being abused and arrange help if needed.
✓   Screen for use of alcohol and other drugs and arrange treatment if needed.
✓   Determine adequacy of living conditions and seek improvement if needed.
✓   Advise about automobile safety and encourage wearing of seatbelts.

Early pregnancy interventions
✓   Repeat the actions and interventions listed above.
✓   Confirm diagnosis of pregnancy and rule out ectopic pregnancy.
✓   Perform general and pregnancy-specific physical exam; note uterine size, perform clinical pelvimetry.
✓   Determine blood type and screen for blood type antibody (Rh, Kell, other blood group sensitization).
✓   Determine hemoglobin or hematocrit, diagnose and treat anemia.
✓   Screen for hepatitis A, B.
✓   Screen for hemoglobinopathy.
✓   Screen for bacteriuria and treat urinary infections.
✓   Screen for syphilis, gonorrhea, chlamydia; treat as needed.

✓ Screen for tuberculosis; evaluate positives and treat as needed.

✓ Screen for HIV, and if positive, offer counseling and treatment, including zidovudine therapy to prevent fetal transmission.

✓ Obtain cervical cytology.

✓ Screen for bacterial vaginosis and treat with systemic antibiotic.

✓ Assess maternal weight and adequacy of nutrition, counsel about diet, obtain additional food sources if needed.

✓ Prescribe nutritional supplements: iron, multivitamins containing folate.

✓ Perform early pregnancy ultrasound to determine duration of pregnancy.

✓ Instruct patient about self care during pregnancy, and signs and symptoms of abnormalities.

✓ Assess adequacy of social supports and offer assistance when needed.

✓ If previous cesarean section, obtain operative report and determine type of uterine incision, and counsel about vaginal birth after cesarean, if appropriate.

Follow-up visits throughout pregnancy

✓ Repeat risk assessment.

✓ Provide 12–14 prenatal visits with monitoring of maternal weight, blood pressure, measurement of uterine fundal height, auscultation of fetal heart rate.

✓ Determine if adequate maternal weight gain is occurring and counsel to improve nutritional status, if appropriate.

✓ Test urine for protein and glucose at each visit.

✓ Test for triple marker (alpha fetoprotein, BHCG, estriol) at 15–17 weeks to screen for Down's syndrome and neural tube defects.

✓ Perform mid-trimester genetic amniocentesis for women over age 35 and others at increased risk.

✓ Perform ultrasound exam at 18–20 weeks to screen for other anomalies.

✓ Perform glucose load test (50 gm glucose, one hour blood sugar) at 24–28 weeks to screen for gestational diabetes.

✓ Administer Rh immune globulin at 28 weeks to Rh negative, unsensitized women.

✓ Rescreen for gonorrhea, chlamydia, syphilis, and group B streptococcus in mid-third trimester.

✓ Instruct about the course of normal pregnancy, warning signs, e.g., decreased fetal movement, rupture of membranes, bleeding, uterine contractions.

✓ Instruct about, or ensure patient receives instruction in, events of labor and delivery, psychoprophylactic preparation for labor pain, education regarding alternatives for pain relief in labor, education in methods of delivery, and indications for intervention.

Detection and management of specific problems (examples; not inclusive)

✓ Rh negative and sensitized: manage with serial antibody titres and amniocentesis, intrauterine transfusion, intentional timed preterm delivery as indicated.

✓ Diabetes screen positive: evaluate with GTT, follow with weekly blood sugars, treat with insulin as indicated.

✓ Hypertension: assess renal, hepatic function, coagulation, advise rest at home, follow

Table 1.2. (*cont.*)

closely, hospitalize when needed for intensive monitoring of mother and fetus, and perform intentional preterm delivery if indicated.

✓   IUGR suspected: evaluate with ultrasound, look for causes, treat if possible, monitor, hospitalize and perform delivery early if indicated.

✓   Post-term pregnancy: conduct weekly ultrasound for amniotic fluid volume, perform twice weekly fetal heart rate monitoring (non-stress testing), consider planned induction of labor.

Sources: Enkin et al., 1996; Johnson et al., 1996; PHS, 1989.

in U.S. prenatal care practice. Some of these conditions, such as heart disease or diabetes mellitus, are made worse by pregnancy. Others are not made worse by pregnancy, but the perceived need for prenatal care brings the patient into the health care system and allows early diagnosis and effective intervention. An example is cancer of the uterine cervix. Cervical cytology, done routinely at first prenatal visits, effectively screens for invasive and preinvasive lesions. These lesions, if untreated, may progress to invasive cancer, but effective therapies exist.

The paradigm: maternal juvenile diabetes mellitus

Diabetes provides an excellent example of the benefits of care for both mother and fetus, before pregnancy, during pregnancy, and after delivery. In contrast to most other maternal illnesses that affect or are affected by pregnancy, the history of pregnancy outcomes of diabetes before modern management has been well documented. Before insulin was discovered, patients of reproductive age usually died within 1–2 years of onset of the illness and pregnancy was very rare. As described by Gabbe (1992), J. Whitridge Williams' 1909 summary of the world literature included only 66 pregnancies in 43 women. Half of the mothers died, either during the pregnancy or within the next 2 years, and the overall pregnancy loss rate was 41%. Then in 1921, insulin was discovered, and by 1922 was being used in diabetic children. Successful pregnancy in three cases of women with diabetes was reported by Dr. Priscilla White of the Joslin Clinic in 1932.

Despite the immediate improvements in maternal survival that occurred when insulin became available, perinatal outcome remained poor. In Kramer's (1936) report of 665 cases, stillbirth occurred in 25% and only 43% of the infants survived. Maternal mortality was 4%. Pregnancy in diabetic women was complicated by a high rate of fetal malformations, sudden fetal death in late pregnancy, pre-eclampsia and eclampsia, death from prematurity, and fetal injury and death from macrosomia.

Over the years since, management of the pregnant diabetic has improved dramatically so that perinatal mortality, with the exception of that from fetal malformations, is close to that of the general population (Landon and Gabbe, 1992). With the reduction in perinatal mortality from intrauterine death and prematurity, neonatal deaths from malformation account for 30–50% of perinatal mortality due to maternal diabetes.

Current management of pregnancy in the diabetic woman is described below. There appears to be no randomized trial of the entire plan of management, nor could withholding of care be ethically acceptable, given the very poor outcome of these pregnancies in the past.

Pre-pregnancy care

Major anomalies are increased about four-fold in women with insulin-dependent diabetes, ranging from 8 to 10% compared with about 2.4% in the general population. Central nervous system anomalies, including anencephaly and myelomeningocele, are increased ten-fold, and major cardiac lesions are increased five-fold. Sacral agenesis is increased 200- to 400-fold (Landon, 1996). These anomalies occur during the first seven weeks of gestation, and have been linked to metabolic abnormalities resulting from poor control of the diabetes. Intensive treatment of the diabetes with insulin before pregnancy reduces the rate of these major malformations from the expected 8% or so to the same rate as non-diabetic women.

Assessing the mother's condition before pregnancy is potentially of great benefit to her as well as to the fetus, because pre-existing vascular disease may contraindicate pregnancy. For example, women with diabetes of long duration may have ischemic heart disease. Myocardial infarction in pregnancy may have a mortality rate as high as 50%. Unfortunately, only about 20% of diabetic women with ischemic heart disease present before pregnancy.

Care during pregnancy

Careful regulation of maternal glucose is essential to a good outcome for mother and fetus. Patients follow a strict diet and are taught to monitor their own glucose control with glucose oxidase impregnated test strips and a glucose reflectance meter, measuring their own glucose with a drop of blood obtained by a finger stick before breakfast, lunch, and dinner, and at bedtime. A mix of regular and intermediate action insulin is given, and two to three injections per day are needed to provide normoglycemia without hypoglycemia. Frequent visits and frequent telephone contact with the providers is needed to adjust the insulin dosage. Ultrasound is performed early in pregnancy to confirm gestational age, again at

18–20 weeks to identify anomalies, and at 4–6 week intervals to confirm normal fetal growth.

Prenatal fetal surveillance is carried out beginning at 32–34 weeks to detect fetuses at risk of sudden intrauterine fetal death. Patients whose glucose has not been well controlled or who have vasculopathy or hypertension are thought to be at increased risk for this calamity, and testing begins earlier for them, at 28 weeks. The non-stress test (NST) appears to be the preferred method for prenatal surveillance in the U.S. The fetal heart rate is detected by Doppler ultrasound and printed on a strip chart. Accelerations of at least 15 beats per minute lasting at least 15 seconds indicate a normal or reactive test. If accelerations are absent, the test is considered non-reactive and abnormal. Further testing with ultrasound biophysical profile or a contraction stress test is then indicated.

Formerly, elective preterm delivery was performed to prevent intrauterine fetal death. The timing was based on the severity and duration of the mother's diabetes. Currently, delivery is usually planned for 38–39 weeks after demonstration of the presence of adequate levels of surfactant in amniotic fluid, and sooner if prenatal surveillance indicates fetal jeopardy. Because fetal macrosomia is common and associated with neonatal injury, elective cesarean delivery is favored if ultrasound estimates of fetal weight exceed 4000 grams.

Renal disease is common in women with insulin dependent diabetes and in 5–10% of pregnant diabetics. Screening with creatinine clearance and testing for proteinuria is therefore routine. The majority of diabetic women with renal disease will develop superimposed pre-eclampsia by late pregnancy, requiring expert management, often with prolonged hospitalization and intentional preterm delivery.

Women with diabetic proliferative retinopathy are at increased risk for progression of this eye disease during pregnancy. An ophthalmologic exam is essential in early pregnancy, and laser therapy is performed as needed. Women with severe retinopathy unresponsive to laser therapy are advised to terminate the pregnancy to avoid permanent severe vision loss (Landon, 1996).

Gestational diabetes

Diabetes develops in 2–3% of pregnancies, but the majority of these new cases will be limited to the duration of the pregnancy, hence the term "gestational" diabetes. In the U.S., universal screening of all pregnant women for diabetes is the norm. This is done with a single blood glucose measurement performed one hour after a 50 gm oral glucose load.

The significance of gestational diabetes and whether it is beneficial to screen for it has been disputed in England (Enkin et al., 1996). Women who have no pre-existing diabetes are probably at little risk during pregnancy. The hazard of gestational diabetes for the fetus is increased risk of macrosomia and related birth injury and neonatal jaundice and hypoglycemia. Risk of macrosomia appears to be reduced by active management of gestational diabetes and insulin therapy if blood glucose levels rise above predetermined levels, but there has been no demonstration that this program reduces neonatal mortality. Further, if gestational diabetes therapy is associated with more cesarean sections for fetal macrosomia, it may increase maternal risk. Regardless of questions about its benefit, however, routine glucose screening has become a part of U.S. practice.

Because as many as 50% of women with gestational diabetes will become overtly diabetic in their later years, screening in pregnancy does provide early identification of a group of women who will benefit from close follow up after pregnancy. Weight loss and exercise may reduce the proportion who will develop overt diabetes and improve their longevity.

Application of the paradigm to other conditions

A variety of other conditions also present opportunities to reduce maternal risk through prenatal interventions. These are discussed below.

Hypertensive disease

Hypertensive disease complicates 5–10% of pregnancies and is therefore the most common medical complication of pregnancy (Sibai, 1996). A variety of hypertensive disorders in pregnancy are recognized. All present a potentially serious risk to the mother and the fetus. These illnesses include chronic hypertension present before pregnancy, pre-eclampsia and eclampsia, and chronic hypertension with superimposed pre-eclampsia. Pregnancy-induced hypertension (PIH) is another term often employed. PIH includes pre-eclampsia or elevated blood pressure alone, presenting for the first time during pregnancy. In addition to the direct effects on the mother, hypertensive illnesses increase the risk of premature separation of the placenta (abruption), which may produce fetal asphyxia and death and places the mother at risk of life-threatening hemorrhage.

Pre-eclampsia

Pre-eclampsia is a systemic vascular disease unique to human pregnancy. It is characterized by hypertension, proteinuria, and edema. It may progress to eclampsia, with convulsions, coma, and death. It also may present as an acute liver disease with associated thrombocytopenia and coagulopathy. This so-called HELLP syndrome (hemolysis, elevated liver enzymes, low platelets) is an especially severe form of pre-eclampsia that can lead to death over 1–2 days if not treated by intentional preterm delivery and expert supportive care.

Reduced maternal perfusion of the uterus, resulting from vasospasm in the uterine arteries, is common with pre-eclampsia and places the fetus at risk for intrauterine growth restriction (IUGR) and sudden fetal death. Pre-eclampsia is more common in first pregnancies, in women with multiple gestations, and women with diabetes. There is familial predisposition. The cause of pre-eclampsia is unknown, but the currently favored theory of etiology is that it results when placental trophoblast cells fail to invade the muscular walls of the uterine arteries and convert them from high-pressure resistance vessels to low-pressure capacitance vessels. This invasion and conversion occurs as part of a normal pregnancy.

Prevention of PIH and pre-eclampsia

Studies of the utility of prenatal care in reducing pregnancy-induced hypertension exist for adolescent women. Adolescents, especially those under age 16, are at increased risk for pregnancy-induced hypertension. A meta-analysis of comprehensive prenatal care versus "traditional care programs," reported in 1994, identified five such trials published between 1972 and 1987. The summary relative risk for PIH with comprehensive prenatal care was 0.59 (95% confidence interval 0.49–0.72), supporting the conclusion that expanded prenatal services do reduce the occurrence of this illness in adolescent women (Scholl et al., 1994). There is considerable current interest in the possibility of preventing pre-eclampsia with medication. For example, calcium supplementation has been tried. Since the disorder has as part of its pathophysiology an excess of synthesis of thromboxane over prostacyclin, partial inhibition of the prostaglandin synthetase system with low-dose aspirin has also been attempted (Dekker, 1995). Unfortunately, as noted in Chapter 4, large randomized studies have found neither calcium supplementation nor low dose aspirin to be of value in preventing pre-eclampsia.

Screening for hypertension in pregnancy

Routine prenatal care includes determination of maternal blood pressure and urinary protein at each visit for all women. Signs and symptoms of pre-eclampsia are looked for at each visit. Women who develop hypertension are followed more closely, and if blood pressure continues to rise and if proteinuria or edema develop, they will be actively managed as described below.

Management of chronic hypertension

In addition to blood pressure and tests for urine protein at each visit, women with a history of pre-existing hypertension receive additional measures: measurement of creatinine clearance to assess initial renal function, and possibly, treatment with antihypertensive agents. The most important risk to the woman with chronic hypertension is the development of superimposed pre-eclampsia. If pre-eclampsia does not supervene, vascular disease does not progress, and there is normal expansion of the intravascular volume, then perinatal outcome is little different from that for normal women. The presence of proteinuria indicates that pre-eclampsia is developing. With superimposed pre-eclampsia, the vascular spasm and reduced vascular volume that are the hallmarks of that illness develop, and the outcome of pregnancy is poor. As summarized by Goldenberg (1992), 10–20% of women with mild chronic hypertension (diastolic BP < 110 mm Hg) developed pre-eclampsia, and in that group, 10% had abruption, 33% had an SGA neonate, and 24% had perinatal mortality. The more severe chronic hypertensives (diastolic BP > 110 mm Hg) had a somewhat greater risk for developing pre-eclampsia (28%). Of these, 78% had an SGA baby, all gave birth prematurely at a mean gestational age of 29 weeks, and perinatal mortality was 48%.

Management of pre-eclampsia

Patients diagnosed as having mild pre-eclampsia are prescribed bed rest at home, and monitored at frequent intervals, usually twice weekly with blood pressure and urine protein measurement. If the condition becomes more severe, the patient is admitted to the hospital for bed rest and assessment of vital signs several times per day, laboratory assessment to look for liver or renal involvement, and fetal monitoring with the non stress test where the fetal heart rate is observed for accelerations. Ultrasound is used to measure fetal dimensions as evidence of appropriate growth, and biophysical parameters are observed. Often, the patient's condition moderates with bed rest in the hospital, and the pregnancy can be allowed to progress for days or even weeks. If either the maternal or fetal condition worsens, labor is induced. Worsening maternal condition might include the development of the HELLP syndrome or progression to eclampsia, which can involve convulsions and coma. This emergency requires seizure prevention with medication, usually intravenous magnesium sulfate in the U.S., and prompt delivery of the infant. Delay in delivery may result in maternal death.

Pre-eclampsia most commonly occurs late in the third trimester, when the fetus is relatively mature and able to survive if intentionally delivered early. However, the condition is also seen early in the third trimester when a favorable fetal outcome is much less certain. Delivery is necessary to cure the illness, but the fetus may die or suffer long-term morbidity from preterm delivery. If delivery is delayed too long, the fetus may die in utero, and the mother may die as well. In this setting, the mother may be managed in an intensive care setting on the labor and delivery unit, with a battery of laboratory tests every few hours, hourly blood pressure measurement, and continuous electronic fetal heart rate monitoring. Glucocorticoids are given to the mother as this has been shown to increase fetal lung production of surfactant, which reduces the risk of respiratory distress syndrome. Any further deterioration in fetal or maternal condition is taken as an indication for induction of labor or immediate delivery by cesarean section.

Poor fetal growth

Poor fetal growth can indicate a fetal abnormality, but it can also indicate underlying maternal illness with resultant poor perfusion of the fetus. Assessment of fetal growth is a part of routine prenatal care. The height of the uterine fundus is measured with calipers or tape measure at each visit and recorded. Progressive growth is expected. If growth is greater or less than expected, an ultrasound examination is obtained. The fetus is imaged with ultrasound and critical dimensions are measured: the biparietal diameter of the fetal head, circumference of abdomen, and length of femur. By comparison to growth charts, these dimensions can be used to predict the gestational age and determine whether fetal size is appropriate. If fetal size is less than expected, a determination is made as to whether there could be an error in dating the pregnancy based on last menstrual period, or whether the problems truly represent a problem in growth. As will be clearly shown in Chapters 6, 7, and 8, it is important to diagnose growth restriction, as it can lead to intrauterine fetal death or long-term morbidity among survivors.

If growth restriction is confirmed, possible causes are sought. Possible maternal illnesses associated with IUGR include hypertensive disease, maternal cardiac disease, pulmonary diseases, renal disease, hemoglobinopathy, connective tissue disease, inflammatory bowel disease, and other severe gastrointestinal disease with maternal starvation, severe diabetes mellitus, and maternal substance abuse (the most common being cigarette smoking) (Carlson, 1988). If maternal illness exists, it should be treated. Generally, when growth restriction is confirmed, women are hospitalized for bed rest, fetal status is monitored with non-stress testing daily or twice weekly, and ultrasound is repeated at two-week intervals to monitor growth.

Cardiovascular disease

Pregnancy produces dramatic changes in the maternal circulatory system. By mid-pregnancy, plasma volume expands by 40%, red cell volume by 30%, and cardiac output rises by as much as 50%, as compared to the nonpregnant state (Hess and Hess, 1992; Landon and Samuels, 1996). Labor poses additional stress, with cardiac output increasing still further. These normal physiologic changes pose a real hazard for the woman with pre-existing cardiac disease.

The prevalence of heart disease in pregnant women ranges from 0.4% to 4.1%

worldwide, with rheumatic heart disease accounting for about 90% and congenital heart disease the rest (Burlew, 1990). In developed countries, rheumatic fever has become much less common, and many fewer women are entering the reproductive years with this disease. Therefore, an increased proportion of cardiac cases are of congenital origin. With the availability of effective surgical therapy for both rheumatic valvular disease and congenital anomalies of the heart, an increased number of women entering pregnancy have had previous surgical repair of their cardiac lesion. This group generally has reduced risk, but may face special problems, as for example, the need for continuous anticoagulation through pregnancy. Examples of some cardiovascular lesions and their effects in pregnancy are given below.

Diagnosis of heart disease before pregnancy and appropriate management can be expected to reduce the risk to mother and baby. However, we have only historical evidence for this. Mortality in the early part of this century for pregnant cardiac patients exceeded 20%, but fell with introduction of specialty clinics after 1920 (Reid et al., 1972). In his paper, Fitzgerald (Fitzgerald et al., 1951) reported a mortality of 0.85% among cardiac patients followed in a special clinic, but 9% among non-clinic patients. Functional class as defined by the New York Heart Association criteria can be used to predict outcome. Women who are class I and II generally do well during the pregnancy, with appropriate care. Women who are class III and IV are at considerable risk, and in one historical series, 30% died within 10 years.

Acquired valvular heart disease

The most common form of acquired valvular heart disease seen in pregnant women is mitral stenosis as a sequel to rheumatic heart fever. About 25% of cases are first diagnosed during pregnancy when women become symptomatic, with tachycardia, fatigue, dyspnea, tachypnea, and orthopnea, as pressure rises in the left atrium and pulmonary veins. With the progression of pregnancy, patients may decompensate suddenly, developing atrial fibrillation or rapid atrial tachycardia and pulmonary edema. Aortic stenosis is much less common, but is associated with a high mortality rate. If the valve area is recognized before pregnancy as being smaller than a critical size, corrective surgery is recommended. Mitral and aortic insufficiencies are usually well tolerated in pregnancy. Mitral valve prolapse without other abnormalities does not increase risk for mother or fetus.

Congenital heart disease

Atrial septal defect is the most common congenital disease in reproductive age women, and if not associated with other lesions, does not adversely effect outcome. However, women who have developed pulmonary hypertension face increased risk (Hess and Hess, 1992).

Patients with Tetralogy of Fallot have pulmonic stenosis, ventricular septal defect, and aortic override. They are cyanotic because of the right to left shunt, and this typically increases during pregnancy. Prognosis is worse if the hematocrit is over 60%, the oxygen saturation is less than 80%, or if the patient already has had syncopal attacks before pregnancy. Patients with the more severe lesions of this type are at risk for sudden death, especially during labor.

Eisenmenger syndrome, characterized by ventricular septal defect associated with progressive pulmonary hypertension and shunt reversal, poses a very great risk. Women with this syndrome have a 30–50% mortality in pregnancy, typically occurring postpartum, and the infant mortality rate is as high as 40%. These women are advised to terminate the pregnancy. If this is refused, or the condition is not recognized until mid-pregnancy, patients are usually hospitalized for the duration of pregnancy, given supplemental oxygen, anticoagulated, and treated for congestive heart failure if it develops.

Marfan's Syndrome is an inherited autosomal dominant disease, affecting connective tissue. The average age at death is 30, secondary to dissection of the aorta and rupture. Measurement by ultrasound of the diameter of the aortic root is of some help in predicting risk. A woman with a root diameter of less than 40 mm has a better prognosis. Termination of pregnancy is generally advised. If refused, patients are managed with β-blocking drugs, careful monitoring of blood pressure and ultrasound measurement of aortic route diameter, limitation of exercise, and generally, hospitalization from mid-pregnancy onward.

Ischemic heart disease

Myocardial infarction (MI) resulting from ischemic heart disease is very rare in women of reproductive age, but if it occurs during pregnancy, there is a risk of death of 40–50%. Women with previous MI are advised to avoid pregnancy. A woman with a history of MI who wishes to undertake a pregnancy should be fully assessed before pregnancy with studies of myocardial contractility and coronary flow, including cardiac catheterization if it has not already been performed. Consideration could be given to angioplasty before pregnancy for patients with significant coronary occlusion. However, there is little information as to how well women do in pregnancy after these procedures. Women with acute MI during pregnancy have occasionally been reported to survive after emergency coronary artery bypass surgery.

Management of women with heart disease

Preconceptional counseling is advised, with full history and physical exam, basic laboratory tests, including an electrocardiogram, and review of previous records of assessment and treatment (Hess and Hess, 1992). Ideally, the patient is evaluated by a team that includes a maternal fetal medicine specialist, cardiologist, cardiac surgeon, anesthesiologist, and genetics counselor. Functional class should be established and stress testing and cardiac ultrasound performed to define the lesion. Specific risks to the patient and the potential child should be discussed with the patient and her family. If the patient is on anticoagulant medication, plans should be made to convert to heparin as soon as pregnancy is confirmed. Patients with rheumatic disease are given prophylactic penicillin to reduce risk of recurrence. When pregnancy occurs, other sources of cardiac stress are reduced as much a possible. Management includes increased rest, restriction of sodium, and the use of diuretics and digitalis preparations. If symptoms worsen, the patient may need to be hospitalized for the duration of the pregnancy for more intensive management. Because poor fetal growth is common, growth is followed by serial ultrasound studies. Fetal surveillance with non-stress testing and ultrasound biophysical profiles is provided in the third trimester.

Maternal smoking

As discussed in Chapter 2 and a number of other chapters, smoking is clearly detrimental to the health of the mother over the long term. Although the most important immediate effect of maternal smoking during pregnancy is an increase in the proportion of infants born at low birth weight, it is also associated with pregnancy complications that can endanger the mother, including placenta previa, placental abruption, and premature rupture of the fetal membranes (Chattinglus, 1992). Smoking is readily detected during prenatal care. In this author's experience, middle-class women typically stop smoking when they become pregnant. Demonstration of effective strategies for smoking cessation in higher-risk, low-income groups is problematic (Kendrick and Merritt, 1996).

Autoimmune diseases

These disorders, mediated by an immunologic response to antigens on normal cells, affect 5–7% of the overall population, and several are more common in women than men.

Myasthenia gravis

This is a rare disorder of neurotransmission across the myoneural junction caused by autoantibodies against the acetylcholine receptors in skeletal muscle. The disease typically undergoes remissions and exacerbations, and commonly exacerbates in pregnancy or postpartum (Floyd and Roberts, 1992). It is treated with with corticosteroids and with quarternary ammonium compounds, which inhibit acetylcholinesterase activity. Acute or chronic respiratory failure with the disease can be life threatening. Anesthesia and surgery present special problems, and expert management is needed during labor and delivery.

Systemic lupus erythematosus (SLE)

SLE is a multi-organ disease characterized by autoantibodies and vasculitis. Maternal autoantibodies produced as a result of SLE may affect the pregnancy. Patients in remission at the beginning of pregnancy and who have not manifested multi-organ disease may do fairly well in pregnancy. However, women with pre-existing lupus nephritis are at serious risk for exacerbation and permanent loss of renal function. Antiphospholipid syndrome also may be seen with lupus, and results in repeated pregnancy losses and markedly increased risk for pre-eclampsia. Although it is difficult to differentiate lupus nephritis from pre-eclampsia, one distinguishing difference is that in lupus nephritis, the levels of serum complement (the system of more than 20 plasma proteins involved in immunomodulation and inflammation) fall, while in pre-eclampsia they remain constant. Women with lupus require expert management and frequent visits through pregnancy, often including prolonged hospitalization in late pregnancy. Slow fetal growth and intrauterine fetal death are a concern, so fetal assessment with ultrasound and non-stress testing should be offered from mid-pregnancy until delivery. High-dose steroids are used to treat exacerbation of the SLE, but because of the overlap with pre-eclampsia, intentional preterm delivery may be needed if the maternal condition worsens.

Antiphospholipid syndrome

This illness is characterized by maternal production of autoantibodies, lupus anticoagulant, and anticardiolipin, and is associated with repeated pregnancy losses from thrombosis in the placental bed, with resulting infarctions of the placenta. It occurs more commonly in women with underlying autoimmune disease, such as SLE, but is also found in women whose only symptom is repeated reproductive failure. It can be successfully treated with low-dose aspirin, and either corticosteroids or low-dose heparin. Both steroids and heparin present special problems in management, and require close follow up and expert management. Even on therapy, these women are at increased risk for superimposed pre-eclampsia and poor fetal growth (Petri, 1997).

Hematologic disorders

Iron deficiency anemia is common in pregnancy because of the increased need for iron from the marked increase in maternal blood volume in later pregnancy and the needs of the fetus. The more severe forms of anemia can lead to high-output congestive heart failure (Perry and Morrison, 1992). Iron supplementation during the prenatal period is routine in this country.

Megaloblastic anemia, resulting from folate deficiency, is also common in pregnancy, and is associated with reduced maternal blood volume, and abruptio placenta. Folate deficiency has recently been implicated in the causation of the common serious fetal neural tube defects called myelomengocele and anencephaly (Rosenberg, 1992). Supplementation with folate is now routine during pregnancy. Food supplementation with folate is to begin in the U.S. as a strategy to prevent neural tube defects.

Hemoglobinopathies

The sickle cell hemoglobinopathies (HbS S, HbS C, and HbS-Thal) are hemolytic anemias characterized by recurrent painful crises, systemic infection, and infarction of various organ systems. HbS S is the most common, and affects approximately one in 708 African Americans. Generally, these diseases are diagnosed in childhood, but sometimes women become symptomatic for the first time during pregnancy. Management during pregnancy requires close follow up and early aggressive treatment of exacerbations. Crises are managed with blood transfusion if symptoms are severe and unresponsive to conservative management with oxygen, hydration, and analgesia. Prophylactic exchange transfusions to prevent crises are also used. Morbidity from pneumonia, pyelonephritis, cholecystitis, pulmonary emboli, retinal hemorrhages, and superimposed pre-eclampsia are considerable (Perry and Morrison, 1992). There is increased risk for fetal death, so care routinely includes ultrasound assessment of fetal growth and prenatal fetal heart rate monitoring.

Standard prenatal screening includes hemoglobin electrophoresis for all African American women in order to detect all forms of hemoglobinopathy. If carrier status is identified, then paternal testing is also needed to allow for appropriate genetic counseling.

Disorders of coagulation

Bleeding

Von Willebrand disease is an inherited disorder of coagulation caused by abnormality of von Willebrand's factor, a carrier for factor VIII in the coagulation cascade. Both autosomal dominant and recessive inheritance patterns are seen. Three major types are recognized, and severity varies with the type. Factor VIII increases in pregnancy, so postpartum hemorrhage from the uterus is not commonly a problem. However, episiotomy may result in hemorrhage, and cesarean section presents a major risk for bleeding from the surgical incision.

Treatment is with desmopressin, which increases complexing of von Willebrand factor with factor VIII, or with recombinant factor VIII. Cryoprecipitate is used less often because of risk for infection.

Thrombosis

Pregnancy and the postpartum period are times of increased risk for venous thrombosis and thromboembolism. Four inherited conditions are now recognized that increase risk of clotting during pregnancy. Antithrombin III, protein S, and protein C are regulatory proteins that inhibit coagulation. Women with deficiencies of these factors are unable to balance the increase in activation of the coagulation system that normally occurs with pregnancy and are at great risk for thrombosis (Trauscht-Van Horn et al., 1992). A recently discovered point mutation in clotting factor V, factor V Leidin, results in a form of factor V that resists destruction by activated protein C. It is found in 3–5% of the population of European ancestry and constitutes the most common form of inherited predisposition to clotting. Women with this condition are also at very great risk for thrombosis during pregnancy. Patients with any of these conditions commonly are given low dose heparin during pregnancy, and if they have previously experienced thrombosis, will receive full anticoagulation throughout pregnancy (Hirsch et al., 1996).

Renal disease

Chronic renal disease often presents as chronic hypertension. This condition was discussed earlier. Pyelonephritis occurs in 1–2% of pregnancies and can rapidly become life threatening (Samuels, 1996). Approximately 10% of young women have asymptomatic bacteriuria, and of these, up to 40% will develop symptomatic urinary infection in pregnancy. Screening urine cultures is routine in prenatal care. Women who test positive are treated with antibiotics to reduce risk for pyelonephritis. A meta-analysis of 11 trials of antibiotic treatment of asymptomatic bacteriuria in pregnancy reported an 80% decrease in odds for developing pyelonephritis (Enkin, 1992).

Neurologic disease

Cerebrovascular disease, though uncommon in young women, is markedly increased with pregnancy. Prompt evaluation of neurologic symptoms and early diagnosis allow more timely intervention and less mortality (Albert and Morrison, 1992).

Pseudotumor cerebri is exacerbated by pregnancy and may lead to blindness from pressure atrophy of the optic nerves. Diagnosis and treatment with carbonic anhydrase inhibitors or steroids can reduce morbidity.

Seizure disorders affect 0.3–0.6% of pregnancies and 35–40% of these women will have an increased frequency of seizures during pregnancy. Congenital anomalies are increased in women with epilepsy, whether or not they are treated with anti-seizure medication. Some of the anti-seizure medications are teratogenic and most depress folate metabolism. Ideally, women with seizures would have pre-pregnancy evaluation, be changed to medications with the least adverse fetal effects, and have close monitoring with dose adjustment in pregnancy to prevent exacerbation of the seizure disorder.

Pregnant spinal cord injury patients are at increased risk for anemia, decubitus ulcers, urinary infections, venous thrombosis, and autonomic hyperreflexia, and require expert management.

Liver disease

Acute fatty liver of pregnancy is rare but until recently was usually fatal. Of unknown cause, the disease begins with nausea, vomiting, and abdominal pain in late pregnancy, progresses to jaundice, then somnolence and coma (Samuels and Landon, 1996). Disseminated intravascular coagulopathy, acidosis, and severe hypoglycemia are important elements of this disease. Management requires correction of coagulopathy with blood products, and treatment of the hypoglycemia with glucose solutions. Delivery is essential, and labor will be induced, or if the cervix is unfavorable, cesarean section is performed after correction of the coagulopathy.

Conclusion

Although this chapter has addressed some of the major illnesses that may complicate pregnancy, increase risk for mother or fetus, or afford opportunities to improve outcome with early diagnosis and management, it is far from exhaustive. Those wishing to know more are referred to current texts of maternal fetal medicine (Gabbe et al., 1996; Sciarra et al., 1997).

The gold standard for evaluating medical interventions has come to be the randomized clinical trial. Meta-analysis of existing randomized trials of components of prenatal care has been very productive in differentiating therapies that are useless, or even harmful, from those that have been proven to be helpful (Enkin et al., 1996). Ideally, any prenatal care for non-life-threatening conditions should be evaluated in this fashion before being adopted into practice. For example, screening for gestational diabetes and its management should be evaluated with a randomized trial. Most of the conditions discussed in this chapter are life-threatening and effective therapy already exists and is in use for them. Therefore, randomized trials to demonstrate the value of prenatal care for these conditions are not ethical. However, the effectiveness of these therapies and their outcomes should still be studied in order to detect opportunities for improved care.

REFERENCES

Albert JR, Morrison JC. Neurologic diseases in pregnancy. Obstetrics and Gynecology Clinics of North America 1992; **19**: 765–79.

Backe B, Nakling J. Effectiveness of antenatal care: a population based study. British Journal of Obstetrics and Gynæcology 1993; **100**: 727–31.

Bahaug H. Problems and prospects in the economic evaluation of antenatal care. International Journal of Technology Assessment in Health Care 1992; **8** (Suppl. 1): 49–56.

Banta HD, Houd S, Suarez OE. Prenatal care – an introduction. International Journal of Technology Assessment in Health Care 1984; **1**: 783–9.

Burlew BS. Managing the pregnant patient with heart disease. Clinical Cardiology 1990; **13**: 757–62.

Carlson DE. Maternal disease associated with intrauterine growth retardation. Seminars in Perinatology 1988; **12**: 17–22.

Cnattingius S. Smoking during pregnancy. International Journal of Technology Assessment in Health Care 1992; **8** (Suppl. 1): 91–5.

Dekker GA. The pharmacologic prevention of pre-eclampsia. Baillières Clinical Obstetrics and Gynæcology 1995; **9**: 509–28.

Eastman NJ, Hellman LM, Pritchard JA. Williams obstetrics. 13th edition. New York: Appleton Century Crofts, 1966: 323–35.

Enkin MW. Randomized controlled trials in the evaluation of antenatal care. International Journal of Technology Assessment in Health Care 1992; **8** (Suppl. 1): 40–5.

Enkin M, Keirse MJNC, Renfrew M, Neilson J. A guide to effective care in pregnancy and childbirth. 2nd edition. New York: Oxford University Press, 1996: 57–9.

Fink A, Yano E, Goya D. Prenatal care programs: what the literature reveals. Obstetrics and Gynecology 1992; **80**: 867–72.

Fitzgerald JE, Webster A, Zummo BP, Williams PC. Evaluation of adequate antepartum care for the cardiac patient. Journal of the American Medical Association 1951; **146**: 910.

Floyd RC, Roberts WE. Autoimmune diseases in pregnancy. Obstetrics and Gynecology Clinics of North America 1992; **19**: 719–32.

Gabbe SG. A story of two miracles: the impact of the discovery of insulin on pregnancy in women with diabetes mellitus. Obstetrics and Gynecology 1992; **79**: 295–9.

Gabbe SG, Niebyl JR, Simpson JL. Obstetrics: normal and problem pregnancies. 3rd edition. New York: Churchill Livingstone, 1996.

Goldenberg RL. Screening for hypertension in pregnancy. International Journal of Technology Assessment in Health Care 1992; **8** (Suppl. 1): 63–71.

Greenberg RS. The impact of prenatal care in different social groups. American Journal of Obstetrics and Gynecology 1983; **145**: 797–803.

Hess DB, Hess LW. Management of cardiovascular disease in pregnancy. Obstetrics and Gynecology Clinics of North America 1992; **19**: 679–95.

Hirsch DR, Mikkola KM, Marks PW, et al. Pulmonary embolism and deep vein thrombosis during pregnancy or oral contraceptive use: prevalence of factor V Leiden. American Heart Journal 1996; **131**: 1145–8.

Johnson TRB, Walker MA, Niebyl JR. Preconception and prenatal care. In: Gabbe SG, Niebyl JR, Simpson JL, eds. Obstetrics: normal and problem pregnancies. 3rd edition. New York: Churchill Livingstone, 1996 161–84.

Kendrick JS, Merritt RK. Women and smoking: an update for the 1990s. American Journal of Obstetrics and Gynecology 1996; **175**: 528–35.

Kramer DW. Diabetes and pregnancy, a survey of 665 cases. Pennsylvania Medicine 1936; **39**: 702–7. Cited in Gabbe SG, 1992.

Landon MB. Diabetes mellitus and other endocrine disease. In: Gabbe SG, Niebyl JR, Simpson JL, eds. Obstetrics: normal and problem pregnancies. 3rd edition. New York: Churchill Livingstone, 1996: 1041.

Landon MB, Gabbe SG. Diabetes mellitus and pregnancy. Obstetrics and Gynecology Clinics of North America 1992; **19**: 633–52.

Landon MB, Samuels P. Cardiac and pulmonary disease. In: Gabbe SG, Niebyl JR, Simpson JL, eds. Obstetrics: normal and problem pregnancies. 3rd edition. New York: Churchill Livingstone, 1996: 997–1024.

Perry KG, Morrison JC. Hematologic disorders in pregnancy. Obstetrics and Gynecology Clinics of North America 1992; **19**: 783–99.

Petri M. Pathogenesis and treatment of the antiphospholipid antibody syndrome. Medical Clinics of North America 1997; **81**: 151–77.

Public Health Service (PHS) Expert Panel on the Content of Prenatal Care. Caring for our future: the content of prenatal care. Washington (DC): U.S. Department of Health and Human Services, Public Health Service, 1989.

Reid DE, Ryan KJ, Benirschke K. Principles and management of human reproduction. Philadelphia: W.B. Saunders Co., 1972: 690.

Rosenberg I. Folic acid and neural tube defects: time for action? Obstetrics and Gynecology Clinics of North America 1992; **327**:1875–7.

Samuels P. Renal disease. In: Gabbe SG, Niebyl JR, Simpson JL, eds. Obstetrics: normal and problem pregnancies. 3rd edition. New York: Churchill Livingstone, 1996: 1025–36.

Samuels P, Landon MB. Hepatic disease. In: Gabbe SG, Niebyl JR, Simpson JL, eds. Obstetrics, normal and problem pregnancies. 3rd edition. New York: Churchill Livingstone, 1996: 1119–26.

Scholl TO, Hediger ML, Belsky DH. Prenatal care and maternal health during adolescent pregnancy: a review and metaanalysis. Journal of Adolescent Health 1994; **15**: 444–56.

Sciarra JJ, Depp R, Eschenback DA, eds. Gynecology and obstetrics. Volume 3, Maternal and fetal medicine. Philadelphia: Harper and Row, 1997.

Sibai BM. Hypertension in pregnancy. In: Gabbe SG, Niebyl JR, Simpson JL, eds. Obstetrics, normal and problem pregnancies. 3rd edition. New York: Churchill Livingstone, 1996: 935–96.

Trauscht-Van Horn JJ, Capeless EL, Easterling TR, Bovill EG. Pregnancy loss and thrombosis with protein C deficiency. American Journal of Obstetrics and Gynecology 1992; **167**: 968–72.

Villar J, Garcia P, Walker G. Routine antenatal care. Current Opinion in Obstetrics and Gynecology 1993; **5**: 688–93.

Williams JW. Obstetrics. New York: D. Appleton Co., 1903: 157–68.

2

Health behaviors during pregnancy: risks and interventions

Lisa L. Paine and Lisa M. Garceau

Introduction

This chapter discusses the risks of and interventions for selected health behaviors during pregnancy and addresses the following questions:

- What are health behavior risks and interventions?
- What does the effectiveness literature about health behavior interventions during pregnancy indicate?
- What gaps in the current literature should be addressed in future research?
- What are the implications of these findings for policy makers, health managers, and health providers?

More specifically, this chapter focuses on the effectiveness of particular interventions in modifying health behaviors within certain sub populations at increased risk of poor outcomes.

Overview

Summary of behavioral change theories

Behavioral change interventions, either explicitly or implicitly, incorporate a theoretical basis for understanding behavior – why individuals act in a specific manner. The field of behavioral sciences offers those interested in developing effective interventions (e.g., clinicians and policy planners) a clearer understanding of what individuals require in order to change undesirable behaviors or to maintain desirable ones (Fishbein and Guinan, 1996).

Behavioral science theory and research suggests that the most effective interventions are those aimed at a specific behavior (Fishbein and Guinan, 1996). Behaviors have unique determinants, and thus require different interventions for change to occur. Identifying the behavior that one wishes to change may well be the most difficult part of developing an intervention. Many interventions are mistakenly directed at increasing the probability that an individual will reach a specific goal or engage in a category of behaviors, rather than increasing the probability that one will engage in a specific behavior. Increasing this probability is more likely to result in successful behavioral change (Fishbein and Guinan, 1996).

This chapter presents the behavior theories that are dominant in the fields of health behavior and health education, including those representing different units of intervention (i.e., the individual, group, and community). In addition, promising theoretical formulations that may guide the field in the future are presented.

The six theories presented are: Social Learning Theory, Theory of Reasoned Action, Health Belief Model, Transtheoretical Stages of Change Theory, Self-in-Relation Theory, and Community Health Model.

Social Learning Theory

Social Learning Theory, one of the most formally developed theories of behavior, emphasizes that an individual's behaviors are motivated by both personal beliefs (cognitive factors) and social factors (community, friends, and family) (Bandura, 1986). Among important personal factors are self-efficacy (the belief that one can perform a particular behavior effectively, with good results, under many different circumstances), behavioral capability (the skill and knowledge to perform a given behavior), and self-control (the regulation of goal-directed behavior). Aspects of the social environment that are important in this theory include observational learning (learning how to perform a specific behavior by watching others do so), and reinforcement (receiving support from others in the environment for practicing certain behaviors) (Perry et al., 1990).

While health care providers who are confronted with the complexities of individual patients might prefer the simplicity provided by a single-variable explanation, Social Learning Theory posits that many relevant concepts must be addressed in an intervention.

Theory of Reasoned Action

The Theory of Reasoned Action states that an individual's behaviors are primarily determined by intentions to perform the behavior (Ajzen and Fishbein, 1980). In turn, one's intentions are determined by attitudes (the overall positive or negative feeling with respect to personally performing the behavior) and subjective norms about the behavior (the perception of normative pressure to perform the behavior in question) (Fishbein and Guinan, 1996). Specifically, one's attitudes about what will result from performing a certain behavior (e.g., that receiving prenatal care will result in a healthy baby) are thought to influence the likelihood that one intends and actually performs a certain behavior, as are the evaluative aspects (e.g., that having a healthy baby is an important and desired outcome). Also important for an understanding of subjective norms is the role of normative beliefs, or beliefs about how others will respond to the behavior (e.g., that others will approve of the keeping of prenatal appointments or attending childbirth classes) and motivations to comply, or the amount of weight given to the others' desires (Carter, 1990).

The Health Belief Model

Developed by Hochbaum (1958) and Rosenstock (1960), the Health Belief Model grew out of concerns with the limited success of various programs supported by the U.S. Public Health Service (Rosenstock, 1990). The Health Belief Model considers a variety of factors thought to influence individuals' health behavior. The three key components of the Health Belief Model are:

- Threat: Perceived susceptibility to a health condition or perceived seriousness of the condition (e.g., if an individual believes she is likely to develop lung cancer, or that her baby will be smaller and less healthy because of her smoking, then she is more likely to stop smoking than if she does not perceive herself to be at risk).
- Outcome expectations: Perceived benefits of specified action or perceived barriers to taking that action (e.g., if an individual perceives that she will have a great deal of difficulty withdrawing from nicotine, or perhaps gain weight when she quits smoking, she may conclude that the costs of quitting smoking are too great).
- Efficacy expectations: One's convictions about the ability to carry out the recommended action (e.g., if an individual believes she will be able to refuse a cigarette under certain circumstances, she may be able to quit, while if she believes she will not be able to refuse, she may not try).

An additional concept that has not been systematically studied but that appears sporadically in the Health Belief Model literature (Larson et al., 1982), is referred to as *cues to action*. These cues prompt individuals to act by reminding them of the need to change their behavior. These stimuli may be internal, such as pain or discomfort, or external, such as advertising campaigns or health practitioners' reinforcement of the health hazards of smoking.

Transtheoretical Stages of Change Model

Because behavior change is a complex process, Prochaska and DiClemente developed a model that describes a series of steps commonly experienced by individuals who are trying to change health-related behaviors. The Transtheoretical Stages of Change Model posits that individuals begin changing behavior after going through distinct stages of readiness (Prochaska and DiClemente, 1986). The first stage is *pre-contemplation*, and represents a time during which an individual is not actively thinking of changing a particular behavior. During the next stage, *contemplation*, an individual begins to think about behavioral change. He or she may think, read, or talk to others about changing a behavior and may become open to health education in preparation for taking actual steps to change behaviors. The *action* stage is when an individual takes steps to change behavior. During this time, individuals are in particular need of support, which may include specific training or education as well as social support from family and friends. It is important to note that not all individuals move through the stages in the same way. Some never proceed to the action stage, for example, while others bypass the contemplation phases and move directly to the action phase.

Assuming that action steps are taken, the individual moves into the *maintenance* stage, where he or she attempts to continue the behavioral change. At this time, it is helpful to identify factors that may tempt a person to relapse, so that they can prevent, avoid, or learn how to cope with these factors. *Relapse*, which is extremely common, occurs when the individual is unable to maintain the changed behavior (Prochaska and DiClemente, 1986). Fishbein and Guinan have described this process of change as sequential, "although people may skip certain stages or relapse (at any stage) and cycle back through the stages repeatedly before achieving long-term maintenance" (1996, p. 8).

Self-in-Relation Theory

In proposing the Self-in-Relation Theory, Miller (1986) presented a theoretical construct applicable to women that stands in sharp contrast to other developmental theories that stress the importance of autonomy and separation. This theory is based on the importance of connection for women, and suggests that the relational self is the basis for growth and development in women. Because of women's basic orientation to others, their relationships and the maintenance of relationships have highly charged meanings (Amaro, 1995). Changes in connections or relationships with others is perceived as a "loss of self." This fear of loss may undermine an intention to change behavior. The Self-in-Relation Theory argues that change can occur only when women examine the quality of their connections rather than act to please others.

Community Health Model

A more recent development in the field of health education is the Community Health (or Public Health) Model. This model proposes programs that are designed to reach populations, not simply individuals. The health of the population may be fostered by developing structures and policies that encourage health-promoting activities by individuals or by reducing or eliminating health hazards in the social and physical environment (Glanz et al., 1990). Concepts central to this approach include:

- *Community empowerment,* "a process by which individuals, communities, and organizations gain mastery over their lives" (Rappaport, 1984).
- *Community competence,* "the ability of a community to engage in effective problem solving" (Iscore, 1980).
- *Community participation,* learning that occurs through doing and with understanding rather than by formula.
- *Issue selection,* effective differentiation between problems and issues.
- *Creating "critical consciousness,"* a process through which group members, with the aid of facilitators, identify root causes of issues (Freire, 1973).

In summary, the six behavioral theories suggest that several factors influence change:

- An individual's perception of personal susceptibility.
- An individual's attitude toward performing a given behavior, which is based on beliefs about the consequences of performing or not performing the behavior.
- The perception that others in the community are also changing their behavior, and that the notion of behavior change is being supported by another person.
- The perception that one can, under varied circumstances, perform a given behavior.
- For women, a connection or a relationship with another person.

Current trends in health behavior

Smoking

In 1965, 33% of U.S. women were cigarette smokers. During 1987–1992, the prevalence of cigarette smoking among reproductive-aged women declined 2.7%, from 29.6% in 1987 to 26.9% in 1992 (CDC, 1994b). However, recent data indicate that the rate of smoking among adolescent females is rising, and has surpassed the rates of smoking among adolescent males (CDC, 1996a). Among women aged 18–24 years, smoking prevalence for black women declined dramatically during 1987–1992, from 21.8% to 5.9%. Among white women in this age group, prevalence was unchanged, 27.8% and 27.2% in 1987 and 1992, respectively (CDC, 1994a). Between 1987–1992, smoking prevalence was inversely related to level of education and was consistently highest among women with less than a high school education (CDC, 1994a).

Since 1972, it has been widely known that women who smoke during pregnancy are adversely affecting the health, development, and functioning of their children, both before and after birth. They are more likely than non-smokers to have babies with low birth weight or who experience intrauterine growth restriction (IUGR) (DHEW, 1973; see also Chapter 7). Smoking during pregnancy is closely linked to an increase in perinatal mortality, higher incidence of spontaneous abortion, greater mortality and morbidity during the first year of an infant's life, a lower rate of growth, and reduction in a child's mental aptitude into late adolescence (Brandt, 1987). However, despite declines in recent years, in 1996 about one in seven (13.6%) women giving birth reported smoking during their pregnancy (Ventura et al., 1998).

Alcohol consumption

Among all childbearing-aged women in 1995, 50.6% reported any drinking, and 12.6% reported frequent drinking. Frequent drinking is defined as consumption of an average of seven or more drinks per week or five or more drinks on at least one occasion. This prevalence is similar to that of 1991 (49.4% any drinking; 12.4% frequent drinking) (CDC, 1997). However, alcohol consumption among pregnant women increased substantially from 1991 to 1995 (CDC, 1997). In 1995, 16.3% of pregnant women reported any drinking during the preceding month, compared with 12.4% in 1991. The rate of frequent drinking among pregnant women was approximately four times higher in 1995 than in 1991 (3.5% in 1995 and 0.8% in 1991) (CDC, 1997).

In 1995, 24% of eighth grade girls and 47% of female high school seniors had consumed alcohol in the previous month. Among these same females, 14% of the eighth graders and 23% of the seniors had at least one episode of binge drinking, defined as five or more drinks in a row at least once in the prior two-week period (CDC, 1996b).

Drug use

The prevalence of drug use among pregnant women, based on state level and hospital-based studies, has been estimated at 7.5% to 15% (Chasnoff et al., 1990). Cocaine use among pregnant women has been estimated at 2.3% to 3.4%; marijuana use during pregnancy is estimated in the range of 3% to 12%; and opiate use during pregnancy is estimated in the range of 2% to 4% (CDC, 1990; Chasnoff et al., 1990).

It is difficult to estimate drug use during pregnancy accurately, because studies suffer from a number of methodologic problems. For example, self-reporting of these illegal activities probably leads to under-reporting. Additionally, samples of pregnant women are often small and nonrepresentative (low-income, urban women who are often in poorer health and under greater stress) (Zuckerman et al., 1989).

Exercise

Close to two-fifths (39%) of all women between the ages of 18 and 64 and nearly one-half of women aged 65 and over do not exercise (Brown et al., 1995). At all ages, women are less likely to exercise than are men; 31% of women exercise three or more days per week compared to 47% of men (Brown et al., 1995). Exercise habits also appear to differ by race; about 50% of Latina and African American women do not exercise, compared with 42% of Asian women and 36% of white women (Brown et al., 1995).

Nutrition/weight

Some 14% of women are underweight (Brown et al., 1995), while more than a quarter (27%) of women are overweight. Overweight problems are more prevalent among low-income women and those without a high school degree than among other women (Brown et al., 1995). Overweight problems also vary among women by ethnicity: 44% of African American women, 33% of Latinas, 25% of white women, and 12% of Asian women are overweight (Brown et al., 1995). Four out of ten women are trying to lose weight (Brown et al., 1995).

Violence

Each year, approximately 1.8 million (3.4%) women in the U.S. are physically assaulted by their partners (CDC, 1994b). In a recent study of violence against women conducted in Alaska, Maine, Oklahoma, and West Virginia, the proportion of women who reported having been physically hurt by their husband or partner during the 12 months preceding childbirth varied among the four states, from 3.8% in Maine to 6.9% in Oklahoma (CDC, 1994b).

In general, in each of these four states, rates of physical violence were higher for women who were less educated (had completed fewer than 12 years of education), of races other than white, aged 19 years or younger, unmarried, living in crowded conditions, had participated in the Women, Infants, and Children (WIC) Program during pregnancy, had delayed or received no prenatal care, or had an unintended pregnancy, than for other women (CDC, 1994a).

Sexual activity as it relates to STDs, HIV, and AIDS

According to a study conducted by the Campaign for Women's Health (1994), two-thirds of women "know almost nothing" about sexually transmitted diseases (STDs) other than HIV and AIDS. Nearly one-half (48%) report being "very uncomfortable" asking a new sex partner to practice safe sex. High-risk sexual activity among men and women in metropolitan areas remains common; 13% of men and 5% of women report two or more heterosexual partners in the last 12 months without consistent condom use (Berrios et al., 1993). In 1995, high-risk sexual behavior also was common among high school students. Nationwide, 53.1% had had sexual intercourse in their lifetime, with 17.8% reporting four or more sexual partners. Just over half (54.4%) reported that a condom was used by them or their partner during their last intercourse (CDC, 1996b). Black teens were more likely than white or Hispanic teens to have had more sexual partners and to have initiated sex at an early age (CDC, 1996b).

National recommendations for selected health behaviors in pregnancy

Prenatal care provides a foundation for improving the health of pregnant women, infants, and families, as well as communities and the population as a whole. As such, the prenatal care system may be understood as a cornerstone of health care delivery in our society. Maternal behaviors before, during, and even after pregnancy may significantly contribute to pregnancy outcomes. Three leading government publications – *Healthy People 2000: National Health Promotion and Disease Prevention Objectives* (DHHS, 1990), *Caring for our Future: The Content of Prenatal Care* (PHS, 1989), and the U.S. Preventive Services Task Force's *Guide to Clinical Preventive Services* (USPSTF, 1996) – have made specific recommendations on selected behaviors during pregnancy, including recommendations on tobacco, alcohol, and drug use; nutrition; sexual activity; exercise; stress reduction; and violence. These recommendations, presented in Table 2.1, are aimed at individual women and health care practitioners and also address goals for the overall population.

Health behavior can be influenced by the characteristics of the woman, the health care provider, and the system of care available. Influences include individual characteristics, such as age, education, ethnicity, family income, motivation, and social support. However, provider characteristics, such as knowledge, skill, and advance preparation, are also important. In addition, service delivery characteristics, such as payment for service, service setting, and visit schedules, may influence health behavior change.

Health behaviors that pose risks in pregnancy

The link between certain behaviors and pregnancy and perinatal outcome has long been a focus of interest to health care providers. Behaviors such as smoking, excessive alcohol use, illicit drug use, overweight, underweight, lack of exercise, and stress place women at increased risk for several acute and chronic illnesses, and have the potential for adversely affecting birth outcomes. Exposure to risky sexual activity and family violence can also negatively affect pregnancy outcome as well as longer-term health.

In 1991, the Commonwealth Fund Commission on Women's Health sponsored a report by the UCLA Center for Health Policy Research to determine the proportions of women engaging in particular risk behaviors and what opportunities existed to help women alter their behaviors (Commonwealth Fund, 1993). The report noted that some behaviors were perceived as a matter of individual choice or responsibility. However, societal factors that determine the level of social, economic, and policy support also could influence these behaviors. Health-related behaviors were found to vary widely according to race/ethnicity, education level, and socioeconomic status.

Specific population groups at risk

As described earlier, specific populations of women with low incomes and a high school education or less are more likely to smoke and be overweight and are less likely to exercise than are other women. Alcohol use increases with income level and education. Alcohol use and smoking are most prevalent among white women, while problems of overweight are most prevalent among African American women (Commonwealth Fund, 1993).

A sizable body of literature exists about the challenges of developing health behavior change in adolescents; some of that literature is relevant to this review. In a study of adolescent pregnancy, Trad (1993) noted that existing interventions seldom take into consideration the emotional upheaval inherent in adolescence. "Previewing" is one intervention that can enable adolescents to overcome their inability to predict long-term outcomes ("it's not going to happen to me"). By predicting and rehearsing adaptive outcomes specific to pregnancy, teens can role play various scenarios that *might* happen to them. In another work, Blankson and colleagues (1993) studied two groups of African American and white adolescents to determine what, if any, differences existed between health behavior and outcomes of sequential pregnancies. He concluded that poorer use of prenatal care and a higher risk for recurrence of adverse outcomes are characteristic of second pregnancies, and that this must be taken into account in providing effective intervention programs.

Advice given by professionals regarding health behavior

The Commonwealth Fund Commission on Women's Health Report (1993) argues that the responsibility of health professionals to improve health-related behaviors lies first in education. Data presented in the report showed that primary health care providers failed to present or discuss information about substance abuse with nearly 80% of women over the age of 18. When such issues were

Table 2.1. National recommendations for selected behaviors in pregnancy

	Healthy People 2000	The Content of Prenatal Care	Guide to Clinical Preventive Services
Smoking	Increase abstinence from tobacco use by pregnant women to at least 90%	Health care providers (HCP) should provide continuing risk assessment and counseling to reduce or eliminate smoking	A complete history of tobacco use, and assessment of nicotine dependence should be obtained. Counseling on the effects of passive smoke and tobacco cessation should be provided
Drug Use	Increase abstinence from cocaine and marijuana by pregnant women by at least 20%	Same as above. In addition, methods should be developed to improve recognition of illicit drug use, creation of appropriate number of effective treatment programs, referral to other programs, and prevention of unwanted pregnancies among drug users	A careful and complete drug use history by trusted clinician. Advise pregnant women of the potential adverse effects on the development of the fetus. Cease drug use during pregnancy
Alcohol use	Increase abstinence from alcohol by pregnant women by at least 20%	Same as drug use	A complete history of alcohol use should be obtained. Routine use of biochemical markers for alcohol consumption not recommended. Limit or cease drinking during pregnancy
Nutrition	Increase to at least 85% the proportion of mothers who achieve the minimum recommended weight gain during their pregnancies	HCP should conduct ongoing nutritional risk assessment, nutritional and breastfeeding counseling, vitamin and iron supplementation, and information on supplemental food programs	Counseling on adequate weight gain during pregnancy, increased requirements for energy and specific nutrients. Multivitamin with folate and iron supplementation as needed. Encourage breastfeeding

Table 2.1. (cont.)

	Healthy People 2000	The Content of Prenatal Care	Guide to Clinical Preventive Services
Sexual activity	Increase to at least 50% the proportion of family practitioners, maternal and child health, STD, TB, drug treatment, and primary care clinics that screen, diagnose, treat, counsel, and provide (or refer for) partner notification services for HIV infection and bacterial STDs*	HCP should conduct sexual risk assessment, provide counseling on safer sex practices, and ongoing sexuality counseling	Counseling on STD prevention, avoidance of high risk sexual behavior, and use of condoms
Exercise	Increase to at least 30% the proportion of people aged 6 and older who engage regularly in light to moderate physical activity for at least 30 minutes per day*	HCP should conduct exercise risk assessment and provide counseling on general health habits, including exercise and muscle toning, and rest and sleep patterns	Counseling to incorporate regular physical activity into daily routine*
Stress	Decrease to no more than 3% the proportion of people aged 18 and older who report experiencing significant levels of stress who do not take steps to reduce or control their stress*	HCP should conduct stress risk assessment and counseling on stress reduction strategies. Referral for social support, housing, etc.	No recommendations
Violence	Reduce physical abuse directed at women by male partners to no more than 27/1000 couples*	HCP should conduct abuse/family violence risk assessment and referrals to safe shelters	Include questions about physical abuse during history taking. Clinicians should be alert to the various presentations of child, spouse, and partner abuse*

*Not specific to maternal and child health populations.
Source: Garceau et al., 1997.

discussed, the most common topic was smoking, followed by diet, exercise, alcohol use, and drug use. The report recommended that more aggressive steps be taken to help women adopt behaviors that promote their health and well-being. Interventions should be especially targeted toward groups that are more vulnerable to health-damaging behaviors, including adolescent, low-income, and minority women.

In 1989, the report of the Public Health Service's Expert Panel on the Content of Prenatal Care provided guidelines for the components of each prenatal visit, including information on the timing of laboratory tests, examinations, and health promotion activities. A further examination of the issue of health promotion was provided in a series of three articles by Kogan and colleagues (1994a,b,c), which examined the relationship between the content of prenatal care and recommended national guidelines, low birth weight, and racial disparities. Using data collected by the 1988 National Center for Health Statistics National Maternal and Infant Health Survey, the authors found the following: Only 56% of the respondents said they received all of the six recommended procedures (blood pressure, urine test, blood test, weight and height measurements, pelvic exam, and pregnancy history) at the first two prenatal visits, and only 32% said they received advice in all seven recommended areas of advice and/or counseling (nutrition; vitamin use; smoking, alcohol, and drug use cessation; breastfeeding; and maternal weight gain). Women receiving their care from private offices were significantly less likely to receive all the procedures and advice than women at publicly funded sites of care. Women who reported not receiving all the types of advice were 38% more likely to have a low birth weight infant compared with women who reported receiving the optimal level of advice. However, there was no difference between women who reported receiving all recommended prenatal care procedures and those who reported not receiving all procedures. African American women were significantly more likely to report not receiving advice from their prenatal care providers about smoking cessation, alcohol use, and breastfeeding than were white, non-Hispanic women.

These data suggest that: (1) women who report receiving sufficient health behavior advice as part of their prenatal care are at lower risk of delivering a low birth weight infant than are women who do not receive such advice; (2) African American women may be at greater risk than white women for not receiving information that could reduce their chances of having an adverse pregnancy outcome; and (3) recommendations of the Public Health Service's expert panel are not being met.

A review of literature on health behavior interventions

Three on-line computerized databases were searched for literature on interventions designed to influence health behavior change during pregnancy: MEDLINE (yielding 54 intervention studies); CINAHL-Comprehensive Index of Nursing and Allied Health Literature (yielding 17 intervention studies); and The Cochrane Database of Systematic Reviews (1995), available on-line from the Cochrane Library. Search terms included "pregnancy" and "health behavior" and each of the following pregnancy-related health behaviors cited in *Healthy People 2000* (DHHS, 1990), the *Content of Prenatal Care* (PHS, 1989), and *Clinical Preventive Services Goals* (USPSTF, 1996) reports: smoking cessation, substance avoidance, alcohol avoidance, maternal nutrition, exercise during pregnancy, stress and social support, sexual behavior, and violence.

Smoking cessation

Although the literature review generated more intervention studies about smoking than any other health behavior, many cessation interventions were too brief, had little follow up, or did not take into account the stage of change that study participants may have been in at the time of the intervention. Researchers have noted some methodologic problems, such as self-report method of testing versus testing urine cotinine concentrations. In a three state, low intensity intervention with women enrolled in the WIC program, self-report did not match urine cotinine levels, and the authors concluded that biochemical verification is essential for an accurate evaluation of smoking cessation (Kendrick et al., 1995).

In 1994, Dolan-Mullen and colleagues assessed the impact of smoking cessation interventions in pregnancy using the available data from randomized clinical trials (RCT). The review, which is published in The Cochrane Database of Systematic Reviews (1995), indicated that behavioral strategies are substantially more effective than advice and feedback on smoking cessation rates; there was no evidence to suggest that counseling is effective (Dolan-Mullen et al., 1994). If effective, interventions aimed at smoking cessation during pregnancy lead to a small increase in mean birth weight and minimal reduction of low birth weight. There does not appear to be a demonstrable effect in the incidence of preterm birth or perinatal mortality (Baric et al., 1976; Bauman et al., 1983; Donovan, 1977; Haddow et al., 1991; Hjalmarson et al., 1991; Lilley and Forster, 1986; Loeb et al., 1983; MacArthur et al., 1987; Mayer et al., 1990; Messimer et al.,1989; Reading et al., 1982; Rush et al., 1992; Sexton and Hebel, 1984; Windsor et al., 1985, 1993).

The Cochrane Database of Systematic Reviews (1995) offers important practice implications, specifically to obstetricians and midwives. Providers should ensure that information on self-help behavioral strategies for smoking cessation are available and accessible to all women in their care, and that these materials are specifically geared toward pregnant women. Because of the limited influence of smoking cessation efforts in pregnancy alone, perinatal health providers are urged to support population-based efforts to reduce overall incidence of smoking (Lumley, 1994). These recommendations were reinforced by O'Campo and colleagues (1995) who noted that even with the most effective individualized counseling, it is increasingly evident that additional strategies are needed to achieve population-wide reductions in smoking and related health conditions. Examples of these efforts include taxation on cigarettes, community-based anti-tobacco programs, and efforts to increase the number of smoke-free environments. Thus, health professionals should take an active role in supporting broad programmatic, legislative, and advocacy efforts, in addition to clinic-based efforts.

Several authors pointed to the importance of understanding the influence of social ties and economic circumstances on smoking behavior. In a study of race differences in the proportion of low birth weight attributable to low-income maternal smoking, Barnett (1995) reported that the impact of smoking on birth weight was two times as great for non-Hispanic whites as for African Americans. Pletsch (1988) offered suggestions for recruiting minority subjects for intervention research, and focused on a smoking cessation study of pregnant Latinas. Lillington and colleagues (1995) evaluated culturally appropriate, low-literacy smoking cessation intervention materials used for low-income African American and Hispanic women. The intervention included a video and one-on-one counseling sessions, a self-help guide, and an incentive contest. The materials used were matched for the cultural, language, and literacy needs of the target populations; the test used self-report and cotinine-validated testing. A positive impact was noted for both pregnancy cessation rates and relapse prevention. Peterson et al.'s (1992) study of smoking reduction showed that a more intensive intervention significantly increased non-smoking postpartum.

Despite the increasing number of women who begin and continue to smoke, little research has been done that focuses on why pregnant women continue to smoke. A knowledge of effects does not seem to exert a major influence on behavior; therefore, education interventions alone do not appear to be sufficient.

Substance abuse

Pregnancy offers a unique opportunity for providers and others to encourage positive health behaviors. However, this opportunity becomes increasingly more complex when the behavior may result in criminal prosecution. Because interventions may be perceived as coercive, the majority of substance abuse interventions focus on education, counseling, and group therapy.

Alemi and colleagues (1996) studied the effect of a voice bulletin board on subject participation in self-help groups, expression of emotional support, use of health care services, and health status. Study subjects were 53 pregnant women who abused drugs. Results found that subjects were eight times more likely to participate in the bulletin board than in individual meetings, and felt a stronger sense of emotional support and connection within the group. Study subjects were less likely to visit outpatient clinics; there was no correlation between number of visits and health status or increased drug use.

A model program integrating theoretical models about changing behavior in women, a focus on ethnic minorities, and the postpartum process of maintaining behavior change has been described by Amaro and Aguiare (1994). Preliminary results of an evaluation of this comprehensive intervention program show improved rates of first trimester prenatal care and entry into drug treatment programs, improved pregnancy outcomes, reduced overall substance use, and decreased experience of violent crime (DHHS/HRSA, 1997).

Alcohol use

In the United States, alcohol abuse is a major cause of birth defects and mental retardation, including dysmorphology, growth restriction, and neurological damage in children with fetal alcohol syndrome. The yearly cost of caring for those affected by alcohol abuse during pregnancy is estimated to be over $30 million.

Although few studies exist to determine their effectiveness, prenatal education and counseling have been advocated as techniques to reduce alcohol use in pregnancy. Interventions have not been rigorously evaluated, and the benefits of any specific approach are unclear. Fox and colleagues (1989) studied the effect of a smoking cessation program on alcohol consumption by pregnant women in prenatal care. Average alcohol intake for all participants decreased before they began prenatal care; smoking decreased during pregnancy for the intervention group, but there was no effect on alcohol intake.

Casiro and colleagues (1994) evaluated the impact of a television public service message about alcohol consumption on 3000 Canadian women aged 15–45 years. After the campaign, more respondents believed that alcohol consumption would put their baby at risk than did before the campaign. The investigators did not note whether there was a change in behavior.

Nutrition

Most nutritional intervention studies focus on nutritional supplementation for women in developing countries, but there are two studies of note among American women.

Graham and colleagues (1992) studied the effectiveness of a home-based intervention for prevention of low birth weight. Of the 154 low-income African

American women studied, no decrease in rate of low birth weight was found for women who received four home visits as compared with women who received no home visits. There was a correlation between the number of home visits received and the number of subsequent prenatal visits. The home visits focused on smoking, drug, and nutrition education and also provided links to community services.

In examining the relationship between pre-pregnancy nutrition intervention and birth weight, Zimmer-Gembeck and Helfand (1996) studied the impact of a psychosocial intervention on 3073 low-income African American, Latina, and white pregnant women. The 45-minute intervention corresponded with a reduced rate of low birth weight for *all* women regardless of risk profile, although the rate remained higher for African American women than for other women, even after adjusting for all maternal biomedical, behavioral, psychosocial, and intervention factors.

Exercise

A minimal amount of information is available about exercise in pregnancy. No intervention studies were reported; therefore, the topic is difficult to assess through the available literature. One small study demonstrated that maintaining an exercise program during pregnancy may affect subcutaneous fat deposition in later pregnancy, but does not appear to affect overall pregnancy weight gain (Clapp and Little, 1995).

Sexual activity

Sexual activity was selected as an important area of women's health behavior due to its relationship with HIV infection and the strength of recent reports linking certain genital tract infections (bacterial vaginosis) and spontaneous preterm births (Goldenberg and Andrews, 1996; Goldenberg et al., 1990, 1996; Hillier et al., 1995; Meis et al., 1995). This is particularly important as it relates to the prevention of prematurity among African American women, who have a substantially higher prevalence of potentially pathogenic organisms than do white, Hispanic, or Asian women. The rate of bacterial vaginosis is 2–3 times higher among African American women than white women (Goldenberg et al., 1990, 1996). This issue is discussed further in Chapter 4.

The literature review yielded little information, identifying only three intervention studies. Smith (1994) evaluated a three-phase teen incentive program (60 freshman at an inner-city high school; 30 in each group) to enhance self-perception and abilities to exercise greater control in their lives, particularly on sexual behavior. Post-test reports showed a decrease in sexual activity (self-report), and an increase in contraceptive use by over 50%. Santelli and colleagues (1995) reported the effect of a community-based intervention program designed to prevent perinatal HIV infection by preventing infection in women. An increase in condom use at the last sexual encounter was significantly higher in the intervention community; condom use was also higher for women exposed to "small media" (e.g., flyers, brochures) with or without "street outreach". One study reported on an intervention plan, but outcomes were not included (Coyle et al., 1996).

Violence

The relationship between abuse and tobacco, alcohol, and illicit drug use has been documented (McFarlane et al., 1992; McFarlane and Wiist, 1996). Amaro and colleagues (1990) found that a woman's alcohol use during pregnancy and her partner's drug use were independently associated with an increased risk of being a victim of violence during pregnancy. The literature review identified no intervention studies about violence.

Stress/social support

Several different definitions of social support are used in the literature evaluating the relationships between maternal stress, maternal anxiety, and social support (Bryce et al., 1988; Cassel, 1974; Cobb, 1974; House, 1981; Norbeck and Tilden, 1983; Nuckolls et al., 1972; Sarason et al., 1978; Thompson, 1990). Although it seems likely that social support is multidimensional, researchers are not yet agreed on this nor on what dimensions are most influential in preventing and/or mediating the effects of stress during pregnancy (Thompson, 1990). The issue of stress and social support during pregnancy is also discussed in Chapter 3.

Many attempts have been made since the early 1970s to link high levels of maternal anxiety as measured by catecholamine levels or state/trait anxiety with negative pregnancy outcomes (low birth weight, longer labor, pregnancy-induced hypertension, and poor parenting). In the classic study by Nuckolls and colleagues (1972) of social support in pregnancy, the concept of "psychosocial assets" was introduced as an intervention that reduced the negative effects of maternal stress.

During the early 1970s, social support was understood to work as a buffer to mediate the relationship between stressful life events and adverse health outcomes. In the mid-1970s, Cassel (1974) and Cobb (1974) suggested that primary group support had health protective effects as well as buffering effects. Currently, there is little agreement as to whether to distinguish between who gives the support and the type of support given. Recent interest in this topic is derived largely from the desire to understand how and why racial and social class differences in birth outcomes have remained. The high rate of preterm delivery among African American women, not adequately accounted for by social class differences, has led some researchers to postulate racism itself as a social stressor.

Observational studies of social support have provided evidence that social support, in particular support from a partner or other close family member, has *main* rather than *buffering* effects, on fetal growth (Collins et al., 1993; Molfese et al., 1987; Reeb et al., 1987; Turner et al., 1990). The association appears stronger among low-income women than among other women.

Hodnett (1997) summarized 11 randomized clinical trials from the 1995 Cochrane Database of Systematic Reviews to assess the effects of additional social support compared with routine care for women in the first or second trimester of pregnancy who were judged to be at risk of having low birth weight babies. Individualized social support (emotional support, counseling, tangible assistance, information/instruction) was provided either in home visits, during regular prenatal clinic visits, or by telephone at several points during pregnancy. Over 8000 women in eight countries were studied. Social support interventions for at-risk pregnant women have not been associated with improvements in any medical outcomes for the index pregnancy. Similarly, only a few improvements in immediate psychosocial outcomes have been found in individual trials.

Hodnett (1997) concluded that pregnant women need and deserve to have the help and support of caring family members, friends, and health professionals. However, such support is unlikely to be powerful enough to overcome the effects of a lifetime of poverty and disadvantage and thereby influence the remaining course of a pregnancy. Pregnant women and their caregivers should be informed that programs that offer additional support during pregnancy are unlikely to prevent the pregnancy from resulting in a preterm or low birth weight baby.

Hodnett's Cochrane Database review suggests no further studies are needed to link social support with a reduction of preterm births. However, she notes that timing, "dosage," length of treatment, and expected benefits are important considerations. An effective support intervention may need to begin before pregnancy and be prolonged and individualized; important health benefits may be long-term rather than immediate.

In their review of the literature, Hoffman and Hatch (1996) concluded that three main findings stand out: (1) there is no convincing evidence that acute life stressors experienced during pregnancy adversely affect fetal growth or gestational length; (2) intimate social support provided by a partner or close family member is associated fairly consistently with improved fetal growth, regardless of a woman's level of stress; and (3) psychosocial factors appear to relate more often to fetal growth than to preterm birth. In another recent study, Kitzman and colleagues (1997) demonstrated positive effects of home visitation by nurses on pregnancy-induced hypertension and subsequent pregnancies among low-income women without previous live births, although no program effects were demonstrated for preterm delivery or low birth weight.

Social support and psychosocial status

Bullock and colleagues (1995) conducted a randomized clinical trial to test the psychosocial benefits of a telephone support program for pregnant women, and concluded that a low-cost health promotion program of telephone support during pregnancy can significantly improve a woman's psychosocial status during pregnancy. The women who experienced intervention reported more use of community resources than did the women in the control group.

Maternal depression has been found to be associated with adverse outcomes in some, but not all, recent studies of social support in pregnancy. Hoffman and Hatch (1996) suggest that maternal depression could be the link between adverse life circumstances and increased obstetric risk. In addition, depressive symptoms have been associated with a greater likelihood of smoking during pregnancy (Prichard, 1994). Women of low socioeconomic status are at an increased risk for smoking and developing depression during pregnancy (Williamson et al., 1989). Further research is needed to determine if depressed smokers are less able to give up smoking or if women who stop smoking are at increased risk for depression. Pursuit of the possible connection between intimate social support and fetal growth is another important area of study. Identifying potential mechanisms for a beneficial effect of social support would increase confidence that the association represents a true effect. It also would assist with the design of new interventions.

Conclusion

The status of research on the topics of health behavior is mixed, with most interventions focusing on smoking cessation. The number of intervention studies is minimal. Research on interventions does not appear to have kept pace with the increased emphasis that has been placed on health behavior in the 1990s.

Gaps in the current literature

There is a distinct discrepancy between knowledge about health behavior in pregnancy and the volume of intervention studies on the topics outlined in national recommendations. Clearly, there is a need for an expanded research effort, with particular emphasis on the evaluation of interventions. In most circumstances, minimal attention has been given to populations at risk. However, it should be noted that in some areas (e.g., drug abuse), the intervention research has been targeted solely to certain populations.

There has been minimal integration of the behavioral intervention theory and research with the study of health behavior in pregnancy. However, there are some examples of this integration that have had positive results, specifically in the areas of substance abuse (Amaro, 1995; Amaro and Aguiare, 1994; Amaro and Hardy-Fanta, 1995; DHHS/HRSA, 1997) and smoking cessation (Mullen et al., 1991). In general, the field would benefit from the integration of research in prenatal care and behavioral science.

Finally, there is currently a weak link between research on primary care for women and research about health behavior in pregnancy. Without this link, frustrations felt by health care providers about the recidivism of women who have made pregnancy-related behavior changes cannot be sufficiently addressed.

Recommendations for policy and practice

To ensure that health outcomes and health care access are optimal, and that health care resources are expended in the most efficient and effective manner, policy makers, health services managers, and providers should give greater attention to behaviors that promote the health of pregnant and nonpregnant women of all ages. Encouraging health-promoting behaviors such as smoking cessation, alcohol and substance avoidance, increased exercise, improved nutrition, and access to social support outlets, must occur at multiple levels of the health system.

Policy makers must be prepared to support broad-based public health approaches to health behavior interventions, including those instituted by programs such as WIC (Kendrick et al., 1995) and through education and outreach services (Petersen et al., 1992; Lillington et al., 1995; Santelli et al., 1995; Smith, 1994). In addition to clinic- and education-based efforts, policy makers must be willing to actively address improvements in health behavior change through such programmatic and legislative strategies as cigarette taxation, community-based anti-tobacco programs, and efforts to increase the number of smoke-free environments (O'Campo et al., 1995).

Managed care and fee-for-service health plans should cover preventive services that have been demonstrated to be effective in improving maternal and fetal health. Physicians, nurses, and other health care professionals must play a more aggressive role in providing counseling on health-promoting behaviors during pregnancy, especially to groups that are more vulnerable to health-damaging behaviors, including adolescent, low-income, and minority women (Commonwealth Fund Report, 1993).

Providers must collaborate to a greater extent if they are to bridge the gap between primary care and pregnancy care. Education of *all* providers of women's health about national health behavior recommendations (PHS, 1989; DHHS, 1990; USPSTF, 1996) should be enhanced, and interventions focused on subpopulations who are at higher risk of poor outcomes related to health-damaging behaviors during pregnancy.

Finally, more pregnant women and their families must be reached through outreach services with accurate information about health-promoting behaviors (Kitzman et al., 1997; Kogan et al., 1994a,b,c; Santelli et al., 1995).

REFERENCES

Ajzen I, Fishbein, M. Understanding attitudes and predicting social behavior. Englewood Cliffs (NJ): Prentice-Hall, 1980.

Alemi F, Mosavel M, Stephens RC, Ghadiri A, Krishnaswamy J, Thakkar H. Electronic self-help and support groups. Medical Care 1996; **34** (Suppl. 10): OS32–44.

Amaro H. Love, sex, and power. American Psychologist 1995; 437–45.

Amaro H, Aguiare M. Programa Mama/MOM's Project: A community-based outreach model for addicted women. A Hispanic/Latino family approach to substance abuse prevention. Rockville (MD): Center for Substance Abuse Prevention, Substance Abuse and Mental Health Services Administration, 1994.

Amaro H, Fried LE, Cabral H. Violence during pregnancy and substance abuse. American Journal of Public Health 1990; **90**: 575–9.

Amaro H, Hardy-Fanta C. Gender relations in addiction and recovery. Journal of Psychoactive Drugs 1995; **27**: 325–37.

Bandura A. Social foundations of thought and action: a social cognitive theory. Englewood Cliffs (NJ): Prentice-Hall, 1986.

Baric L, MacArthur C, Sherwood M. A study of health education aspects of smoking in pregnancy. International Journal of Health Education 1976; **19S**: 1–17.

Barnett E. Race differences in the proportion of low birth weight attributable to maternal cigarette smoking in a low-income population. American Journal of Health Promotion 1995; **10**: 105–10.

Bauman KE, Bryan ES, Dent CW, Koch GG. The influence of observing carbon monoxide level on cigarette smoking by public prenatal patients. American Journal of Public Health 1983; **73**: 1089–91.

Berrios DC, Hearst N, Coates RJ, et al. HIV antibody testing among those at risk for infection. The national AIDS behavioral surveys. Journal of the American Medical Association 1993; **270**: 1576–80.

Blankson ML, Cliver SP, Goldenberg RL, Hickey CA, Jin J, Dubard MB. Health behavior and outcomes in sequential pregnancies of black and white adolescents. Journal of the American Medical Association 1993; **269**: 1401–3.

Brandt EN. Smoking and reproductive health. In: Rosenburg MJ, ed. Smoking and reproductive health. Littleton (MA): PSG Publishing, 1987.

Brown ER, Wyn R, Cumberland WG, et al. Women's health-related behaviors and use of clinical preventive services. New York: The Commonwealth Fund, 1995.

Bryce RL, Stanley FJ, Enkin MW. The role of social support in the prevention of preterm birth. Birth 1988; **15**: 19–23.

Bullock LF, Wells JE, Duff GB, Hornblow AR. Telephone support for pregnant women:

outcome in late pregnancy. New Zealand Medical Journal 1995; **108**: 476–8.

Campaign for Women's Health and American Medical Women's Association. Women and sexually transmitted diseases: the dangers of denial. Executive summary. Washington (DC): American Medical Women's Association, 1994.

Carter W. Health behavior as a rational process: theory of reasoned action and multiattribute utility theory. In: Glanz K, Lewis F, Rimer B, eds. Health behavior and health education: theory, research, and practice. San Francisco: Jossey-Bass, 1990.

Casiro OG, Stanwick RS, Pelech A, Taylor V. Public awareness of the risks of drinking alcohol during pregnancy: the effects of a television campaign. Canadian Journal of Public Health. Revué Canadienne de Santé Publique 1994; **85**: 23–7.

Cassel J. Psychosocial processes and "stress": theoretical formulations. International Journal of Health Services 1974; **4**: 471–82.

Centers for Disease Control and Prevention (CDC). Statewide prevalence of illicit drug use by pregnant women – Rhode Island. Morbidity and Mortality Weekly Report 1990; **39**: 225–7.

Centers for Disease Control and Prevention (CDC). Physical violence during the 12 months preceding childbirth, Alaska, Maine, Oklahoma, and West Virginia, 1990–1991. Morbidity and Mortality Weekly Report 1994a; **43**: 132–7.

Centers for Disease Control and Prevention (CDC). Cigarette smoking among women of reproductive age: United States 1987–1992. Morbidity and Mortality Weekly Report 1994b; **43**: 789–97.

Centers for Disease Control and Prevention (CDC). Cigarette smoking among adults: United States, 1994. Morbidity and Mortality Weekly Report 1996a; **45**: 588–90.

Centers for Disease Control and Prevention (CDC). Youth risk behavior surveillance: United States, 1995. CDC Surveillance Summaries. 1996b; **45(SS-4)**: 1–91.

Centers for Disease Control and Prevention (CDC). Alcohol consumption among pregnant and childbearing-aged women – United States, 1991 and 1995. Morbidity and Mortality Weekly Report 1997; **46**: 346–50.

Chasnoff IJ, Landress HJ, Barett ME. The prevalence of illicit-drug or alcohol use during pregnancy and discrepancies in mandatory reporting in Pinellas County, Florida. New England Journal of Medicine 1990; **322**: 1202–6.

Clapp JF, Little KD. Effect of recreational exercise on pregnancy weight gain and subcutaneous fat deposition. Medicine and Science In Sports and Exercise 1995; **27**: 170–7.

Cobb S. A model for life events and their consequences. In: Dohrenwend BS, Dohrenwend BP, eds. Stressful life events. New York: Wiley, 1974.

The Cochrane Database of Systematic Reviews. Oxford: Cochrane Collaboration, 1995.

Collins NL, Dunkel-Schetter C, Lobel M, Scrimshaw SC. Social support in pregnancy: psychosocial correlates of birth outcomes and postpartum depression. Journal of Personality and Social Psychology 1993; **65**: 1243–58.

The Commonwealth Fund Women's Health Study. New York: Louis Harris and Associates, 1993.

Coyle K, Kirby D, Parcel G, et al. Safer choices: a multicomponent school-based HIV/STD and pregnancy prevention program for adolescents. Journal of School Health 1996; **66**: 89–94.

Dolan-Mullen P, Ramirez G, Groff JY. Obstetrics: a meta-analysis of randomized trials of prenatal smoking cessation interventions. American Journal of Obstetrics and Gynecology 1994; **171**: 1328–34.

Donovan JW. Randomised controlled trial of anti-smoking advice in pregnancy. British Journal of Social Medicine 1977; **31**: 6–12.

Fishbein M, Guinan, M. Behavioral science and public health: a necessary partnership for HIV prevention. Public Health Reports 1996; **111**: 5–10.

Fox NL, Sexton M, Hebel JR, Thompson B. The reliability of self-reports of smoking and alcohol consumption by pregnant women. Addictive Behaviors 1989; **14**: 187–95.

Freire, P. Education for critical consciousness. New York: Seabury Press, 1973.

Garceau LM, Paine LL, Barger MK. Population-based primary care for women: an overview for midwives. Journal of Nurse Midwifery 1997; **42**: 465–77.

Glanz K, Lewis F, Rimer B, eds. Health behavior and health education: theory, research, and practice. San Francisco: Jossey-Bass, 1990.

Goldenberg RL, Andrews WW. Editorial: intrauterine infection and why preterm prevention programs have failed. American Journal of Public Health 1996; **86**: 220–2.

Goldenberg RL, Davis RO, Copper RL, Corliss DK, Andrews JB, Carpenter AH. The Alabama preterm birth prevention project. Obstetrics and Gynecology 1990; **75**: 933–9.

Goldenberg RL, Klebanoff MA, Nugent R, Krohn MA, Hillier S, Andrews WW. Bacterial colonization of the vagina during pregnancy in four ethnic groups. Vaginal Infections and Prematurity Study Group. American Journal of Obstetrics and Gynecology 1996; **174**: 1618–21.

Graham AV, Frank SH, Zyzanski SJ, Kitson GC, Reeb KG. A clinical trial to reduce the rate of low birth weight in an inner-city black population. Family Medicine 1992; **24**: 439–46.

Haddow JE, Knight GJ, Kloza FM, Palomaki GE, Wald NJ. Cotinine-assisted intervention in pregnancy to reduce smoking and low birthweight delivery. British Journal of Obstetrics and Gynæcology 1991; **98**: 859–65.

Hillier SL, Nugent RP, Eschenbach DA, et al. Association between bacterial vaginosis and preterm delivery of a low-birth-weight infant. New England Journal of Medicine 1995; **333**: 1737–42.

Hjalmarson AIM, Hahn L, Svanberg B. Stopping smoking in pregnancy: effect of a self-help manual in controlled trial. British Journal of Obstetrics and Gynæcology 1991; **98**: 260–6.

Hochbaum G. Public participation in medical screening programs: a sociopsychological study. Washington (DC): Public Health Service, U.S. Department of Health, Education and Welfare. Publication No. 572, 1958.

Hodnett ED. Support from care-givers during at-risk pregnancy. In: Neilson JP, Crowther CA, Hodnett ED, Hofmeyer GJ, Keirse MJNC, eds. Pregnancy and childbirth module of the Cochrane database of systematic reviews [Updated March 1997]. Available in the Cochrane Library. The Cochrane Collaboration; Issue 2. Oxford: Update Software, 1997. Updated quarterly.

Hoffman S, Hatch MC. Stress, social support and pregnancy outcome: a reassessment based on recent research. Paediatric and Perinatal Epidemiology 1996; **10**: 381–405.

House J. Work, stress, and social support. Reading (MA): Addison-Wesley, 1981.

Iscore I. Community psychology and the competent community. American Psychologist 1980; **29**: 607–13.

Kendrick JS, Zahniser SC, Miller N, Salas N, Stine J, Gargiullo PM, et al. Integrating smoking cessation into routine public prenatal care: the smoking cessation in pregnancy project. American Journal of Public Health 1995; **85**: 217–22.

Kitzman H, Olds DL, Henderson CR Jr, Hanks C, Cole R, Tatelbaum R, et al. Effect of prenatal and infancy home visitation by nurses on pregnancy outcomes, childhood injuries, and repeated childbearing. A randomized clinical trial. Journal of the American Medical Association 1997; **278**: 644–52.

Kogan MD, Alexander GR, Kotelchuck M, Nagy DA. Relation of the content of prenatal care to the risk of low birth weight. Maternal reports of health behavior advice and initial prenatal care procedures. Journal of the American Medical Association 1994a; **271**: 1340–5.

Kogan MD, Alexander GR, Kotelchuck M, Nagey DA, Jack BW. Comparing mothers' reports on the content of prenatal care received with recommended national guidelines for care. Public Health Reports 1994b; **109**: 637–46.

Kogan MD, Kotelchuck M, Alexander GR, Johnson WE. Racial disparities in reported prenatal care advice from health care providers. American Journal of Public Health 1994c; **84**: 82–8.

Larson EB, Bergman J, Heidrich F, Alvin BL, Schneeweiss R. Do postcard reminders improve influenza vaccination compliance? Medical Care 1982; **20**: 639–48.

Lilley J, Forster DP. A randomized controlled trial of individual counseling of smokers in pregnancy. Public Health 1986; **100**: 309–15.

Lillington L, Royce J, Novak D, Ruvalcaba M, Chlebowski R. Evaluation of a smoking cessation program for pregnant minority women. Cancer Practice 1995; **3**(3): 157–63.

Loeb BK, Waage G, Bailey JW. Smoking intervention in pregnancy. Proceedings of 5th World Conference on Smoking and Health, Winnipeg, Manitoba, Canada, 1983: 389–95.

Lumley J. Strategies for reducing smoking in pregnancy. In: Enkin MW, Keirse MJNC, Renfrew MJ, Neilson JP, eds. Pregnancy and childbirth module. Cochrane Database of Systematic Reviews: Review No. 03312 2 October 1993. Published through Cochrane Updates on Disk, Oxford: Update Software 1994. Disk Issue I.

MacArthur C, Newton JR, Knox EG. Effect of anti-smoking health education on infant size at birth: a randomized controlled trial. British Journal of Obstetrics and Gynæcology 1987; **94**: 295–300.

Mayer JP, Hawkins B, Todd R. A randomized evaluation of smoking cessation interventions for pregnant women at a WIC clinic. American Journal of Public Health 1990; **80**: 76–8.

McFarlane J, Parker B, Soeken K, Bullock L. Assessing for abuse during pregnancy. Severity and frequency of injuries and associated entry into prenatal care. Journal of the American Medical Association 1992; **267**: 3176–8.

McFarlane J, Wiist WW. Documentation of abuse to pregnant women: a medical chart audit in public health clinics. Journal of Women's Health 1996; **5**: 137–42.

Meis PJ, Goldenberg RL, Mercer B, et al. The National Institute of Child Health and Human Development Maternal–Fetal Medicine Units Network. The preterm prediction study: significance of vaginal infections. American Journal of Obstetrics and Gynecology 1995; **173**: 1231–5.

Messimer SR, Hickner JM, Henry RC. A comparison of two antismoking interventions among pregnant women in eleven private primary care practices. Journal of Family Practice 1989; **28**: 283–8.

Miller JB. Toward a new psychology of women. Boston: Beacon Press, 1986.

Molfese VJ, Thomson BK, Beadnell B, Bricker MC, Manion LG. Perinatal risk screening and infant outcome. Can predictions be improved with composite scales? Journal of Reproductive Medicine 1987; **32**: 569–76.

Mullen PD, Carbonari JP, Tabak ER, Glenday MC. Improving disclosure of smoking by pregnant women. American Journal of Obstetrics and Gynecology 1991; **165**: 409–13.

Norbeck JS, Tilden VP. Life stress, social support and emotional disequilibrium in complications of pregnancy: a prospective, multivariate study. Journal of Health and Social Behavior 1983; **24**: 30–46.

Nuckolls KB, Cassel J, Kaplan BH. Psychological assets, life crises and the prognosis of pregnancy. American Journal of Epidemiology 1972; **95**: 431–41.

O'Campo P, Davis PMV, Geilen AC. Smoking cessation intervention for pregnant women: review and future directions. Seminars in Perinatology 1995; **19**: 279–85.

Perry C, Baranowski T, Parcel G. How individuals, environments, and health behavior interact: social learning theory. In: Glanz K, Lewis F, Rimer B, eds. Health behavior and health education: theory, research, and practice. San Francisco: Jossey-Bass, 1990.

Petersen L, Handel J, Kotch J, Podenworny T, Rosen A. Smoking reduction during pregnancy by a program of self-help and clinical report. Obstetrics and Gynecology 1992; **79**: 924–30.

Pletsch PK. Substance use and health activities of pregnant adolescents. Journal of Adolescent Health Care 1988; **9**: 38–45.

Prichard CW. Depression and smoking in pregnancy in Scotland. Journal of Epidemiology and Community Health 1994; **48**: 377–82.

Prochaska JO, DiClemente CO. Toward a comprehensive model of change. In: Miller DR, Healther N, eds. Treating addictive behaviors. New York: Plenum Press, 1986.

Public Health Service (PHS) Expert Panel on the Content of Prenatal Care. Caring for our future: the content of prenatal care. Washington (DC): U.S. Department of Health and Human Services, Public Health Service, 1989.

Rappaport J. Studies in empowerment: introduction to the issue. Preventive Human Services 1984; **3**: 1–7.

Reading AE, Campbell S, Cox DN, Sledmore CM. Health beliefs and health care behavior in pregnancy. Psychological Medicine 1982; **12**: 379–83.

Reeb KA, Graham AV, Ayzanski SJ. Predicting low birthweight and complicated labor in urban black women: a biopsychosocial perspective. Social Science and Medicine 1987; **25**: 1321–7.

Rosenstock IM. What research in motivation suggests for public health. American Journal of Public Health 1960; **50**: 295–301.

Rosenstock IM. The health belief model: explaining health behavior through expectancies. In: Glanz K, Lewis F, Rimer B, eds. Health behavior and health education: theory, research, and practice. San Francisco: Jossey-Bass, 1990.

Rush D, Orme J, King J, Eiser JR, Butler NR. A trial of health education aimed to reduce cigarette smoking among pregnant women. Paediatric and Perinatal Epidemiology 1992; **6**: 285–97.

Santelli JS, Celentano DD, Rozsenich C, et al. Interim outcomes for a community-based program to prevent perinatal HIV transmission. AIDS Education and Prevention 1995; **7**: 210–20.

Sarason IG, Johnson JH, Siegel JM. Assessing the impact of life changes: development of the life experiences survey. Journal of Consulting and Clinical Psychology 1978; **46**: 932–46.

Sexton MJ, Hebel JR. A clinical trial of change in maternal smoking and its effect on birth weight. Journal of the American Medical Association 1984; **251**: 911–15.

Smith MAB. Teen incentives program: evaluation of a health promotion model for adolescent pregnancy prevention. Journal of Health Education 1994; **25**: 24–9.

Thompson JE. Maternal stress, anxiety, and social support during pregnancy; possible directions for prenatal intervention. In: Merkatz IR, Thompson JE, eds. New perspectives on prenatal care. New York: Elsevier, 1990.

Trad PV. Adolescent pregnancy: an intervention challenge. Child Psychiatry and Human Development 1993; **24**: 99–113.

Turner RJ, Grindstaff CF, Phillips N. Social support and outcome in teenage pregnancy. Journal of Health and Social Behavior 1990; **75**: 341–5.

U.S. Department of Health, Education, and Welfare (DHEW). The health consequences of smoking. Washington (DC): U.S. Government Printing Office, Publication No. DHEW/HSM 73–8704, 1973.

U.S. Department of Health and Human Services (DHHS). Healthy people 2000: national health promotion and disease prevention objectives. Washington (DC): U.S. Government Printing Office, DHHS Publication No., (PHS) 91–50212, 1990.

U.S. Department of Health and Human Services (DHHS/HRSA). Models that work: MOM's Project strategy transfer guide. Rockville (MD): Health Resources and Services Administration, Bureau of Primary Health Care, 1997.

U.S. Preventive Services Task Force. Guide to clinical preventive services, 2nd edition. Baltimore (MD): Williams & Wilkins, 1996.

Ventura SJ, Martin JA, Curtin SC, Mathews TJ. Report of final natality statistics, 1996. Monthly vital statistics report. Hyattsville (MD): National Center for Health Statistics. 1998; **46** (Suppl. 11).

Williamson DF, Serdula MK, Kendrick JS, Binkin NJ. Comparing the prevalence of smoking in pregnant and nonpregnant women, 1985 to 1986. Journal of the American Medical Association, 1989; **261**: 70–4.

Windsor RA, Cutter G, Morris J, et al. The effectiveness of smoking cessation methods for smokers in public health maternity clinics: a randomized trial. American Journal of Public Health 1985; **75**: 1389–92.

Windsor RA, Lowe JB, Perkins LL, Smith-Yoder D, et al. Health education for pregnant smokers: its behavioral impact and cost benefit. American Journal of Public Health 1993; **83**: 201–6.

Zimmer-Gembeck MJ, Helfand M. Low birthweight in a public prenatal care program: behavioral and psychosocial risk factors and psychosocial intervention. Social Science and Medicine 1996; **43**: 187–97.

Zuckerman B, Amaro H, Bauchner H, Cabral H. Depressive symptoms during pregnancy: relationship to poor health behaviors. American Journal of Obstetrics and Gynecology 1989; **160**: 1107–11.

Part II

Preventing Prematurity

3

Causes of prematurity

David A. Savitz and Lisa M. Pastore

Introduction

The causes of preterm delivery can be viewed from a number of different perspectives. Similarly, the concept of "prevention of preterm delivery" can be approached in different ways. Causes can be conceptualized along the spectrum from macro-level social and political forces all the way to immediate biological antecedents of the event (Figure 3.1). Contributing causes of preterm delivery in an individual case could be poverty, cocaine use, and placental abruption, comprising a cascade of events that ultimately requires medical intervention and delivery before term. In principle, interventions to interrupt that cascade can be considered at any of the points along the way.

This chapter considers only a subset of possible determinants of preterm delivery. For those processes operating at the societal level, such as poverty and geography, the comments will be brief. Although the ultimate determinants of preterm delivery may be based on these societal forces, societal changes occur slowly, and preventive measures are urgently needed. Thus, our focus is on individual attributes and behaviors, with a particular focus on those that can be modified, such as tobacco use or physical exertion.

To lay a foundation for the chapter, we first discuss some concepts of causality as they relate to preterm delivery; then we describe key sociodemographic patterns associated with prematurity, as presented in Berkowitz and Papiernik's comprehensive 1993 review. We then define several markers of risk that are not amenable to intervention, though they may be of great value in the intensive clinical monitoring of warning signs of preterm delivery. These attributes include height, history of adverse pregnancy outcomes, and other markers used in risk scoring systems. This portion of the chapter is followed by a detailed discussion of a number of behavioral, or "lifestyle," factors that are more likely to be influenced by an intervention and, as such, could constitute a primary avenue for the prevention of preterm delivery.

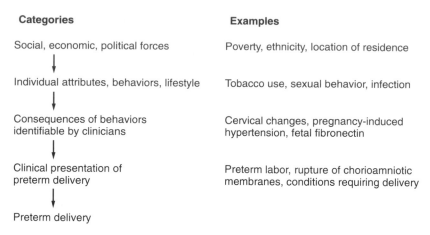

Categories	Examples
Social, economic, political forces	Poverty, ethnicity, location of residence
↓	
Individual attributes, behaviors, lifestyle	Tobacco use, sexual behavior, infection
↓	
Consequences of behaviors identifiable by clinicians	Cervical changes, pregnancy-induced hypertension, fetal fibronectin
↓	
Clinical presentation of preterm delivery	Preterm labor, rupture of chorioamniotic membranes, conditions requiring delivery
↓	
Preterm delivery	

Figure 3.1   Conceptual model of causes of preterm delivery.

Concept of "cause" applied to preterm delivery

Some basic notions of causality articulated by Rothman (1976) are worthy of brief summary as they apply to preterm delivery. First, there are often a variety of causal pathways, that is, more than one constellation of component causes leading to the same outcome, preterm delivery. For example, the outcome of preterm delivery may be caused by factors such as severe hypertension that result in medically indicated preterm delivery, or by quite different factors that result in preterm labor. Determinants of premature rupture of the chorioamniotic membranes before term may be different from those causing preterm labor (Savitz et al., 1991a), although this is not necessarily the case (Klebanoff and Shiono, 1995). Conceptually, if we can isolate distinctive causal pathways, our ability to identify the contributors to those pathways will be enhanced, and we will be better able to ascertain the role of these factors in preterm delivery in the aggregate. For example, a specific exposure may double the risk of the subset of preterm delivery resulting from membrane rupture, even though we might observe only a 30% increased risk for preterm delivery in the aggregate. The associations we can observe are thus stronger if we are able to isolate and study the portion of those deliveries truly affected by the exposure of interest.

Another important consideration with regard to causality is that a given risk factor can and often does contribute to more than one causal pathway. For example, tobacco use might restrict fetal growth, which could affect preterm delivery. Tobacco may also suppress immune function to facilitate changes in the vaginal flora resulting in bacterial vaginosis, thus contributing to the pathway mediated by insufficient fetal growth and to the pathway mediated by membrane rupture.

The division between modifiable individual attributes and those signs detectable by clinicians is not distinct. For example, symptomatic genital tract infection might be included in the category of patient characteristics, although asymptomatic infection – which is also a consequence of individual behaviors (e.g., sexual activity, douching) – is detectable only by the clinician. We will discuss genital tract infection in some detail, despite this ambiguity. On the other hand, some markers are distinctive to clinical detection, such as cervical changes and fetal fibronectin. Because patients cannot act specifically on these markers, they will not be considered as "causes" of preterm delivery for this discussion.

A major challenge to identifying causes of preterm delivery is a lack of knowledge about the time course of exposure and outcome. Some determinants may be established long before the pregnancy, even at the time of the mother's birth in the case of genetic or anatomic factors. Other exposures operating early in pregnancy may affect the formation and function of the placenta. Finally, some exposures are thought to affect preterm delivery over a brief time course, so that the woman's experience days or even hours before delivery are most critical. In the face of such variety and uncertainty, it is important to be explicit about the hypothesized causal pathway under study. Implicating or exonerating an exposure at one time during the pregnancy does not mean that this exposure is necessarily implicated or exonerated at other points in time.

Our review is guided by two concerns: the adequacy of the epidemiologic literature as a basis for intervention, and the research needed to resolve whether a causal association is present and, thus, one for which intervention would be warranted. We will not consider the feasibility of interventions once such a linkage is made, for example, the practical barriers to persuading pregnant women to refrain from smoking. Our review is not comprehensive, but we have focused on the most recent literature, particularly from 1987 to the present, and considered what we believe to be the methodologically strongest studies.

Sociodemographic patterns

The review by Berkowitz and Papiernik (1993) provides a complete and insightful summary of the literature up to the early 1990s. Except for potential risk factors that are of special interest because they can be changed, we will rely largely on that review.

Socioeconomic status

Most studies cited by Berkowitz and Papiernik (1993) reported an increased risk of preterm delivery associated with lower socioeconomic status, though there have been some contradictory reports (Shiono and Klebanoff, 1986). Measures of socioeconomic status in different studies are based on education, income, occupation, or some combination of those attributes, and the magnitude of association with preterm delivery is not likely to be consistent across those indicators. Because socioeconomic status acts as an indirect marker of some more proximal determinants, such as behaviors or health care, the strength and consistency of association will depend on the adequacy of the social class indicator as a marker. This phenomenon may help to account for the inconsistent magnitudes of social class associations across distinctive subpopulations. For example, there is a stronger social class gradient for whites than for African Americans (Kleinman and Kessel, 1987).

Race and ethnicity

Research has consistently shown an increased risk of preterm delivery among African American as compared to white women (Berkowitz and Papiernik, 1993). The relative risks are typically in the range of 2.0 to 2.5 for all preterm deliveries, but the relative risks tend to be higher, in the range of 2.5 to 3.5 for preterm deliveries at the lowest gestational ages (Blackmore et al., 1995; National Center for Health Statistics, 1988). A number of studies have attempted to identify the explanatory factors accounting for this pattern, but with limited success. In fact, racial differences may well reflect a complex constellation of factors with no single explanation. At present, race is best viewed as a marker of risk and an important clue to etiology that has not been adequately elucidated. In particular, it is clearly *not* a marker of genetics or some immutable biological attribute, but rather a socially based construct with a wide range of correlates. Considering the differences in culture, economics, health care, and lifestyles experienced by African Americans compared to whites, as well as the diversity among African Americans, there are an extensive set of possible mediators of the observed pattern of preterm delivery.

Other major ethnic groups in the United States have been studied far less extensively. In one study, the occurrence of preterm delivery among Mexican Americans tended to be intermediate between African Americans and whites and similar in Asian Americans and whites (Shiono and Klebanoff, 1986).

Age

The traditional "j-shaped" pattern of reproductive risk in relation to age, with increases below age 20 and over age 35, is thought to hold for preterm delivery (Berkowitz and Papiernik, 1993). Like race, age at pregnancy is correlated with many other social and behavioral traits, and thus it is actually quite difficult to isolate the true impact of age per se. The literature on risks to adolescents (as reviewed by Berkowitz and Papiernik, 1993) is quite mixed, perhaps reflecting heterogeneity among adolescents as a function of age, social conditions, and accompanying risk factors. There is no reason to expect adolescents of 18 or 19 to be biologically disadvantaged, though as one moves to younger and younger ages, biological factors may account for increased risks (Scholl et al., 1992b). Analogously, the evidence for increased risk of premature delivery among older women also is inconsistent. This is a sharp contrast to the clear reduction in fecundity and fetal survival that accompanies advanced maternal age (Kline et al., 1989).

Marital status

Berkowitz and Papiernik (1993) report a consistent observation, not explained by socioeconomic factors, of increased risk of preterm delivery associated with being unmarried. Like the other attributes considered above, there are a wide range of more proximal risk factors suggested by marital status, including economic, psychological, and behavioral considerations.

Other markers of risk

Beyond sociodemographic attributes, a number of other traits are potential markers of risk of preterm delivery but are not amenable to intervention. As for the previous factors, our review relies largely on the assessment by Berkowitz and Papiernik (1993).

Height

Short maternal stature has been reported in some studies to be associated with increased risk of preterm delivery, possibly as an indicator of nutritional deprivation in early life. However, an equal or greater number of studies do not find this association, once the effect of height is isolated from the effect of weight.

Prepregnancy weight

Low maternal weight before pregnancy is associated with an increased risk of preterm delivery, independent of weight gain (Kramer et al., 1995; Lang et al., 1996; Siega-Riz et al., 1996). Although prepregnancy weight is, in principle, amenable to modification, the intervention of having women gain weight before conception poses substantial logistical challenges. The magnitudes of relative risks vary in the range of 1.5 to 2.5, but the relationship shows a clear threshold in which only the lowest weight women are at increased risk, rather than a continuous diminution in risk with increasing prepregnancy weight.

Parity

Based on a series of studies reviewed by Berkowitz and Papiernik (1993), there is consistent evidence against a large impact of parity on preterm birth. The patterns are not consistent across studies, and the magnitude of association is always modest within individual studies.

History of adverse pregnancy outcomes

Perhaps no marker of risk is more strongly or consistently related to risk of preterm delivery than a prior preterm delivery. Relative risks are of the order of 3.0 and sometimes higher across a substantial number of studies (Berkowitz and Papiernik, 1993). Furthermore, a dose–response relationship is seen between the number of prior preterm deliveries and the risk of a subsequent preterm delivery (Bakketeig et al., 1979).

Previous spontaneous abortions are less consistently or strongly related to risk of preterm delivery (Berkowitz and Papiernik, 1993). A pooled estimate of the relative risk was 1.6 for prior spontaneous abortion (Kramer, 1987). Some studies have suggested the magnitude of association is stronger with multiple spontaneous abortions and with second rather than first trimester spontaneous abortions (Berkowitz and Papiernik, 1993).

Multiple gestation

Multiple gestation (e.g., twins or triplets) is strongly predictive for preterm delivery (Berkowitz and Papiernik, 1993). Based on estimates of 25 to 50% of multiple gestations being born before term, the relative risks are of the order of 3 to 6 compared to singleton gestations.

"Lifestyle" factors

Because behavioral factors are more likely to be amenable to intervention, and because modification of those behaviors would constitute primary prevention of preterm delivery, the evidence linking lifestyle factors to preterm delivery is discussed in much more detail than the preceding material.

Smoking

The literature on the effect of smoking on prematurity is not consistent, in sharp contrast to the evidence relating cigarette smoking to low birth weight or small-for-gestational-age births (IOM, 1985). In general, the studies of smoking and preterm delivery show a moderate, positive association, with risk estimates mostly within the 1.2–1.6 range (Table 3.1). Some of the variation among studies is probably due to differing study entry criteria (for example, some studies were restricted to singleton births, some studies are mostly confined to one racial or social class group). In general, no association has been found for women who stop

Table 3.1. Summary of selected publications on cigarette smoking and preterm delivery

Author and publication year	Study design	PT count	Outcome measure	Exposure measurement	Primary results (relative risk)
Van den Berg 1977	Cohort	558	PT	15 + cigarettes/day	1.6 ($P < 0.05$)
	Cross-sectional	7100	PT	Any smoking	1.3
Wen et al. 1990	Retrospective cohort	Total $n = 15\,539$	PT	Any smoking	1.4–2.0 ($P < 0.05$, for age > 25)
Ahlborg & Bodin 1991	Prospective cohort	200	PT	Any smoking	1.5–2.2 (mostly $P < 0.05$)
				Passive smoking	No association
Virji & Cottington 1991	Case-control	775	PT	Any smoking	1.3 (1.1–1.6)
McDonald et al. 1992	Cross-sectional	2830	PT	Any smoking	1.2–1.4 ($P < 0.05$)
Chattingius et al. 1993	Retrospective cohort	29 937	≤ 36 wks	Any smoking	1.4–1.8 ($P < 0.05$, ages 20–34), 2.3 ($P < 0.05$, age ≥ 35)
Li et al. 1993	Randomized clinical trial	180	PT	Non-quitters	1.6 (1.1–2.3)
				Early quitters	No association
Mainous & Hueston 1994	Retrospective cohort	305	≤ 36 wks	Smokers who quit in 1st trimester	No association
				Smoking beyond 1st trimester	1.6 (1.2–2.1)
Kliegman et al. 1994	Cohort	73	PT	Any smoking	1.9 (0.7–5.5)
Shiono et al. 1995	Prospective cohort	896	PT	Any smoking	No association
Peacock et al. 1995	Prospective cohort	113	PT	Any smoking	2.0 (1.3–2.9) (< 32 wks GA)
					No association (32–36 wks GA)
Wisborg et al. 1996	Prospective cohort	178	PT	Smoking among heavy caffeine consumers	6–10 cig/day: 2.9 ≥ cig/day: 4.9
Kisten et al. 1996	Retrospective cohort	1400	PT	Any smoking, non-drug users	1.4 ($P < 0.05$)
Nordentoft et al. 1996	Cohort	212	PT	Any smoking	No association

PT, preterm delivery < 37 weeks; GA, gestational age; P, probability.

Table 3.2. Summary of selected publications on alcohol consumption and preterm delivery

Author and publication year	Study design	PT count	Exposure measurement	Primary Results (relative risk)
Van den Berg 1977	Cohort	558	Any alcohol use	No association
Virji & Cottington 1991	Case-control	775	2 drinks/day	1.4 (0.7–3.0)
McDonald et al. 1992	Cross-sectional	2830	1–2 drinks/wk in 1st trimester	0.9 ($P < 0.05$)
Lazzaroni et al. 1993	Retrospective cohort	123	Alcohol use in 1st trimester	1–10 g/day: 0.6 (0.3–1.2)
				11–20 g/day: 1.7 ($P > 0.05$)
				> 20 g/day: 2.4 ($P > 0.05$)
Verkerk et al. 1993	Cohort	120	Drinking 3 months before pregnancy and 3rd trimester	Modest inverse associations ($P > 0.05$)
Borges et al. 1993	Case-control	227	Any alcohol use	0.7 (0.4–1.1) frequent, heavy drinking: 2.2 (0.4–12.3)
Kliegman et al. 1994	Cohort	73	Any alcohol use	No association
Peacock et al. 1995	Prospective cohort	113	Any alcohol use	No association
Windham et al. 1995	Retrospective cohort	n/a	Any alcohol use	No association
Shiono et al. 1995	Prospective cohort	896	Any alcohol use	No association

PT, preterm delivery; P, probability.
All publications above defined prematurity as < 37 weeks.

smoking within the first trimester (Li et al., 1993; Mainous and Hueston, 1994), which offers clear promise for interventions. There is some suggestion of a stronger association of smoking and preterm delivery with increasing maternal age (Cnattingius et al., 1993; Wen et al., 1990). A dose–response relationship between intensity of smoking and risk of preterm delivery was found in only two reports (Van den Berg, 1977; Wisborg et al., 1996).

Alcohol use

Our review of the literature found no meaningful association between alcohol use during pregnancy and preterm delivery (Table 3.2). Weak inverse associations have been reported (Lazzaroni et al., 1993; McDonald et al., 1992; Verkerk et al., 1993), as well as two-fold, non-significant associations with the highest levels of drinking (Borges et al., 1993; Lazzaroni et al., 1993). Overall, however, alcohol consumption is not likely to be a strong determinant of preterm delivery.

Illicit drug use

Most studies have examined cocaine or crack exposure (Table 3.3), although a few reports addressing marijuana were located. Prior research has generally found a positive association between cocaine/crack and prematurity, with a relative risk of approximately 2 for users as compared to non-users. Prenatal care appears to reduce the association, but a positive association remains even among cocaine-using women with prenatal care interventions (MacGregor et al., 1989).

Despite the consistency noted in reviews (Holzman and Paneth, 1994), there are several issues that need to be considered in evaluating whether the literature should be interpreted as suggesting a causal influence of illicit drug use. Probably the most important factors are confounding by use of other drugs and other behaviors and accurate measurement of drug use. Women who use one drug, such as cocaine, are much more likely to be using other illicit drugs, as well as tobacco and alcohol, so that the ideal comparison between women using only cocaine and women using no illicit substances is difficult to achieve. In addition, women who are heavy drug users may exchange sex for drugs, with the concomitant risk of sexually transmitted diseases, and are likely to have poor nutrition, inadequate prenatal care, be subject to violence, and have other risk factors for preterm delivery. Isolation of drug use from these other factors is challenging.

A second, major challenge is accurate measurement of drug use. Studies rely either on self-report of use or urine screens. Both methods are known to be highly fallible (Kline et al., 1997). Self-reports are subject to misrepresentation, and urine drug screens reflect drug use over a very limited time period. It may be argued that previous studies have identified only the heaviest users and that, as a result, their findings should be interpreted as indicating the association for heavy drug use and

Table 3.3. Summary of selected publications on illicit drug use and preterm delivery

Author and publication year	Study design	PT count	Outcome measure	Exposure measurement	Primary results (relative risk)
MacGregor et al. 1987	Case-control	19	PT	Cocaine use	Association ($P < 0.01$)
				Cocaine vs. polydrug use	Association ($P > 0.05$)
Cherukuri et al. 1988	Case-control	37	⩽ 37 weeks	Crack use only	3.1 (1.7–5.6)
MacGregor et al. 1989	Case-control	44	n/a	Cocaine use	w/ PNC interventions: 2.8 (1.2–6.3)
					w/o PNC: 20.0 (6.6–61)
Witter & Neibyl 1990	Retrospective cohort	1437	PT	Marijuana use only	No association
Handler et al. 1991	Retrospective cohort	1587	PT	Cocaine use	2.4 (1.9–3.1)
Spense et al. 1991	Retrospective cohort	63	PT	Cocaine use at delivery	Association ($P < 0.001$)
Singer et al. 1994	Case-control	62	PT	Cocaine use at delivery	Association ($P < 0.01$)
Kliegman et al. 1994	Cohort	73	PT	Cocaine use	13.4 (1.2–145)
				Marijuana use	1.9 (0.3–10.5)
Eyler et al. 1994	Case-control	126	⩽ 37 weeks	Cocaine use	Association ($P < 0.05$)
Feldman et al. 1992	Cohort	79	PT	Illicit drug use	2.6 (1.2–5.8)
Shiono et al. 1995	Prospective cohort	896	PT	Marijuana	No association
			PT	Cocaine	1.3 (0.9–2.0)
Kisten et al. 1996	Retrospective cohort	1400	PT	Non-smoking cocaine use	4.0 (2.3–7.0)
Reviewed by Holzman and Paneth (1994):					
Chouteau et al. 1988			< 34 weeks	Cocaine use	2.0 ($P < 0.05$)

Study	Study type	n	PT/FT	Exposure	OR (CI)
Gillogley et al. 1990			PT	Cocaine use	2.3 ($P < 0.05$)
Bateman et al. 1993			PT	Cocaine/polydrug use	2.9
Reviewed by Slutsker (1992):					
Ryan et al. 1987	Case-control	7	PT	Cocaine/methodone	2.7 (0.4–21.6)
Oro & Dixon 1987	Case-control	17	FT	Cocaine/polydrug use	4.0 (1.1–6.4)
Chasnoff et al. 1989	Case-control	21	< 38 weeks	Cocaine vs. methodone use	8.2–17.3 (wide CIs)
Keith et al. 1989	Case-control	34	PT	Cocaine use	4.2 (1.2–6.8)
				Cocaine/polydrug use	5.1 (1.6–16.6)
Mastrogiannis et al. 1990	Case-control	34	PT	Cocaine use	2.8 (1.1–7.6)

PT, preterm delivery < 37 weeks; *P*, probability; CI, confidence interval; PNC, prenatal care.

Table 3.4. Summary of selected publications on the association of caffeinated beverages and preterm deliveries

Author and publication year	Method (cases/controls)	PT count	Exposure measurement*	Primary results (relative risk)
Weathersbee et al. 1977	Cross-sectional	15	≥ 300 mg/day coffee, tea, cola among husband or wife	6.4 (1.7–24.1)
Van den Berg 1977	Cohort	558	Coffee	2–6 cups/day: 1.3 (1.0–1.7) ≥ 7 cups/day: 1.8 (1.7–2.0)
Berkowitz et al. 1982	Case-control	166	3rd tri. coffee: 3 cups/day 3rd tri. tea: ≥ 4 cups/day	1.5 (0.7–3.0) 1.5 (0.8–3.1)
Linn et al. 1982	Retrospective cohort	1204	Coffee – 1st trimester	Association with PROM for ≥ 4 cups/day: 1.5 (1.0–2.2) No association with PT
Fenster et al. 1991	Case-control	n/a	Heavy use of coffee, tea, or soft drinks	1.7 (0.7–4.2)
Olsen et al. 1991	Case-control	370	Any coffee Any tea	No association 1.6 (1.0–2.7)
Williams et al. 1992	Nested case-control	307 PROM, 488 non-PROM	≥ 3 cups/day of coffee Tea	2.0 (1.4–2.7) No association
McDonald et al. 1992	Cross-sectional	2830	Coffee in 1st trimester	No association
Fortier et al. 1993	Retrospective cohort	391	Any coffee, tea, cola, or chocolate	No association
Pastore & Savitz 1995	Case-control	408	Any coffee, tea, cola, or caffeinated non-cola	No association
Peacock et al. 1995	Prospective cohort	113	Caffeine (mg/week)	No association
Wisborg et al. 1996	Prospective cohort	178	≥ 400 mg/day coffee, tea, cola or chocolate	1.8 (among smokers)

* Ascertainment of decaffeinated coffee or decaffeinated tea is not listed.

All publications above defined prematurity as < 37 weeks.

PROM, premature rupture of membranes; PT, preterm delivery.

preterm delivery. However, there is the possibility that reporting inaccuracy is distorting the measured association with preterm delivery, either upward or downward. Also, our knowledge regarding the effects of intermittent use, which is poorly captured by self-report or urine screens, is quite limited.

Caffeine

The 12 studies that have been published in English on the association between caffeine and preterm delivery have contradictory results (Table 3.4), with a preponderance reporting no association and approximately equal numbers finding positive and negative associations. The studies are limited because most used retrospective designs, and all but three (Olsen et al., 1991, Peacock et al., 1995; Wisborg et al., 1996) obtained caffeine consumption data after delivery. Of the seven studies that considered consumption by trimester (Berkowitz et al., 1982; Fenster et al., 1991; Linn et al., 1982; McDonald et al., 1992; Olsen et al., 1991; Pastore and Savitz, 1995; Williams et al., 1992), three ascertained only first trimester consumption (Fenster et al., 1991; Linn et al., 1982; Williams et al., 1992) and the remainder, with two exceptions (Berkowitz et al., 1982; Pastore and Savitz, 1995), appear to have averaged across trimesters. The variation in the sources of caffeine examined (coffee, tea, soda, chocolate) in these studies may also explain the differing findings.

Prenatal weight gain

There are a number of reports on the impact of weight gained during pregnancy and preterm delivery (Table 3.5), nearly all of which reported a positive association between low weight gain and preterm delivery (adjusted relative risks in the range of 1.5 to 2.5). There are methodologic concerns with the measurement of weight (self-report versus weight on a scale at prenatal care visits) and the definition of adequate weight gain (an absolute figure or relative to pregravid weight or body mass index). Perhaps the most compelling question is whether inadequate weight gain is a causal factor in preterm delivery or rather an indicator of problems in the course and progress of the pregnancy.

Sexual intercourse and orgasm

The literature on the association between prematurity and sexual intercourse and orgasm is inconsistent, with reports of sexual activity associated with increased risk, decreased risk, and no association (Table 3.6). Of the 11 manuscripts reviewed, all analyzed frequency of intercourse and four evaluated orgasm. Three authors reported an inverse association between frequency of intercourse and prematurity (Klebanoff et al., 1984; Kurki and Ylikorkala, 1994; Read and Klebanoff, 1993), that is, the women who were sexually active later in pregnancy

Table 3.5. Summary of selected publications on prenatal weight gain and preterm delivery

Author and publication year	Study design	PT count	Outcome measurement	Exposure measurement	Primary results (relative risk)
Frentzen et al. 1987	Case-control	30	26–37 wks	Lower weight gain at wk 30	Association ($P < 0.04$)
Hediger et al. 1989	Cohort	190	PT	Inadequate weight gain after 24 wks ($<$ 400 g/wk)	1.6(1.1–2.3)
				Total inadequate weight gain ($<$ 4.3 kg $\leq$ 24 wks)	2.6(1.6–4.3)
Scholl et al. 1989	Cohort	n/a	PT	Inadequate weight gain by GA	1.5 (1.1–2.0)
Abrams et al. 1989	Cohort	118	$<$ 38 wks	Low weight gain ($<$ 0.27 kg/wk)	2.5 (1.5–4.9)
Ketterlinus et al. 1990	Cohort	n/a	PT	Low pregravid weight and prenatal weight gain	Slightly higher risk of PT
Virji & Cottington 1991	Case-control	775	PT	Weight gain $\leq$ 20 lbs	2.1(1.8–2.5)
Kramer et al. 1992	Retrospective cohort	770	PT	Low overall weight gain ($<$ 0.27 kg/wk)	No association
Siega-Riz et al. 1994	Cohort	n/a	PT	$<$ 80% IOM recommendations	Increased risk
				$>$ 200% IOM recommendations	Increased risk
				$<$ 60% IOM recommendations in 3rd trimester	2 +

PT, preterm delivery $<$ 37 weeks; GA, gestational age; P, probability; IOM, Institute of Medicine.

Table 3.6. Summary of selected publications on sexual intercourse/orgasm and preterm delivery

Author and publication year	Study design	PT count	Outcome measurement	Exposure measurement	Primary results (relative risk)
Puch & Fernandez 1953	Cohort	68	Preterm labor	Time between last I and delivery	Association with more recent coitus (but not believed by authors)
					No association with PROM
Solberg et al. 1973	Cohort	19	< 37 wks or < 2500 g	I or O in months 7 +	No association
Perkins 1979	Cohort	27	< 38 wks	Any sex experience in last 24 hrs	3.3 (1.1–9.6)
				Sex activity in last 2 months	No association
				Orgasm	No association
Rayburn & Wilson 1980	Case-control	111	PT	No. of I in last week	Association with idiopathic preterm labor
Mills et al. 1981	Cohort	1191	PT	I in 3rd trimester	No association with PROM
Georgakopoulos et al. 1984	Case-control	58	PT	Frequency of I	No association
				Frequency of O	No association
Klebanoff et al. 1984	Cohort	n/a	n/a	Less frequent I	Association ($P < 0.001$)
Neilson 1989	Case-control	52	PT	No. of I in last wk preg.	No association
Ekwo et al. 1993	Case-control	359	PT	Orgasm	1.9 (1.0–3.9) preterm PROM
				Male superior position in last 4 wks preg.	Preterm PROM, 2.4 (1.2–5.0); preterm w/o PROM, 1.8 (1.0–3.2)
Kurki & Ylikorkala 1994	Cohort	23	PT	Less frequent I	Association
Read & Klebanoff 1993	Cohort	1527	PT	Less than 1 I/wk	1.2 (1.0–1.3)

I, intercourse; O, orgasm; PT, preterm delivery < 37 weeks; P, probability; PROM, premature rupture of membranes.

Table 3.7. Summary of selected publications on stress and preterm delivery

Author and publication year	Study design	PT count	Outcome measurement	Exposure measurement	Primary results (relative risk)
Newton et al. 1979	Cross-sectional	49 (37%)	Moderate PT 33–37 wks very PT < 33 wks	Cochrane–Robinson Life Events Inventory (mean number, number in week before delivery)	Association
Berkowitz & Kasl 1983	Case/control	166	PT	Holmes & Rahe Social Readjustment Rating Q (life events)	Whites only: OR > 2.0 for ≥ 4 events For highly desired pregnancies: 2.0
Newton & Hunt 1984	Nested case-control	12	PT	Life Events Inventory (objective major life event)	Association (P < 0.001)
Molfese et al. 1987	Cohort	n/a	GA at delivery	Spielberger's State Anxiety Index State–trait Anxiety Inventory Beck Depression Inventory Mediators: Life events, I-E scale, maternal attitude toward pregnancy, social support	No association No association No association
Stein et al. 1987	Cohort	14	PT	Life events over prior 12 months British state psychiatric exam	No association No association
Pagel et al. 1990	Cohort	n/a total n = 100	GA at delivery	20-item RAND life events index Smilkstein Family APGAR measure Spielberger's State Anxiety scale	No association No association No association
Osborn et al. 1990	Cohort	14	< 38 wks PT labor w/o delivery	Stress from being a MD resident	1.8 (P > 0.05) 12.3 (2.4–61.6) (premature labor among whites)
Mutale et al. 1991	Case(LBW) control	62	PT	Brown & Harris Life Events and Difficulty Schedule	Association with severe life event/difficulty
Bryce et al. 1991	Randomized clinical trial	273	20–36 wks	Half of high risk women offered social support from midwives	Inverse association with social support program (P=0.038) No association among women in lowest social class No association among women who lived alone
Lobel et al. 1992	Cohort	22	GA at delivery	Perceived Stress Scale Speilberger State Anxiety Inventory Problem Oriented Perinatal Risk Assessment System	Association with stress No association with life events

Study	Design	N	PT definition	Instrument	Findings
MacDonald et al. 1992	Cohort	37	n/a	General Health Q (depression); Paykel Life Events Inventory	No association; No association
Steer et al. 1992	Cohort	75	PT	Beck Depression Inventory	No association (adolescents); 1.06 (per point increase in BDI among adults); 3.39 (among clinically depressed adults)
Villar et al. 1992	Randomized clinical trials	264	PT	Half of high risk women offered social support	No association
Perkin et al. 1993	Cohort	109	≤36 wks	General Health Q (anxiety); Eysenck Personality Q (depression)	No association; No association
Wadhwa et al. 1993	Cohort	12	PT	Holmes & Rahe Schedule of Recent Life Events; Hopkins Symptom Checklist (strain); Perceived Stress Scale; DeLongis Daily Hassles Q anxiety (unique scale)	Each unit increase in anxiety = 3-day decrease in GA; No association otherwise
Hedegaard et al. 1993	Cohort	207	< 259 days	General Health Q (distress)	1.22 for moderate distress and 1.75 for high distress
Honnor et al. 1994	Randomized clinical trial	133	PT	Women's Interview Schedule for Life Events; Half of high-risk women offered social support	No association
Orr & Miller 1995	Cohort	177	PT	Center for Epidemiologic Studies Depression Scale	Association with high depression scores among black women ($P=0.06$)
Hedegaard et al. 1996	Cohort	207	PT	Modified Life Events Inventory perceived stress, social support; General Health Q	1.6–1.8 (1.1–2.7) (highly stressful events in wk 30); No association with social support
Copper et al. 1996	Cohort	101	Spontaneous PT following PT labor or PROM < 35 wks	Abbreviated Scale for Assessment of Psychosocial Status	1.16 ($P = 0.003$) (per point increase on stress scale); No association with anxiety, self-esteem, depression, or mastery

PT, preterm delivery < 37 weeks; GA, gestational age; P, probability; PROM, premature rupture of membranes; Q, questionnaire; LBW, low birth weight.

were less likely to deliver before term. Three authors reported a positive association between intercourse and prematurity (Ekwo et al., 1993 (association with male superior position); Perkins, 1979 (association with intercourse in 24 hours before labor onset); Rayburn and Wilson, 1980). The remaining five reports generally did not find any association between coitus and preterm delivery. In terms of orgasm, three reports found no association with prematurity (Georgakopoulos et al., 1984; Perkins, 1979; Solberg et al., 1973), while one reported a non-significant positive association (Ekwo et al., 1993).

Isolating the influence of sexual activity per se on risk of preterm delivery is quite challenging. There are several reasons to expect maintenance of a sexual relationship to serve as a marker of reduced risk of adverse outcome: such behavior indicates a continuing partner with the potential associated social and economic advantages, as well as a state of feeling well enough to sustain sexual activity. Isolating the biological consequences of sexual activity from the social and psychological context is very difficult. The biological consequences are quite diverse, including potential links with sexually transmitted infections, physiologic effects of orgasm, and influence of exposure to semen. In addition, the personal nature of sexual behavior makes it difficult to be confident that reporting is accurate.

Stress and pregnancy

The effect of stress and related psychological factors during pregnancy, including anxiety, depression, and coping skills, has been the subject of many studies (Table 3.7). Interpretation of this literature is hampered by methodologic concerns, including small sample sizes, poorly defined measures of stress, varying definitions of stress, enrollment so late in pregnancy that some preterm births are missed, and restriction to special populations. In several studies, medical and behavioral factors were not considered as potential confounders or mediators of the impact of stress (Berkowitz and Kasl, 1983; Falorni et al., 1977; Newton et al., 1979; MacDonald et al., 1992; Osborn et al., 1990; Stein et al., 1987). Also, as reviewed by Orr and Miller (1995), assessment of certain disorders, such as depression, is complicated in the pregnant population because symptoms of depression, such as fatigue, are common and normal during pregnancy. If the investigator uses cut-points determined among non-pregnant women, then the psychological assessment of the pregnant women may be invalid.

Finally, and perhaps most important, an adverse outcome itself could well result in recall of a stressful pregnancy. Among the many risk factors that can only be assessed by self-report, perhaps none is more demanding of prospective ascertainment than psychological status.

Studies variably emphasize "objective events" or stressful stimuli (e.g., Life

Events Inventory), perceptions of locus of control (Perceived Stress Scale), or emotional response (State and Trait Anxiety Scales). Other factors studied in connection with stress are depression, social support, anxiety, self-esteem, attitudes toward pregnancy, strain, daily hassles, and family functioning, though some of these factors could be viewed as stressors and some as mediating factors. For this brief review, the stress-related factors will be divided into five categories: social support, life events, anxiety, depression, and general stress.

Prior research has not found a consistent association between social support and preterm delivery (Hedegaard et al., 1996; Norbeck and Tilden, 1983; Villar and Repke, 1990); these investigations include randomized clinical trials of social support interventions. The one report that found reduced prematurity among the entire population given social support intervention found no association among women in the lowest social class and no association among women who lived alone (Bryce et al., 1991).

Life events generally were not associated with increased risk of preterm delivery (Honnor et al., 1994; Lobel et al., 1992; MacDonald et al., 1992; Pagel et al., 1990; Stein et al., 1987), although three publications did report positive associations (Berkowitz and Kasl, 1983 (white mothers only); Newton et al., 1979; Newton and Hunt, 1984). "Severe" life events were associated with an increased risk of prematurity in two reports (Hedegaard et al., 1996 (events reported at week 30 only); Mutale et al., 1991).

Anxiety states were generally found not to be associated with preterm birth (Copper et al., 1996; Molfese et al., 1987; Newton and Hunt, 1984; Pagel et al., 1990; Perkin et al., 1993), although one publication reported a three-day decrease in gestational age for every unit increase in anxiety (Wadhwa et al., 1993).

The literature generally does not support an association between depression and preterm delivery (Copper et al., 1996; MacDonald et al., 1992; Molfese et al., 1987; Orr and Miller, 1995; Perkin et al., 1993; Steer et al., 1992). The only positive association was found among clinically depressed adults (Steer et al., 1992).

Stress in general has been associated with preterm delivery when measured by the Perceived Stress Scale (Lobel et al., 1992), the General Health Questionnaire (Hedegaard et al., 1993), the British state psychiatric exam (Stein et al., 1987), and the Abbreviated Scale for Assessment of Psychosocial Status in Pregnancy (Copper et al., 1996). The stress related to being a medical school resident was not found to increase preterm delivery relative to male residents' wives (Klebanoff et al., 1990b).

In addition to the literature on stress in general, there are a small number of studies focused on occupational stress and preterm delivery (Brandt and Nielsen, 1992; Brett et al., 1997; Henriksen et al., 1994). The studies have generally found small increases in risk, with relative risks typically in the range of 1.2 to 1.5 for high stress compared to low stress workers. Within this range, it is difficult to judge whether an association is truly present.

Diet

This brief review of the literature on dietary factors and preterm delivery focuses on several specific micronutrients, namely zinc, folate, calcium, and ascorbic acid (with only one report identified for each of the latter two) and anemia, as a diet-related medical condition (Table 3.8). The study of diet and preterm delivery poses several methodologic challenges. Measurement is very difficult, and without clear biologic mechanisms, it is unclear what the relevant time frame is for dietary assessment. A number of these dietary factors are also discussed in Chapter 4.

Of the six reports located on the association of zinc and prematurity, half were cohort studies and half were clinical trials of zinc supplementation. Generally, the literature did not find an association with either low zinc levels or zinc supplementation and risk of preterm delivery, although two reports found an increased risk of very preterm deliveries (less than 33 weeks gestation) among women with low zinc (Scholl et al., 1993) or women without zinc supplementation (Jameson, 1993).

The Recommended Dietary Allowance for folate for pregnant women is 400 μg/day, twice the level recommended for non-pregnant women of reproductive age. This increased intake is recommended for pregnant women because folate is needed for cell replication, which is increased during pregnancy because of fetal growth, placental development, uterine expansion, and increased blood volume (NAS, 1990), and because folate deficiency during pregnancy is associated with neural tube defects (Werler et al., 1993). The potential connection between folate and preterm delivery, however, has not been extensively considered. Of the five publications identified, three found an association between low folate (or no folate supplementation) and increased risk of prematurity (Blot et al., 1981; Scholl et al., 1996; Tchernia et al., 1982). Two found no association (Czeizel et al., 1994; Rolschau et al., 1979). Notable is the fact that the large, well-designed randomized trial by Czeizel and colleagues (1994) found that folate supplementation was not associated with a reduced risk of preterm delivery.

The literature on anemia and iron-deficiency anemia uses varying definitions of these conditions. Often, anemia is defined by a combination of hemoglobin and ferritin levels, but the cut-points are not consistent. At other times, studies analyze levels of hemoglobin or hematocrit without using the term "anemia." The literature is inconsistent and sparse regarding the association between anemia and preterm delivery: a positive association was reported by Klebanoff and colleagues (1991) for anemia in the second trimester and no association was reported by Scholl and colleagues (1992a). Two studies reported a positive association between prematurity and iron-deficiency anemia (Scholl et al., 1992a, 1993), although the association in the second reference was restricted to very preterm births (< 33 weeks). Of the four publications that examined hemoglobin levels as predictors of preterm delivery, three found a positive association with high hematocrit (Garn et al., 1981; Knottnerus et al., 1990; Lieberman et al., 1987).

The one publication we located on calcium (Villar and Repke, 1990) reported that calcium supplementation reduced the risk of preterm delivery. The one study located on ascorbic acid (Caldwell et al., 1988) implied an association between high levels of ascorbic acid and very preterm births (≤ 34 weeks), but did not control for smoking, which was a likely confounder.

Physical exertion

The isolation of effects of physical activity on preterm birth, whether during occupational or leisure time, has proven to be quite challenging for a number of reasons. Overall, employment during pregnancy appears to be a marker of reduced risk of a range of adverse outcomes (Saurel-Cubizolles and Kaminski, 1986), presumably because employed women are healthier and have socioeconomic, behavioral, and health care advantages relative to women not employed (Savitz et al., 1991b). However, a number of studies, particularly in Europe, have suggested that strenuous work may be associated with increased risk of preterm delivery (Mamelle et al., 1984; Marbury, 1992). Associations have also been reported with specific components of workplace physical activity, including prolonged standing, lifting, and long working hours (reviewed by Berkowitz and Papiernik, 1993 and summarized in Table 3.9). This literature is notably inconsistent, with high quality studies reporting no association somewhat more often than positive associations. The multiple dimensions of "exertion" also need to be considered, with prolonged standing, lifting, and strenuousness each having a potentially distinctive contribution to the risk of preterm delivery.

Leisure time physical activity is also challenging to isolate from the favorable health status that is a prerequisite for engaging in such activities. Reviews (Dye and Oldenettel, 1996; Lokey et al., 1991) have found the literature inconclusive with regard to potential adverse or beneficial effect of leisure time activity on preterm delivery. The range of physical activity under consideration extends from moderate energy expenditure in walking, for example, to intensive competition at the level of Olympic athletes. Both adverse and beneficial effects are plausible, but neither has been identified with any certainty.

Occupational and environmental chemical and physical agents

Among the diverse array of potentially toxic environmental agents, lead has received the greatest amount of attention as a potential risk factor for preterm

Table 3.8. Summary of selected publications on dietary factors and preterm delivery

	Author and publication year	Study design	PT count	Outcome measure	Exposure measurement	Primary Results (relative risk)
Zinc	Higashi et al. 1988	Cohort	10	PT	Maternal blood zinc at delivery	No association
					Zinc levels in cord blood	Association ($P < 0.05$)
	Bro et al. 1988	Cohort	34	PT	Maternal zinc vs. non-pregnant women	No association
					Zinc level in cord blood	No association
	Cherry et al. 1989	Randomized clinical trial	117	< 38 wks	30 mg zinc supplement among normal weight women	Inverse association
	Jameson 1993	Clinical trial	82	PT	22.5 mg zinc supplement (some variation in dose)	No association (all PT) 0.15 ($P < 0.01$, PT < 33 wks)
	Scholl et al. 1993	Cohort	803	very PT < 33 wks	Low zinc ($\leqslant 6$ mg/day)	1.9 (1.1–3.1) (all PT); 3.3 (1.8–6.3) (very PT)
	Johnsson et al. 1996	Randomized clinical trial	82	$\leqslant 36$ wks	44 mg zinc supplement	No association
Calcium	Villar & Repke 1990	Randomized clinical trial	91	PT	Calcium supplement 2.0 g/day	Reduced PT ($P < 0.007$)
Iron, anemia	Garn et al. 1981	Cohort	8510	$\leqslant 37$ wks	High and low levels of Hb or Ht	Association
	Lieberman et al. 1987	Cohort	495	PT	Increased Ht	1.22 for a 1–point change
	Knottnerus et al. 1990	Cohort	34	PT	High Hb ($\geqslant 8.0$ mmol/l) High Ht ($\geqslant 38\%$)	2.4 (1.0–5.6) 2.6 (1.2–5.9)

	Study type	Sample size	Outcome	Definition	Result
Lu et al. 1991	Cohort	2160	PT	Ht 30–36% High Ht (≥ 43%)	Association ($P < 0.05$, all PT) Association ($P < 0.05$, PT 26–37 wks)
Klebanoff et al. 1991	Case-control	n/a	n/a	Anemia ≤ 10th percentile in 2nd tri.	1.9 (1.2–3.0)
Scholl et al. 1992a	Cohort		PT	Anemia ≤ 5th percentile by GA Iron-def. anem. = anemia + ferritin < 12 µg/l	No association 2.7 (1.2–6.2)
Scholl et al. 1993	Cohort	803	very PT < 33 wks	Iron def. anemia (Hb < 11 g/dl, serum ferritin < 12 ng/ml)	1.9 (0.6–5.6)
Ascorbic acid					
Caldwell et al. 1988	Cohort	24	≤ 34 wks vs. > 37 wks	Serum ascorbic acid at delivery	Association ($P < 0.03$)
Folate					
Scholl et al. 1996	Cohort	112/167	PT	Low serum folate at 28 wks (< 240 µg/day)	1.9(1.2–3.2) – 3.4(1.8–6.1)
Tchernia et al. 1982	Clinical trial	9	38 wks	350 µg/day folate supplement	0.3 (0.1–1.3)
Czeizel et al. 1994	Randomized clinical trial	344	n/a	0.8 mg folate in multivitamin preconception to week 12	No association
Rolschau et al. 1979	Clinical trial	n/a	n/a	5 mg/day folate from wk 21	No association
Blot et al. 1981	Randomized clinical trial	3	GA	350 µg/day folate	40.7 mean GA with supplement vs. 39.9 without

PT, preterm delivery < 37 weeks; GA, gestational age; P, probability; Hb, hemoglobin; Ht, hematocrit.

Table 3.9. Summary of selected publications on physical activity and preterm delivery

Author and publication year	Study design	PT count	Exposure measurement	Primary results (relative risk)
McDonald et al. 1988	Cohort	109	Lifting heavy weights	1.3 ($P < 0.01$)
McDonald et al. 1988	Cohort	158	Other physical effort	1.1 ($P < 0.05$)
McDonald et al. 1988	Cohort	204	Standing > 8 hours/day	1.1 ($P < 0.05$)
Nurminen et al. 1989	Case-control	21	Standing work	0.5 (3 exposed cases)
Nurminen et al. 1989	Case-control	21	Moderate/high work load	0.5 (6 exposed cases)
Klebanoff et al. 1990	Cohort	138	Medical resident	1.2 (0.8–1.7)
Ahlborg et al. 1990	Cohort	197	Lifting at work	1.0 (0.6–1.7)
Ahlborg et al. 1990	Cohort	197	Lifting outside work	1.0 (0.6–1.5)
Teitelman et al. 1990	Cohort	29	Standing (vs. active)	2.7 (1.2–6.0)
Teitelman et al. 1990	Cohort	36	Sedentary (vs. active)	1.4 (0.5–2.8)
Launer et al. 1990	Cohort	368	Standing (vs. sitting)	1.6 (1.0–2.6)
Launer et al. 1990	Cohort	368	Walking (vs. sitting)	1.3 (0.9–2.1)
Homer et al. 1990	Cohort	46	High exertion job	2.0 (1.1–3.9)
Klebanoff et al. 1990a	Cohort (VIP)	n/a	Long hours standing	1.3 (1.0–1.7)
Klebanoff et al. 1990a	Cohort (VIP)	n/a	Heavy work	1.0 (0.8–1.4)
Ramirez et al. 1990	Cohort	604	Occupational exertion	1.8 (1.1–2.8)
Saurel-Cubizolles et al. 1991	Cohort	44	Strenuous work	1.4 (0.6–3.1)
Magann et al. 1996	Cohort	n/a	Occupational exertion	Approx. 0.8

P, probability; PT, preterm delivery; VIP, Vaginal Infection Prematurity Study.
All publications defined prematurity as < 37 weeks.

delivery (Andrews et al., 1994). Although the studies are not perfectly consistent, in the aggregate they do suggest that blood lead levels are higher in preterm as compared to term deliveries. Relative risks of 1.5 or greater have been found in a number of studies, with seven providing at least partial support for an association between elevated lead exposure and preterm delivery.

The other types of studies have examined occupational groups broadly for associations with preterm delivery (McDonald et al., 1988; Sanjose et al., 1991; Savitz et al., 1989, 1996). Both maternal and paternal occupation have been considered, and individual jobs, industrial sectors, and imputed exposure to specific agents have been evaluated. As noted above, women's employment per se tends to be associated with reduced risk of preterm delivery, presumably due to the favorable selection for employment. There is no clear, consistent pattern of increased risk associated with specific occupations of women, but more than one study has implicated food services, textiles, and cleaning services. A number of studies have found an absence of association for preterm delivery, even if other effects, such as spontaneous abortion or size for gestational age, have been identified. Paternal exposures have received less attention, but some associations have been reported for textile workers (Savitz et al., 1989) and for solvent and lead exposure (Kristensen et al., 1993). For this line of investigation to lead to opportunities for prevention, researchers must identify the specific, alterable aspects of work, if any, that are associated with increased risk. Should specific chemical or physical agents, physical exertion, or psychological stress emerge as causative factors, then changes in the work setting or in the placement of pregnant workers would be worthy of consideration.

Genitourinary tract infection

Among the potential modifiable causes of preterm delivery, genitourinary tract infections are among the leading contenders. These infections arise through a range of biological and social events, including sexual transmission, compromised immune function, and anatomic factors favoring ascension of lower genital tract infections. The role of infection in the etiology of preterm delivery has been reviewed extensively (Gibbs et al., 1992; McGregor and French, 1991; Romero and Mazor, 1988), with thorough consideration of biological mechanisms and pathways linking infection to preterm delivery.

The focus in this brief review will be on the empirical epidemiologic evidence, including clinical trials. Because of the capability of randomized controlled clinical trials to isolate any causal effect of the agent (or at least persistence of the agent), results from such studies have a distinct advantage over those obtained from observational studies. More than most potential causes of preterm delivery,

Table 3.10. Summary of selected publications on genital tract infections and preterm delivery

	Author and publication year	Study design	PT count	Outcome definition	Results (relative risk)
Bacterial vaginosis	Gravett et al. 1986	Cohort	36	PT labor	2.0 (1.1–3.5)
	Gravett et al. 1986	Cohort	32	PPROM	2.0 (1.1–3.7)
	Martius et al. 1988	Case-control	61	PT	2.3 (1.1–5.0)
	Elliott et al. 1990	Case-control	166	PT & LBW	1.0 (0.5–2.1)
	McDonald et al. 1991	Case-control	428	PT labor	2.9 (1.5–5.5)
	Kurki et al. 1992	Cohort	17	PT	6.9 (2.5–18.8)
	Read & Klebanoff 1993	Cohort (VIP)	1527	PT	0.9 (0.7–1.2) (infrequent sex)
	Read & Kelbanoff 1993	Cohort (VIP)	1527	PT	1.2 (1.0–1.4) (frequent sex)
	Riduan et al. 1993	Cohort	61	PT	2.0 (1.0–3.9)
	Hay et al. 1994	Cohort	26	PT	2.8 (1.1–7.4)
	Morales et al. 1994	RCT	24	PT	2.4 (1.0–6.3) (placebo) (referent)
	McGregor et al. 1994	Cohort	18	PT	3.3 (1.2–9.1)
	Joesoef et al. 1995	RCT	97	PT	1.1 (0.7–1.7)
	Hillier et al. 1995	Cohort	368	PT & LBW	1.4 (1.1–1.8)
	Hauth et al. 1995	RCT	178	PT	1.4 (1.1–1.8) (placebo) (referent)
	Meis et al. 1995	Cohort	111	PT < 35 wks	1.4 (0.9–2.1) (24 wks)
	Meis et al. 1995	Cohort	111	PT < 35 wks	1.8 (1.2–3.0) (28 wks)
Group B streptococcus	Sweet et al. 1987	Cohort	55	PT	1.2 (0.8–1.8)
	Alger et al. 1988	Case-control	52	PPROM	8.0 ($P = 0.007$)
	Matorras et al. 1989	Cohort	163	PT	0.9 (0.5–1.5)
	Elliott et al. 1990	Case-control	166	PT & LBW	1.0 (0.5–2.1)
	McDonald et al. 1991	Case-control	428	PT labor	0.9 (0.6–1.4)

Reference	Study design	N	Outcome	Odds ratio (CI)
Klebanoff & Shiono 1995	RCT	109	PT	1.1 (0.9–1.7)
Regan et al. 1996	Cohort (VIP)	1188	PT	1.0 (0.8–1.2)
Regan et al. 1996	Cohort (VIP)	1188	PT & LBW	1.5 (1.1–1.9)
Chlamydia				
Gravett et al. 1986	Cohort	48	PT labor	4.3 (2.1–8.8)
Gravett et al. 1986	Cohort	34	PPROM	2.4 (1.1–5.4)
Sweet et al. 1987	Cohort	55	PT	1.0 (0.7–1.6)
Berman et al. 1987	Cohort	23	PT & LBW	2.0 (0.9–4.8)
Martius et al. 1988	Case-control	61	PT	5.4 (1.3–23.4)
Alger et al. 1988	Case-control	52	PPROM	7.7 ($P < 0.001$)
Johns Hopkins U. 1989	Cohort	106	PT	1.6 (1.0–2.5)
Elliott et al. 1990	Case-control	166	PT & LBW	0.7 (0.4–1.4)
Ngassa & Egbe 1994	Case-control	63	PT labor	2.8 (1.1–7.0)
Claman et al. 1995	Cohort	11	PT	4.0 (1.1–14.6)
Trichomonas				
Minkoff et al. 1984	Cohort	40	PPROM	1.4 ($P < 0.03$)
Read & Klebanoff 1993	Cohort (VIP)	1527	PT	1.0 (0.8–1.2) (infrequent sex)
Read & Klebanoff 1993	Cohort (VIP)	1527	PT	1.5 (1.2–1.8) (frequent sex)
Meis et al. 1995	Cohort (VIP)	111	PT < 35 wks	1.5 (0.1–1.8) (24 wks)
Meis et al. 1995	Cohort (VIP)	111	PT < 35 wks	0.9 (0.2–3.6) (28 wks)
Gonorrhea				
Elliott et al. 1990	Case-control	166	PT & LBW	3.2 (1.3–8.4)

PT, preterm delivery < 37 weeks; *P*, probability; VIP, Vaginal Infection and Prematurity Study; PROM, premature rupture of membranes; PPROM, preterm premature rupture of membranes; LBW, low birth weight; RCT, randomized clinical trial.

genital tract infections have been subjected to randomized controlled trials of treatment.

Bacterial vaginosis

As discussed in Chapter 4 and summarized here in Table 3.10, a number of observational studies and a few randomized trials have considered the role of bacterial vaginosis in the etiology of preterm delivery. The evidence is fairly consistent in identifying an association, with most studies yielding relative risks in the range of 1.4 to 2.4. Risk estimates close to the null have also been generated. Some of the potential influences in the association are suggested in Table 3.7 as well, including the concomitant level of sexual activity and the timing in pregnancy when the infection is assessed. Two clinical trials that support the inferences from the numerous observational studies lend added credibility to the overall body of evidence.

Based on the epidemiologic data alone, the evidence for an association between bacterial vaginosis and preterm delivery is strong but not overwhelming, due to the inconsistency across studies as well as the relatively modest strength of association in most studies. However, the notably high prevalence of bacterial vaginosis, in the range of 10 to 40 percent of reproductive age women (French and McGregor, 1997), argues strongly for further examination of the implications for prevention.

Chlamydia

Compared to the literature on bacterial vaginosis, the size and quality of the studies of chlamydia and preterm delivery is less impressive (Table 3.10). Nonetheless, six of the nine individual studies noted showed relative risks of 1.6 or higher, with five having relative risks of 2.0 or higher. Although a number of these were case-control studies, with chlamydia assessed during or after delivery, the fact that chlamydia is not naturally present, suggests it was present in late pregnancy as well, even if it is not identified until after delivery. The studies to date are consistent in suggesting a moderately strong association between infection with chlamydia and preterm delivery.

Trichomonas

The only major study noted in Table 3.10 that provides epidemiologic evidence on trichomonas and preterm delivery is the Vaginal Infection and Prematurity Study (Meis et al., 1995; Read and Klebanoff, 1993). Accompanied by frequent sexual activity or based on assessment earlier in gestation, modest positive associations have been found (relative risks of 1.5). Other subgroups or assessment times do not show such associations, leaving the overall epidemiologic evidence rather tenuous at present.

Group B streptococcus

A number of studies have examined group B streptococcus infection and preterm delivery (Table 3.10), and there is some consistency in the finding of a lack of association. Of the seven individual studies noted, one found a small association for preterm low birth weight deliveries (relative risk of 1.5) and an earlier case-control study of preterm premature rupture of the membranes reported an eight-fold increased risk. All other relative risk estimates ranged from 0.8 to 1.2, leaving the evidence for a positive association very weak at this time.

Urinary tract infection

The literature regarding urinary tract infections and prematurity (Table 3.11) is complicated by several factors: (1) differing severity of infections in the reports, ranging from the most mild, asymptomatic bacteriuria, to the most serious, pyelonephritis; (2) differing time in pregnancy at which the infection is diagnosed, ranging from the first prenatal visit to time of delivery; (3) the impact of antibiotics prescribed for the infection; and (4) the changes over time in the typical clinical protocol for prescribing antibiotics. Research during the 1960s so strongly linked untreated asymptomatic bacteriuria on the first prenatal visit to pyelonephritis later in pregnancy that antibiotics are now routinely given to pregnant women with asymptomatic bacteriuria. In comparison to earlier decades, there has been relatively little research on urinary tract infections during pregnancy since the mid-1970s.

As reviewed by Dodson and Fortunato (1988), strong associations were reported between pyelonephritis and prematurity in the era before antibiotics (publication years 1902–1936). Between 20% and 55% of women with prenatal pyelonephritis delivered prematurely. Since that time, there have been many studies of pyelonephritis and low birth weight, but few have examined preterm delivery. Wren (1969) found that 15% of women treated for bacteriuria or pyelonephritis delivered before term, versus 4.6% in women without either bacteriuria or pyelonephritis. Others have found no association. More recently, Schieve and colleagues (1994) reported an unadjusted odds ratio of 1.9 for preterm delivery among women whose prenatal urinary tract infection progressed to pyelonephritis, while Fan and colleagues (1987) found no association.

The association of cystitis and preterm delivery is not consistent in the literature. Four reports contained in Table 3.11 found positive associations ranging from elevated risks of 1.3 to 3.7 (Kramer et al., 1992; McGrady et al., 1985; McKenzie et al., 1994; Schieve et al., 1994), but two other reports reviewed by Romero and Mazor (1988) found no association between cystitis and prematurity.

There is inconsistency in studies of the association between bacteriuria and preterm delivery as well. In a summary of 19 studies by Sweet and Gibbs (1984), there was a 2.3% overall increased risk of preterm delivery in pregnancies with

Table 3.11. Summary of selected publications on urinary tract infection and preterm delivery

Author and publication year	Study design	PT count	Outcome measurement	Exposure measurement	Primary results (relative risk)
Henderson et al. 1962	Cohort	97	< 36 wks	Bacteriuria at delivery	1.3 ($P > 0.05$)
Layton 1964	Case-control	13	< 37 wks	Untreated ASB	0.8 (0.3–2.9)
Patrick 1967	Cohort	29	PT	Treated ASB	1.6 (0.6–4.6)
				Untreated ASB	1.3 (0.5–3.6)
Robertson et al. 1968	Cohort	78	< 36 wks	Treated ASB	0.6 (0.2–1.9)
				Untreated ASB	2.0 (1.1–3.6)
Wren 1969	Cohort	224	PT	Treated ASB	0.9 (0.4–2.1)
				Untreated ASB	2.6 (1.5–4.6)
				Symptomatic UTI	2.2 (1.0–5.1)
Williams et al. 1978	Case-control	25	< 36 wks	Treated bacteriuria	3.0 (1.2–7.3)
McGrady et al. 1985	Case-control	94	PT	Vital Statistics record of UTI	1.8 (1.3–2.6)
Fan et al. 1987	Case-control	27	PT	Pyelonephritis	No association
Kramer et al. 1992	Retrospective cohort	770	PT	Self-report of UTI	3.7 (1.1–12.3) (stronger association for very PT)
McKenzie et al. 1994	Cohort	138	PT	Urine culture $\geqslant 10^5$/ml	2.4 ($P = 0.02$)
Schieve et al. 1994	Cohort	2839	PT	Urine culture $\geqslant 10^5$/ml or positive diagnosis	1.3 (1.1–1.4)
				Pyelonephritis	1.9 (1.3–2.9)

PT, preterm delivery < 37 weeks; *P*, Probability; UTI, urinary tract infection; ASB, asymptomatic bacteriuria.

bacteriuria compared to those that were nonbacteriuric. Romero and Mazor (1988) reviewed four cohort studies conducted in the 1960s and found that when the data from the four studies were pooled, untreated asymptomatic bacteriuria was associated with twice the risk of prematurity. In two other studies contained in the table, one found that treated bacteriuric women had three times the risk of preterm birth (Williams et al., 1978), while the second found no association between prematurity and bacteriuria at delivery (Henderson et al., 1962).

Conclusion

Increasing the understanding of the pathophysiology of preterm delivery is important. However, the primary goal should be to identify modifiable factors that, if removed through prenatal interventions, would prevent at least some cases of preterm delivery. Although a formal evaluation to identify the strategies most likely to be effective in preventing preterm delivery is beyond the scope of this review, some considerations relevant to establishing priorities to reduce the occurrence of preterm delivery are described here.

First, it is important to consider whether modifying a specific exposure will truly modify the risk of preterm delivery. Many potential risk factors are part of a cluster of adverse circumstances and behaviors that are associated with preterm delivery. These include, for example, sexually transmitted infection, inadequate diet, tobacco use, and illicit drug use. If a component of such a cluster were removed, say illicit drug use, it is not clear that the risk of preterm delivery would change. Because many of these factors have been studied only or mostly in observational research, it is difficult to establish with certainty that their association with preterm delivery is truly causal.

Next, it is important to consider whether a specific attribute is amenable to modification. The challenges in modifying addictive behaviors are well known, for example. Even if these behaviors are known to cause preterm delivery, current approaches to modifying them may have limited impact on modifying the exposure, and thus limited effect on preterm delivery. Even in the case of habitual exposures, such as diet, the means by which an attribute could be modified is far from clear.

If an attribute is both causal and modifiable, one must still assess its potential to have a substantial impact on preterm delivery. The concept of attributable fraction (i.e., the proportion of disease that might be removed through changing exposure) is critical. Even if a certain exposure has a large impact on those who are exposed, if the number of women who have the exposure is small, the potential impact of an intervention directed at that exposure is limited. This is the case, for example, for an exposure like heavy cocaine use, which is relatively rare in the population of pregnant women. Research on other exposures, such as anemia or tobacco use, that may well have a less dramatic impact on preterm delivery but that are more prevalent in the population, may lead to interventions resulting in a greater overall reduction in preterm delivery.

The literature offers few examples of exposures that are clearly established to cause preterm delivery, that are amenable to modification, and that would have a large benefit in reducing preterm delivery if acted upon. There are indeed promising leads worthy of research or intervention trials, but the need to better understand the exogenous causes of preterm delivery is critical.

Among the exposures that we have considered, the most promising targets for prevention strategies appear to be tobacco use, iron stores and anemia, bacterial vaginosis, chlamydia, and psychosocial stress. In addition to these, high priorities for further research include studies directed to improving our understanding of the effects of dietary vitamin C and folate, illicit drug use, and physical activity.

REFERENCES

Abrams B, Newman V, Key T, et al. Maternal weight gain and preterm delivery. Obstetrics and Gynecology 1989; **74**: 577–83.

Ahlborg G Jr, Bodin L. Tobacco smoke exposure and pregnancy outcome among working women: a prospective study at prenatal care centers in Orebro County, Sweden. American Journal of Epidemiology 1991; **133**: 338–47.

Ahlborg G Jr, Bodin L, Hogstedt C. Heavy lifting during pregnancy – a hazard to the fetus? A prospective study. International Journal of Epidemiology 1990; **19**: 90–7.

Alger LS, Lovchik JC, Hevel JR, et al. The association of *Chlamydia trachomatis, Neisseria Gonorrhoeae*, and group B streptococci with preterm rupture of the membranes and pregnancy outcome. American Journal of Obstetrics and Gynecology 1988; **159**: 397–404.

Andrews KW, Savitz DA, Hertz-Picciotto I. Prenatal lead exposure in relation to gestational age and birth weight: a review of epidemiologic studies. American Journal of Industrial Medicine 1994; **26**: 13–32.

Bakketeig LS, Hoffman HJ, Harley EE. The tendency to repeat gestational age and birth weight in successive births. American Journal of Obstetrics and Gynecology 1979; **135**: 1086–103.

Bateman DA, Ng SK, Hansen CA, et al. The effects of intrauterine cocaine exposure in newborns. American Journal of Public Health 1993; **83**: 190–3.

Berkowitz GS, Holford TR, Berkowitz RL. Effects of cigarette smoking, alcohol, coffee and tea consumption on preterm delivery. Human Development 1982; **7**: 239–50.

Berkowitz GS, Kasl SV. The role of psychosocial factors in spontaneous preterm delivery. Journal of Psychosomatic Research 1983; **27**: 283–90.

Berkowitz GS, Papiernik E. Epidemiology of preterm birth. Epidemiologic Reviews 1993; **15**: 414–43.

Berman SM, Harrison HR, Boyce WT, et al. Low birth weight, prematurity, and postpartum endometritis. Association with prenatal cervical mycoplasma hominis and *Chlamydia trachomatis* infections. Journal of the American Medical Association 1987; **257**: 1189–94.

Blackmore CA, Savitz DA, Edwards LJ, et al. Racial differences in the patterns of preterm delivery in central North Carolina. Pædiatric and Perinatal Epidemiology 1995; **9**: 281–95.

Blot I, Papiernik E, Kaltwasser JP, et al. Influence of routine administration of folic acid and iron during pregnancy. Gynecologic and Obstetric Investigation 1981; **12**: 294–304.

Borges G, Lopez-Cervantes M, Medina-Mora ME, et al. Alcohol consumption, low birth weight and preterm delivery in the National Addiction Survey (Mexico). International Journal of Addictions 1993; **28**: 355–68.

Brandt LPA, Nielsen CV. Job stress and adverse outcome of pregnancy: a causal link or recall bias? American Journal of Epidemiology 1992; **135**: 302–11.

Brett KM, Strogatz DS, Savitz DA. Employment, job strain, and preterm delivery among women in North Carolina. American Journal of Public Health 1997; **87**: 199–204.

Bro S, Berendtsen H, Norgaard J, et al. Serum zinc and copper concentrations in maternal and umbilical cord blood. Relation to course and outcome of pregnancy. Scandinavian Journal of Clinical and Laboratory Investigation 1988; **48**: 805–11.

Bryce RL, Stanley FJ, Garner JB. Randomized controlled trial of antenatal social support to prevent preterm birth. British Journal of Obstetrics and Gynæcology 1991; **98**: 1001–8.

Caldwell EJ, Carlson SE, Palmer SM, et al. Histamine and ascorbic acid: a survey of women in labor at term and significantly before term. International Journal for Vitamin and Nutrition Research 1988; **58**: 319–25.

Chasnoff I, Griffith D, MacGregor S, et al. Temporal patterns of cocaine use in pregnancy. Journal of the American Medical Association 1989; **261**: 1741–4.

Cherry FF, Sandstead HH, Rojas P, et al. Adolescent pregnancy: associations among body weight, zinc nutriture, and pregnancy outcome. American Journal of Clinical Nutrition 1989; **50**: 945–54.

Cherukuri R, Minkoff H, Feldman J, et al. A cohort study of alkaloid cocaine ("crack") in pregnancy. Obstetrics and Gynecology 1988; **72**: 147–51.

Chouteau M, Namerow PB, Leppert P. The effect of cocaine abuse on birth weight and gestational age. Obstetrics and Gynecology 1988; **72**: 351–4.

Claman P, Toye B, Peeling RW, et al. Serologic evidence of *Chlamydia trachomatis* infection and risk of preterm birth. Canadian Medical Association Journal 1995; **153**: 259–62.

Cnattingius S, Forman MR, Berendes HW, et al. Effect of age, parity, and smoking on pregnancy outcome: a population-based study. American Journal of Obstetrics and Gynecology 1993; **168**: 16–21.

Copper RL, Goldenberg RL, Das A, et al. The preterm prediction study: maternal stress is associated with spontaneous preterm birth at less than thirty-five weeks' gestation. American Journal of Obstetrics and Gynecology 1996; **175**: 1286–92.

Czeizel AE, Dudas I, Merneki J. Pregnancy outcomes in a randomized controlled trial of periconceptional multivitamin supplementation. Archives of Gynecology and Obstetrics 1994; **255**: 131–9.

Dodson MG, Fortunato SJ. Microorganisms and premature labor. Journal of Reproductive

Medicine 1988; **33**(Suppl. 1): 87–96.

Dye TD, Oldenettel D. Physical activity and the risk of preterm labor: an epidemiological review and synthesis of recent literature. [review]. Seminars in Perinatology 1996; **20**: 334–9.

Ekwo EE, Gosselink CA, Woolson R, et al. Coitus late in pregnancy: risk of preterm rupture of amniotic sac membranes. American Journal of Obstetrics and Gynecology 1993; **168**: 22–31.

Elliott B, Brunham RC, Laga M, et al. Maternal gonococcal infection as a preventable risk factor for low birth weight. Journal of Infectious Diseases 1990; **161**: 531–6.

Eyler FD, Behnke M, Conlon M, et al. Prenatal cocaine use: a comparison of neonates matched on maternal risk factors. Neurotoxicology and Teratology 1994; **16**: 81–7.

Falorni ML, Fornasarig A, Stefanile C. Research about anxiety effects on the pregnant woman and her newborn child. In: Carenza L, Zichella L, eds. Emotion and reproduction. Fifth International Congress of Psychosomatic Obstetrics and Gynecology, Rome, 1977. Proceedings of the Serono Symposia. New York: Academic Press. Vol 20B: 1147–53.

Fan YD, Pastorek JG, Miller JM, et al. Acute pyelonephritis in pregnancy. American Journal of Perinatology 1987; **4**: 324–6.

Feldman JG, Minkoff HL, McCalla S, et al. A cohort study of the impact of perinatal drug use on prematurity in an inner-city population. American Journal of Public Health 1992; **82**: 726–8.

Fenster L, Eskenazi B, Windham GC, et al. Caffeine consumption during pregnancy and fetal growth. American Journal of Public Health 1991; **81**: 458–61.

Fortier I, Marcoux S, Beaulac-Baillargeon L. Relation of caffeine intake during pregnancy to intrauterine growth retardation and preterm birth. American Journal of Epidemiology 1993; **137**: 931–40.

French JI, McGregor JA. Bacterial vaginosis: history, epidemiology, microbiology, sequelae, diagnosis, and treatment. In: Borschardt KA, Noble MA, eds. Sexually transmitted diseases. Epidemiology, pathology, diagnosis, and treatment. Boca Raton(FL): CRC Press, 1997: 3–39.

Frentzen BH, Johnson JWC, Simpson S. Nutrition and hydration: relationship to preterm myometrial contractility. Obstetrics and Gynecology 1987; **70**: 887–91.

Garn SM, Ridella SA, Petzold AS, et al. Maternal hematologic levels and pregnancy outcomes. Seminars in Perinatology 1981; **5**: 155–62.

Georgakopoulos PA, Dodos D, Mechleris D. Sexuality in pregnancy and premature labour. British Journal of Obstetrics and Gynæcology 1984; **91**: 891–3.

Gibbs RS, Romero R, Hillier SL, et al. A review of premature birth and subclinical infection. American Journal of Obstetrics and Gynecology 1992; **166**: 1515–28.

Gillogley KM, Evans AT, Hansen RL. The perinatal impact of cocaine, amphetamine, and opiate use detected by universal intrapartum screening. American Journal of Obstetrics and Gynecology 1990; **163**: 1535–42.

Gravett MG, Nelson HP, DeRouen T, et al. Independent associations of bacterial vaginosis and *Chlamydia trachomatis* infection with adverse pregnancy outcome. Journal of the American Medical Association 1986; **256**: 1899–903.

Handler A, Kistin N, Davis F, et al. Cocaine use during pregnancy: perinatal outcome. American Journal of Epidemiology 1991; **133**: 818–25.

Hauth JC, Goldenberg RL, Andews WW, et al. Reduced incidence of preterm delivery with metronidazole and erythromycin in women with bacterial vaginosis. New England Journal of

Medicine 1995; **333**: 1732–6.

Hay PE, Lamont RF, Taylor-Robinson D, et al. Abnormal bacterial colonisation of the genital tract and subsequent preterm delivery and late miscarriage. British Journal of Medicine 1994; **308**: 295–8.

Hedegaard M, Henriksen TB, Sabroe S, et al. Psychological distress in pregnancy and preterm delivery. British Journal of Medicine 1993; **307**: 234–9.

Hedegaard M, Henriksen TB, Secher NJ, et al. Do stressful life events affect duration of gestation and risk of preterm delivery? Epidemiology 1996; **7**: 339–45.

Hediger ML, Scholl TO, Belsky DH, et al. Patterns of weight gain in adolescent pregnancy: effects on birth weight and preterm delivery. Obstetrics and Gynecology 1989; **74**: 6–12.

Henderson M, Entwisle G, Tayback M. Bacteriuria and pregnancy outcome: preliminary findings. American Journal of Public Health 1962; **52**: 1887–93.

Henriksen TB, Hedegaard M, Secher NJ. The relation between psychosocial job strain, and preterm delivery and low birthweight for gestational age. International Journal of Epidemiology 1994; **23**: 764–74.

Higashi A, Tajiri A, Matsukura M, et al. A prospective survey of serial maternal serum zinc levels and pregnancy outcome. Journal of Pediatric Gastroenterology and Nutrition 1988; **7**: 430–3.

Hillier SL, Nugent RP, Eschenbach DA, et al., for the Vaginal Infections and Prematurity Study Group. Association between bacterial vaginosis and preterm delivery of a low-birth-weight infant. New England Journal of Medicine 1995; **333**: 1737–42.

Holzman C, Paneth N. Maternal cocaine use during pregnancy and perinatal outcomes. Epidemiologic Reviews 1994; **16**: 315–34.

Homer CJ, Beresford SAA, James SA, et al. Work-related physical exertion and risk of preterm, low birthweight delivery. Paediatric and Perinatal Epidemiology 1990; **4**: 161–74.

Honnor MJ, Zubrick SR, Stanley FJ. The role of life events in different categories of preterm birth in a group of women with previous poor pregnancy outcome. European Journal of Epidemiology 1994; **10**: 181–8.

Institute of Medicine (IOM), Committee to Study the Prevention of Low Birthweight. Preventing low birthweight. Washington (DC): National Academy Press, 1985.

Investigators of the Johns Hopkins Study of Cervicitis and Adverse Pregnancy Outcome. Association of *Chlamydia trachomatis* and *Mycoplasma hominis* with intrauterine growth retardation and preterm delivery. American Journal of Epidemiology 1989; **129**: 1247–57.

Jameson S. Zinc status in pregnancy: the effect of zinc therapy on perinatal mortality, prematurity, and placental ablation. Annals of the New York Academy of Science 1993; **678**: 178–92.

Joesoef MR, Hillier SL Wiknjosastro G, et al. Intravaginal clindamycin treatment for bacterial vaginosis: effects on preterm delivery and low birth weight. American Journal of Obstetrics and Gynecology 1995; **173**: 1527–31.

Johnsson B, Hauge B, Larsen MF, et al. Zinc supplementation during pregnancy: a double blind randomised controlled trial. Acta Obstetricia et Gynecologica Scandinavica 1996; **75**: 725–9.

Keith L, MacGregor S, Friedell S, et al. Substance abuse in pregnant women: recent experience at the Perinatal Center for Chemical Dependence of Northwestern Memorial Hospital. Obstetrics and Gynecology 1989; **73**: 715–20.

Ketterlinus RD, Henderson SH, Lamb ME. Maternal age, sociodemographics, prenatal health and behavior: influences on neonatal risk status. Journal of Adolescent Health Care 1990; **11**: 423–31.

Kisten N, Handler A, Davis F, Ferre C. Cocaine and cigarettes: a comparison of risks. Pædiatric and Perinatal Epidemiology 1996; **10**: 269–78.

Klebanoff MA, Nugent RP, Rhoads GG. Coitus during pregnancy: is it safe? Lancet 1984; **2**: 914–17.

Klebanoff MA, Shiono PH. Top down, bottom up and inside out: reflections on preterm birth. Pædiatric and Perinatal Epidemiology 1995; **9**: 125–9.

Klebanoff MA, Shiono PH, Carey JC. The effect of physical activity during pregnancy on preterm delivery and birth weight. American Journal of Obstetrics and Gynecology 1990a; **163**: 1450–6.

Klebanoff MA, Shiono PH, Rhoads GG. Outcomes of pregnancy in a national sample of resident physicians. New England Journal of Medicine 1990b; **323**: 1040–5.

Klebanoff MA, Shiono PH, Selby JV, et al. Anemia and spontaneous preterm birth. American Journal of Obstetrics and Gynecology 1991; **164**: 59–63.

Kleinman JC, Kessel SS. Racial differences in low birth weight: trends and risk factors. New England Journal of Medicine 1987; **317**: 749–53.

Kliegman RM, Madura D, Kiwi R, et al. Relation of maternal cocaine use to the risks of prematurity and low birth weight. The Journal of Pediatrics 1994; **124**: 751–6.

Kline J, Ng SKC, Schittini M, et al. Cocaine use during pregnancy: sensitive detection by hair assay. American Journal of Public Health 1997; **87**: 352–8.

Kline J, Stein Z, Susser M. Conception to birth: epidemiology of prenatal development. Vol 14. New York: Oxford University Press, 1989.

Knottnerus JA, Delgado LR, Knipschild PG, et al. Hæmatologic parameters and pregnancy outcome: a prospective cohort study in the third trimester. Journal of Clinical Epidemiology 1990; **43**: 461–6.

Kramer MS. Determinants of low birth weight: methodological assessment and meta-analysis. Bulletin of the World Health Organization 1987; **65**: 663–737.

Kramer MS, Coates AL, Michoud M-C, et al. Maternal anthropometry and idiopathic preterm labor. Obstetrics and Gynecology 1995; **86**: 744–8.

Kramer MS, McLean FH, Eason EL, et al. Maternal nutrition and spontaneous preterm birth. American Journal of Epidemiology 1992; **136**: 574–83.

Kristensen P, Irgens LM, Daltveit AK, et al. Perinatal outcome among children of men exposed to lead and organic solvents in the printing industry. American Journal of Epidemiology 1993; **137**: 134–44.

Kurki T, Sivonen A, Renkonen O-V, et al. Bacterial vaginosis in early pregnancy and pregnancy outcome. Obstetrics and Gynecology 1992; **80**: 173–7.

Kurki T, Ylikorkala O. Coitus during pregnancy is not related to bacterial vaginosis or preterm birth. American Journal of Obstetrics and Gynecology 1994; **169**: 1130–4.

Lang JM, Lieberman E, Cohen A. A comparison of risk factors for preterm labor and term small-for-gestational-age birth. Epidemiology 1996; **7**: 369–76.

Launer LJ, Villar J, Kestler E, et al. The effect of maternal work on fetal growth and duration of pregnancy: a prospective study. British Journal of Obstetrics and Gynæcology 1990; **97**: 62–70.

Layton R. Infection of the urinary tract in pregnancy: an investigation of a new routine in antenatal care. British Journal of Obstetrics and Gynæcology 1964; **71**; 927–33.

Lazzaroni F, Bonassi S, Magnani M, et al. Moderate drinking and outcome of pregnancy. European Journal of Epidemiology 1993; **9**: 599–606.

Li CQ, Windsor RA, Perkins L, et al. The impact on infant birth weight and gestational age of cotinine-validated smoking reduction during pregnancy. Journal of the American Medical Association 1993; **269**: 1519–24.

Lieberman E, Ryan KJ, Monson RR, et al. Risk factors accounting for racial differences in the rate of premature births. New England Journal of Medicine 1987; **317**: 743–8.

Linn S, Schoenbaum SC, Monson RR, et al. No association between coffee consumption and adverse outcomes of pregnancy. New England Journal of Medicine 1982; **306**: 141–5.

Lobel M, Dunkel-Schetter C, Scrimshaw SC. Prenatal stress and prematurity: a prospective study of socioeconomically disadvantaged women. Health Psychology 1992; **11**: 32–40.

Lokey EA, Tran ZV, Wells CL, et al. Effects of physical exercise on pregnancy outcomes: a meta-analytic review. Medicine and Science In Sports and Exercise 1991; **23**: 1234–9.

Lu ZM, Goldenberg RL, Cliver SP, et al. The relationship between maternal hematocrit and pregnancy outcome. Obstetrics and Gynecology 1991; **77**: 190–4.

MacDonald LD, Peacock JL, Anderson HR. Marital status: association with social and economic circumstances, psychological state and outcomes of pregnancy. Journal of Public Health Medicine 1992; **14**: 26–34.

MacGregor SN, Keith LG, Bachicha JA, et al. Cocaine abuse during pregnancy: correlation between prenatal care and perinatal outcome. Obstetrics and Gynecology 1989; **74**: 882–5.

MacGregor SN, Keith LG, Chasnoff IJ, et al. Cocaine use during pregnancy: adverse perinatal outcome. American Journal of Obstetrics and Gynecology 1987; **157**: 686–90.

Magann EF, Evans SFE, Newnh P. Employment, exertion, and pregnancy outcome: assessment by kilocalories expended each day. American Journal of Obstetrics and Gynecology 1996; **175**: 182–7.

Mainous AG, Hueston WJ. The effect of smoking cessation during pregnancy on preterm delivery and low birthweight. Journal of Family Practice 1994; **38**: 262–6.

Mamelle N, Laumon B, Lazar P. Prematurity and occupational activity during pregnancy. American Journal of Epidemiology 1984; **119**: 309–22.

Marbury MC. Relationship of ergonomic stressors to birthweight and gestational age. Scandinavian Journal of Work, Environment and Health 1992; **18**: 73–83.

Martius J, Krohn MA, Hillier SL, et al. Relationships of vaginal lactobacillus species, cervical *Chlamydia trachomatis*, and bacterial vaginosis to preterm birth. Obstetrics and Gynecology 1988; **71**: 89–95.

Mastrogiannis D, Decavalas G, Verma U, et al. Perinatal outcome after recent cocaine usage. Obstetrics and Gynecology 1990; **76**: 8–11.

Matorras R, Perea AG, Omenaca F, et al. Group B streptococcus and premature rupture of membranes and preterm delivery. Gynecologic and Obstetric Investigation 1989; **27**: 14–18.

McDonald AD, Armstrong BG, Sloan M. Cigarette, alcohol, and coffee consumption and prematurity. American Journal of Public Health 1992; **82**: 87–90.

McDonald AD, McDonald JC, Armstrong B, et al. Prematurity and work in pregnancy. British Journal of Industrial Medicine 1988; **45**: 56–62.

McDonald HM, O'Loughlin JA, Jolley P, Vigneswaran R, McDonald PJ. Vaginal infection and preterm labour. British Journal of Obstetrics and Gynæcology 1991; **98**: 427–35.

McGrady GA, Daling JR, Peterson DR. Maternal urinary tract infection and adverse fetal outcomes. American Journal of Epidemiology 1985; **121**: 377–81.

McGregor JA, French JI. *Chlamydia trachomatis* infection during pregnancy. American Journal of Obstetrics and Gynecology 1991; **164**: 1782–9.

McGregor JA, French JI, Jones W, et al. Bacterial vaginosis is associated with prematurity and vaginal fluid mucinase and sialidase: results of a controlled trial of topical clindamycin cream. American Journal of Obstetrics and Gynecology 1994; **170**: 1048–60.

McKenzie H, Donnet ML, Howie PW, et al. Risk of preterm delivery in pregnant women with group B streptococcal urinary infections or urinary antibodies to group B streptococcal and *E. coli* antigens. British Journal of Obstetrics and Gynæcology 1994; **101**: 107–13.

Meis PJ, Goldenberg RL, Mercer B, et al. and the National Institute of Child Health and Human Development Maternal–Fetal Medicine Units Network. The preterm prediction study: significance of vaginal infections. American Journal of Obstetrics and Gynecology 1995: 173: 1231–5.

Mills JL, Harlap S, Harley EE. Should coitus late in pregnancy be discouraged? Lancet 1981; **2**: 136–8.

Minkoff H, Grunebaum AN, Schwarz RH, et al. Risk factors for prematurity and premature rupture of membranes: a prospective study of the vaginal flora in pregnancy. American Journal of Obstetrics and Gynecology 1984; **150**: 965–72.

Molfese VJ, Bricker MC, Manion LG, et al. Anxiety, depression and stress in pregnancy: a multivariate model of intra-partum risks and pregnancy outcomes. Journal of Psychosomatic Obstetrics and Gynæcology 1987; **7**: 77–92.

Morales WJ, Schorr S, Albritton J. Effects of metronidazole in patients with preterm birth in preceding pregnancy and bacterial vaginosis: a placebo-controlled, double-blind study. American Journal of Obstetrics and Gynecology 1994; **171**: 345–9.

Mutale T, Creed F, Marech M, et al. Life events and low birthweight – analysis by infants preterm and small for gestational age. British Journal of Obstetrics and Gynæcology 1991; **98**: 166–72.

National Academy of Sciences (NAS). Nutrition during pregnancy. Part I. Weight gain. Part II. Nutrient supplements. Washington (DC): National Academy Press, 1990.

National Center for Health Statistics. Vital Statistics of the United States 1988. Vol 1. Natality. Hyattsville (MD): National Center for Health Statistics, 1988.

Neilson JP, Mutambira M. Coitus, twin pregnancy, and preterm labor. American Journal of Obstetrics and Gynecology 1989; **160**: 416–18.

Newton RW, Hunt LP. Psychosocial stress in pregnancy and its relation to low birth weight. British Journal of Medicine 1984; **288**: 1191–4.

Newton RW, Webster PAC, Binu PS, et al. Psychological stress in pregnancy and its relation to the onset of premature labour. British Journal of Medicine 1979; **2**: 411–13.

Ngassa PC, Egbe JA. Maternal genital *Chlamydia trachomatis* infection and the risk of preterm labor. International Journal of Gynecology and Obstetrics 1994; **47**: 241–6.

Norbeck JS, Tilden VP. Life stress, social support, and emotional disequilibrium in complications of pregnancy: a prospective, multivariate study. Journal of Health and Social Behavior 1983; **24**: 30–46.

Nordentoft M, Lou H, Hansen D, et al. Intrauterine growth retardation and premature delivery: the influence of maternal smoking and psychosocial factors. American Journal of Public Health 1996; **86**: 347–54.

Nurminen T, Lusa S, Ilmarinen J, et al. Physical work load, fetal development and course of pregnancy. Scandinavian Journal of Work, Environment and Health 1989; **15**: 404–14.

Olsen J, Overvad K, Frische G. Coffee consumption, birthweight, and reproductive failures. Epidemiology 1991; **2**: 370–4.

Oro A, Dixon S. Perinatal cocaine and methamphetamine exposure: maternal and neonatal correlates. The Journal of Pediatrics 1987; **111**: 571–8.

Orr ST, Miller CA. Maternal depressive symptoms and the risk of poor pregnancy outcome: review of the literature and preliminary findings. Epidemiologic Reviews 1995; **17**: 165–71.

Osborn LM, Harris DL, Reading JC, et al. Outcome of pregnancies experienced during residency. Journal of Family Practice 1990; **31**: 618–22.

Pagel MD, Smilkstein G, Regen H, et al. Psychosocial influences on newborn outcomes: a controlled prospective study. Social Science and Medicine 1990; **30**: 597–604.

Pastore LM, Savitz DA. A case-control study of caffeinated beverages and preterm delivery. American Journal of Epidemiology 1995; **141**: 61–9

Patrick MJ. Influence of maternal renal infection on the fetus and infant. Archives of Disease in Childhood 1967; **42**: 208–13.

Peacock JL, Bland JM, Anderson HR. Preterm delivery: effects of socioeconomic factors, psychological stress, smoking, alcohol, and caffeine. British Journal of Medicine 1995; **311**: 531–5.

Perkin MR, Bland JM, Peacock JL, et al. The effect of anxiety and depression during pregnancy on obstetric complications. British Journal of Obstetrics and Gynæcology 1993; **100**: 629–34.

Perkins RP. Sexual behavior and response in relation to complications of pregnancy. American Journal of Obstetrics and Gynecology 1979; **134**: 498–505.

Puch WE, Fernandez FL. Coitus late in pregnancy: a follow-up study of the effects of coitus on pregnancy, delivery, and the puerperium. Obstetrics and Gynecology 1953; **2**: 636–42.

Ramirez G, Grimes RM, Annegers JF, et al. Occupational physical activity and other risk factors for preterm birth among US Army primigravidas. American Journal of Public Health 1990; **80**: 728–9.

Rayburn WF, Wilson EA. Coital activity and premature delivery. American Journal of Obstetrics and Gynecology 1980; **137**: 972–4.

Read JS, Klebanoff MA, for the Vaginal Infections and Prematurity Study Group. Sexual intercourse during pregnancy and preterm delivery: effects of vaginal microorganisms. American Journal of Obstetrics and Gynecology 1993; **168**: 514–19.

Regan JA, Klebanoff MA, Nugent RP, et al., for the VIP Study. Colonization with group B streptococci in pregnancy and adverse outcome. American Journal of Obstetrics and Gynecology 1996; **74**: 1354–60.

Riduan JM, Hillier SL, Utomo B, et al. Bacterial vaginosis and prematurity in Indonesia: association in early and late pregnancy. American Journal of Obstetrics and Gynecology 1993; **169**: 175–8.

Robertson JG, Livingstone JRB, Isdale MH. The management and complications of asymptomatic bacteriuria in pregnancy. British Journal of Obstetrics and Gynæcology 1968; **75**: 59–65.

Rolschau J, Date J, Krostoffersen K. Folic acid supplement and intrauterine growth. Acta Obstetricia et Gynecologica Scandinavica 1979; **58**: 343–6.

Romero R, Mazor M. Infections and preterm labor. Clinical Obstetrics and Gynecology 1988; **31**: 553–84.

Rothman KJ. Causes. American Journal of Epidemiology 1976; **104**: 587–92.

Ryan L, Ehrlich S, Finnegan L. Cocaine abuse in pregnancy: effects on the fetus and newborn. Neurotoxicology and Teratology 1987; **9**: 295–9.

Sanjose S, Roman E, Beral V. Low birthweight and preterm delivery, Scotland, 1981–1984: effect of parents' occupation. Lancet 1991; **338**: 428–31.

Saurel-Cubizolles MJ, Kaminski M. Work in pregnancy: its evolving relationship with perinatal outcome (a review). Social Science and Medicine 1986; **22**: 431–42.

Saurel-Cubizolles MJ, Subtil D, Kaminski M. Is preterm delivery still related to physical working conditions in pregnancy? Journal of Epidemiology and Community Health 1991; **45**: 29–34.

Savitz DA, Blackmore C, Thorp JM. Epidemiology of preterm delivery: etiologic heterogeneity. American Journal of Obstetrics and Gynecology 1991a; **164**: 467–71.

Savitz DA, Olshan AF, Gallagher K. Maternal occupation and pregnancy outcome. Epidemiology 1996; **7**: 269–74.

Savitz DA, Whelan EA, Kleckner RC. Effect of parents' occupational exposures on risk of stillbirth, preterm delivery, and small-for-gestational-age infants. American Journal of Epidemiology 1989; **129**: 1201–18.

Savitz DA, Whelan EA, Rowland AS, et al. Maternal employment and reproductive risk factors. American Journal of Epidemiology 1991b; **133**: 123–32.

Schieve LA, Handler A, Hershow R, et al. Urinary tract infection during pregnancy: its association with maternal morbidity and perinatal outcome. American Journal of Public Health 1994; **84**: 405–10.

Scholl TO, Hediger ML, Fischer RL, et al. Anemia vs iron deficiency: increased risk of preterm delivery in a prospective study. American Journal of Clinical Nutrition 1992a; **55**: 985–8.

Scholl TO, Hediger ML, Huang J, et al. Young maternal age and parity: influences on pregnancy outcome. Annals of Epidemiology 1992b; **2**: 565–75.

Scholl TO, Hediger ML, Salmon RW, Belsky DH, Ances IG. Influence of prepregnant body mass and weight gain for gestation on spontaneous preterm delivery and duration of gestation during adolescent pregnancy. American Journal of Human Biology 1989; **1**: 657–64.

Scholl TO, Hediger ML, Schall JI, et al. Dietary and serum folate: their influence on the outcome of pregnancy. American Journal of Clinical Nutrition 1996; **63**: 520–5.

Scholl TO, Hediger ML, Schall JI, et al. Low zinc intake during pregnancy: its association with preterm and very preterm delivery. American Journal of Epidemiology 1993; **137**: 1115–24.

Shiono PH, Klebanoff MA. Ethnic differences in preterm and very preterm delivery. American

Journal of Public Health 1986; **76**: 1317–21.

Shiono PH, Klebanoff MA, Nugent RP, et al. The impact of cocaine and marijuana use on low birth weight and preterm birth: a multicenter study. American Journal of Obstetrics and Gynecology 1995; **172**: 19–27.

Siega-Riz AM, Adair LS, Hobel CJ. Institute of Medicine maternal weight gain recommendation and pregnancy outcome in a predominantly Hispanic population. Obstetrics and Gynecology 1994; **84**: 565–73.

Siega-Riz AM, Adair LS, Hobel CJ. Maternal underweight status and inadequate rate of weight gain during the third trimester of pregnancy increases the risk of preterm delivery. Journal of Nutrition 1996; **126**: 146–53.

Singer L, Arendt R, Song LY, et al. Direct and indirect interactions of cocaine with childbirth outcomes. Archives of Pediatrics and Adolescent Medicine 1994; **148**: 959–64.

Slutsker L. Risks associated with cocaine use during pregnancy. Obstetrics and Gynecology 1992; **79**: 778–89.

Solberg DA, Butler J, Wagner NN. Sexual behavior in pregnancy. New England Journal of Medicine 1973; **288**: 1098–103.

Spense MR, Williams R, DiGregorio GJ, et al. The relationship between recent cocaine use and pregnancy outcome. Obstetrics and Gynecology 1991; **78**: 326–9.

Steer RA, Scholl TO, Hediger ML, et al. Self-reported depression and negative pregnancy outcomes. Journal of Clinical Epidemiology 1992; **45**: 1093–9.

Stein A, Campbell EA, Day A, et al. Social adversity, low birth weight, and preterm delivery. British Journal of Medicine 1987; **295**: 291–3.

Sweet RL, Gibbs RS. Urinary tract infection. In: Sweet RL, ed. Infectious diseases of the female genital tract. Baltimore: Williams & Wilkins, 1984; 293–313.

Sweet RL, Landers DV, Walker C, et al. *Chlamydia trachomatis* infection and pregnancy outcome. American Journal of Obstetrics and Gynecology 1987; **156**: 824–33.

Tchernia G, Blot I, Rey A, et al. Maternal folate status, birthweight and gestational age. Developmental Pharmacology and Therapeutics 1982; **4**: 58–65.

Teitelman AM, Welch LS, Hellenbrand KG, et al. Effect of maternal work activity on preterm birth and low birth weight. American Journal of Epidemiology 1990; **131**: 104–13.

Van den Berg BJ. Epidemiological observations of prematurity: effects of tobacco, coffee and alcohol. In: Reed DM, Stainley FJ, eds. The epidemiology of prematurity. Baltimore: Urban & Schwarzenberg, 1977: 157–77.

Verkerk PH, van Noord-Zaadstra BM, Florey C, et al. The effect of moderate maternal alcohol consumption on birth weight and gestational age in a low risk population. Early Human Development 1993; **32**: 121–9.

Villar J, Farnot U, Barros F, et al. A randomized trial of psychosocial support during high-risk pregnancies. New England Journal of Medicine 1992; **327**: 1266–71.

Villar J, Repke JT. Calcium supplementation during pregnancy may reduce preterm delivery in high-risk populations. American Journal of Obstetrics and Gynecology 1990; **163**: 1124–31.

Virji SK, Cottington E. Risk factors associated with preterm deliveries among racial groups in a national sample of married mothers. American Journal of Perinatology 1991; **8**: 347–53.

Wadhwa PD, Sandman CA, Porto M, et al. The association between prenatal stress and infant birth weight and gestational age at birth: a prospective investigation. American Journal of Obstetrics and Gynecology 1993; **169**: 858–65.

Weathersbee PS, Olsen LK, Lodge JR. Caffeine and pregnancy: a retrospective study. Postgraduate Medicine 1977; **62**: 64–9.

Wen SW, Goldenberg RL, Cutter GR, et al. Smoking, maternal age, fetal growth, and gestational age at delivery. American Journal of Obstetrics and Gynecology 1990; **162**: 53–8.

Werler MM, Shapiro S, Mitchell AA. Periconceptional folic acid exposure and risk of occurrent neural tube defects. Journal of the American Medical Association 1993; **269**: 1257–61.

Williams JD, Reeves, DS, Condie AP, et al. Significance of bacteriuria in pregnancy. In: Kass EH, Brumfitt W, eds. Infections of the urinary tract: proceedings of the third international symposium on pyelonephyritis. Chicago: University of Chicago Press, 1978: 1–7.

Williams MA, Mittendorf R, Stubblefield PG, et al. Cigarettes, coffee, and preterm premature rupture of the membranes. American Journal of Epidemiology 1992; **135**: 895–903.

Windham GC, Fenster L, Hopkins B, et al. The association of moderate maternal and paternal alcohol consumption with birthweight and gestational age. Epidemiology 1995; **6**: 591–7.

Wisborg K, Henriksen TB, Hedegaard M, et al. Smoking during pregnancy and preterm birth. British Journal of Obstetrics and Gynæcology 1996; **103**: 800–5.

Witter FR, Neibyl JR. Marijuana use in pregnancy and pregnancy outcome. American Journal of Perinatology 1990; **7**: 36–8.

Wren BG. Subclinical renal infections and prematurity. Medical Journal of Australia 1969; **2**: 596–600.

4

Interventions to prevent prematurity

Robert L. Goldenberg and Dwight J. Rouse

Introduction

In the United States, 10% of all pregnancies end prematurely, that is, before 37 weeks' gestational age. Prematurity is responsible for a large majority of neonatal mortality among normally formed infants and as much as 50% of birth-attributable major neurologic disability, including cerebral palsy (McCormick, 1985). In addition, due to organ system immaturity, preterm infants are subject to a host of acute medical morbidities. Much of this mortality and morbidity is concentrated in the very lowest birth weight (< 1500 gm) or early gestational age infants (< 32 weeks), who represent between 10 and 20% of preterm births (only 1–2% of all births) (Copper et al., 1993; Robertson et al., 1992). In contrast, preterm birth at relatively more advanced gestational ages (35 and 36 weeks) represents 50% or more of all preterm births and, on an individual basis, infrequently results in severe morbidity or death.

This chapter builds upon the previous chapter by reviewing the evidence on interventions currently practiced to prevent prematurity or improve its outcomes. As the discussions of these interventions – prenatal care, risk scoring, behavior change interventions, early identification of preterm labor, nutrition interventions, tocolytic drugs, bed rest, maternal hydration, cerclage for incompetent cervix, progestins, antibiotic treatment for infections, and interventions for premature rupture of the membranes – will show, few prevent preterm delivery. However, the development of effective antibiotic treatment strategies for bacterial vaginosis has great potential for improving some important outcomes associated with early spontaneous preterm birth in high-risk women. An improved understanding of the mechanisms leading to preterm birth will do much to foster more rational and effective approaches to intervention.

Prematurity rates in the United States

Over the last 10 or 15 years, vital statistics data from individual states, as well as national data, suggest that both the total preterm birth rate, and the very early preterm birth rate, are slowly rising (Creasy, 1993). In contrast, the low birth weight rate (< 2500 gm) is actually slowly declining because fewer full-term infants are of low birth weight (Kleinman and Kessel, 1987). Low birth weight term infants (and term infants born weighing less than the 10th percentile for their gestational age) have a small increased risk of both mortality and short and long-term morbidity (Goldenberg et al., 1996b,c). In contrast to those infants born at very early gestational ages, these full-term "small-for-gestational-age" births contribute relatively little to the overall number of infants with adverse outcomes.

Most commonly, preterm birth is categorized as resulting from spontaneous labor (50% of preterm births), or spontaneous preterm rupture of membranes (PROM) (25% of preterm births), or intentionally for fetal or maternal benefit (25% of preterm births), in which case the delivery is classified as "indicated" (Tucker et al., 1991). In predominantly African American populations, a higher proportion of preterm births follows spontaneous rupture of the membranes, with correspondingly fewer births in the two other categories (Kempe et al., 1992; Savitz et al., 1991). Interventions aimed at reducing preterm delivery have generally been targeted to one of these three categories.

A number of risk factors have been identified for predicting preterm birth. The most consistent, aside from multiple gestation, is African American race (Gardner and Goldenberg, 1995a; Goepfert and Goldenberg, 1996; Shiono et al., 1986; Wen et al., 1990a). Regardless of the geographic area in the United States, African American women have an approximately two-fold increased risk of preterm birth and a three-fold increased risk of early preterm birth. It is this discrepancy in preterm, and especially very early preterm, birth rates that is predominantly responsible for the two-fold difference in infant mortality seen between African Americans and whites in the United States.

Although there is some difference in preterm birth rates among specific Hispanic and Asian groups, in general, the risk of prematurity for most Hispanic women is approximately the same as for white women, while Asian women are generally at lower risk of preterm birth (Gardner and Goldenberg, 1995a; Shiono et al., 1986; Starfield et al., 1991). Within these groups, higher levels of income and education are usually associated with lower preterm birth rates (Creasy et al., 1980; Goepfert and Goldenberg 1996; Mercer et al., 1996; Savitz et al., 1991; Wen et al., 1990a). Lifestyle factors, such as smoking and alcohol and drug use, which are clearly associated with an increased risk of a small-for-gestational-age infant, have not been consistently associated with an increased risk of preterm birth (Goldenberg, 1994; Kramer, 1987; Wen et al., 1990a). Finally, although 50% or more of the births of small for gestational age infants are explained by known risk factors, once multiple births have been considered, few preterm births are explained by known risk factors.

Prevention of preterm birth is not an end unto itself. Preterm birth is consequential only if there is an associated increase in mortality or short- or long-term morbidity, or if there is an associated increase in cost. For example, if an infant is born at 36 rather than 37 weeks, does not die or experience any morbidity, and does not have a prolonged hospital stay, being born preterm is of little consequence. It may even be that a preterm birth of a healthy infant will represent an improvement over a term birth of an infant who dies or suffers neurologic damage as a result of a late pregnancy insult. The fact that 20–25% of preterm births occur because the physician believes the outcome of pregnancy would be improved suggests that at least some of these indicated preterm births may be associated with less morbidity and mortality in the mother or infant than if the pregnancy had been allowed to progress to term. While delaying births until term is desirable in most circumstances, in some situations an increase in preterm births may actually improve outcome.

Strategies to improve the outcome of prematurity

There are essentially two types of strategies used to reduce adverse outcomes associated with prematurity: (1) attempts to either delay or prevent preterm birth; and (2) attempts to prevent or ameliorate the morbidity and mortality that result from preterm birth (Goldenberg, 1994). Strategies of the latter type have been aimed at specific acute medical morbidities, such as respiratory distress syndrome, necrotizing enterocolitis, intraventricular hemorrhage, and sepsis. Because the mortality associated with prematurity has lessened, one or more of the strategies aimed at reducing mortality most likely has been successful. However, because the preterm delivery rate has not declined, it is not clear if any of the strategies aimed at reducing preterm birth have been effective.

This chapter does not review the strategies used to prevent morbidity and mortality in preterm newborns in detail. However, among them, the most successful in improving outcome has been the introduction of regionalized newborn intensive care, with the result that most very preterm infants are now delivered at the site of a newborn intensive care unit (Goldenberg, 1994). As noted in Dr. Milliez's description of the French perinatal care system in Chapter 16, systems that do not yet regionalize newborn intensive care recognize the effectiveness of this approach. The individual medical interventions associated with this improvement in outcome also cannot be discussed in detail, but certainly include improved methods of ventilation, the use of surfactant, liberal and appropriate antibiotic treatment, better fluid and electrolyte management, and many other interventions that now comprise routine care in the newborn intensive care units. From the obstetric perspective, it appears that the increased use of prenatal corticosteroids, antibiotic strategies to reduce the risk of neonatal group B streptococcal sepsis, and a lowered tolerance for fetal hypoxia may have all contributed to the reduction in morbidity and mortality of early preterm infants (Crowley, 1995; Gardner and Goldenberg, 1995b; Paul et al., 1979; Rouse et al., 1994).

Certainly, active attempts by obstetricians and neonatologists to salvage very low birth weight fetuses and newborns are associated with an improvement in outcomes (Bottoms et al., 1997; Rouse et al., 1995b). In 1000–1500 gm infants, mortality has decreased from about 50% in the early 1960s to a little more than 5% today. Similarly, improvements have been achieved in infants of even lower birth weight. In the early 1960s, 500–1000 gm infants had a mortality of about 95%, while today in most newborn intensive care units, these infants have only a 20% risk of mortality (Hack et al., 1991). Despite these tremendous improvements in survival, approximately 50–60% of all neonatal mortality still occurs in the babies born weighing less than 1000 gm. It should be emphasized again that the remarkable improvement in survival in very early gestational age newborns has not been accompanied by a reduction in their occurrence, nor has the improvement in survival been accompanied by a substantial reduction, if any, in the associated risk of long-term neurologic handicap.

Indicated preterm birth

The majority of indicated preterm births result from the development of pre-eclampsia, leading to the judgment that either the mother or the fetus is at unacceptable risk for an adverse outcome should the pregnancy continue (Meis et al., 1998; Tucker et al., 1991). A number of different approaches to reduce the rate or severity of pre-eclampsia have been tried. Because one of the pathways leading to pre-eclampsia seems to involve an over-production of thromboxane and an underproduction of prostacyclin (both prostaglandins), it has been hypothesized that using low-dose aspirin to selectively inhibit thromboxane production might reduce the risk of pre-eclampsia (Beaufils et al., 1985; Hauth et al., 1993; Schiff et al., 1989; Wallenburg et al., 1986; Walsh, 1985). Several early studies seemed to support this hypothesis (Beaufils et al., 1985; Hauth et al., 1993; Schiff et al., 1989; Wallenburg et al., 1986). However, in recent years, several large multi-center randomized trials have not confirmed benefit for this intervention and it now appears that low-dose aspirin has minimal, if any, benefit in reducing the risk of pre-eclampsia or the preterm births associated with this condition (Caritis, 1997; CLASP, 1994; ECPPA, 1996; Sibai et al., 1993).

Calcium supplementation has been observed to lower blood pressure, and in several small trials also seemed to be associated with a reduction in pre-eclampsia (Belizan et al., 1991; Bucher et al., 1996). However, in the largest placebo-controlled, randomized multi-center U.S. study that evaluated the effect of two grams of supplemental calcium per day, no reduction in pathologically elevated blood pressure or in the risk of pre-eclampsia was observed (Levine et al., 1996, 1997). Many other strategies, including the use of bed rest, anti-hypertensive medications, diuretics, and salt restriction, which at one time or another have been used in an attempt to reduce the risk of pre-eclampsia or to reduce its severity (thus reducing the risk of associated indicated preterm delivery) have not been shown to improve pregnancy outcome (Crowther et al., 1992; Crowther and Chalmers, 1989; Goldenberg, 1994; 1995; Goldenberg et al., 1990b, 1994; Laurin and Persson, 1987; Levine et al., 1997).

The principal fetal-specific reason for indicated preterm delivery is impaired fetal growth, usually associated with poorly characterized placental dysfunction, resulting in failure to appropriately oxygenate or nutritionally sustain the fetus. Infrequent fetal indications for early delivery include progressive worsening of some congenital malformation, such as hydrocephaly, or worsening disease processes, such as erythroblastosis fetalis. In each of these situations, the physician may make the decision that the risks of prematurity are lower than the risks associated with continuation of the pregnancy (fetal death or delivery of a compromised infant) (Goldenberg, 1995; Goldenberg et al., 1990b). Severe or life-threatening maternal disease affecting such organs as the heart, lung, or liver may also lead to preterm delivery.

A large number of infants with presumed fetal growth restriction are delivered prematurely each year due to the physician's belief that these infants are at an increased risk for intrauterine death or neurologic impairment if left undelivered. Since the risk factors associated with fetal growth restriction are better understood than those associated with spontaneous preterm birth, a number of strategies have evolved to reduce the maternal risk factors associated with fetal growth restriction. These include smoking, alcohol, and drug reduction programs, bed rest, supplemental maternal oxygen administration, mineral corticoid administration, and various types of nutrition intervention programs, including counseling and supplementation (Floyd et al., 1993; Goldenberg et al., 1994; Kramer, 1993; Nicolaides et al., 1987; Laurin and Persson, 1987).

Although these types of interventions may have a marginal impact on the risk for fetal growth restriction, they have been associated with little or no reduction in prematurity. In initial studies, low-dose aspirin appeared to have an independent effect on fetal growth restriction distinct from its effect on pre-eclampsia (Goldenberg et al., 1995a; Uzan et al., 1991). However, in the most recent large randomized trials, there was no impact of this treatment strategy on either the rate of fetal growth restriction or on the risk of indicated preterm birth (Caritis, 1997; CLASP, 1994; ECPPA, 1996; Sibai et al., 1993).

At present, the overall strategy for improving outcome associated with pre-eclampsia, and other clinical situations in which the fetus may be at increased risk of death or disability, is one that attempts to identify fetuses at imminent risk of death through the use of such techniques as non-stress or contraction stress test monitoring, biophysical profile (using electronic fetal monitoring and ultrasound observation of the fetus), Doppler blood flow measurements (usually in the umbilical artery), or fetal movement counting (Goldenberg et al., 1990b; Goldenberg and Bronstein, 1994; Goldenberg, 1995). If the fetus is deemed to be at immediate risk of death or felt to be at risk of damage due to ongoing oxygen or other substrate deprivation, options include early delivery (with or without fetal lung maturity testing to determine the risk of respiratory distress syndrome) or heightened fetal surveillance and corticosteroid administration to lessen fetal morbidity in the event that delivery occurs. There is little evidence to suggest that there has been a reduction in long-term neurologic handicap associated with these strategies. It also is not conclusively established that the increase in neonatal morbidity and mortality associated with iatrogenic preterm birth is less than the combined fetal mortality and neonatal morbidity and mortality that would have resulted had the pregnancies been left undelivered. However, the substantial reduction in third trimester stillbirths over the last two decades suggests that this strategy of fetal assessment and indicated delivery may have had a substantial impact in reducing the stillbirth component of adverse pregnancy outcomes (Goldenberg et al., 1987).

Therefore, although the 20–25% of preterm births that occur as a result of a physician's decision to effect delivery represent an inviting target for reducing the preterm birth rate, at present there are few, if any, interventions that are proven to result in a reduction in the underlying conditions leading to indicated preterm birth, and more importantly, none that is proven to result in a reduction in indicated preterm births themselves.

An evaluation of strategies used to reduce spontaneous preterm birth

In this section, the definition of spontaneous preterm birth includes those that result from both spontaneous labor and spontaneous rupture of membranes. Although often thought of as two distinct entities, there is considerable evidence that the risk factors for both conditions are similar, and that the distinction between the two entities is not as clear as many believe (Guinn et al., 1995). Many women have intermittent contractions and small degrees of cervical change, sometimes diagnosed as spontaneous preterm labor and sometimes not. During this process, the membranes may rupture spontaneously. Whether the rupture of membranes is a component of the spontaneous preterm labor, or precedes or follows it, is often not clear. For this discussion, we have considered the two as a single entity.

There are many ways of characterizing the interventions aimed at reducing spontaneous preterm birth. Perhaps the most straightforward is to examine the strategies associated with prenatal care in asymptomatic women versus those strategies designed to treat suspected or established preterm labor in symptomatic women. The next section therefore examines prenatal care as a general strategy for reducing preterm birth, then examines various candidate strategies for reducing preterm birth that could be included as components of prenatal care.

Prenatal care

Liberal provision of prenatal care is often advocated as an effective means of reducing the rate of spontaneous preterm birth (Alexander and Cornely, 1987; Buescher et al., 1988, 1991; Donaldson and Billy, 1984; Fink et al., 1992; Fiscella, 1995a; Hulsey et al., 1991; Kogan et al., 1994; Korenbrot, 1984; Main et al., 1985; McDuffie et al., 1996; Scholl et al., 1987). Support for this intervention centers on the observation that women who have more prenatal visits or enroll earlier in prenatal care have a lowered risk of preterm birth. This association has been confirmed in virtually every vital statistics data set ever evaluated. However, for two reasons, causality cannot be inferred from this association. First, self-selection plays a large role in this association: women at low risk of preterm birth avail themselves of prenatal care more frequently. The second reason that causality should be doubted is arithmetic: women who deliver early will necessarily have fewer prenatal care visits because prenatal visits are concentrated in late pregnancy.

Other types of studies that have related prenatal care to a reduction in preterm births include: (1) the introduction of standard prenatal care (however that may be defined) into a geographic area where previously there was little or no prenatal care available; and (2) the introduction of some sort of enhanced or more intensive prenatal care in which a comparison is made to routine prenatal care (Buescher et al., 1988). The volume of literature describing both types of studies is very large, and the individual reports are too numerous to cite in this chapter. Nevertheless, an overall evaluation of this literature suggests that the introduction of more prenatal care into an area where there was little or none, thereby making prenatal care available to more women, or making more visits available to the same number of women, has not generally been associated with a reduction in the prematurity rate (Buescher et al., 1988; Fiscella, 1995a).

There are many studies in which a specific new prenatal care program has been established in a geographic area and some, but not all, area residents enrolled. The women who enroll in these programs often have lower rates of preterm birth than women who choose not to enroll. These types of studies all suffer the common bias of self-selection, and few, if any, have analyzed the data geographically to determine if the apparent reduction in prematurity in the enrolled women translated into an overall reduction in preterm births in the geographic area. Most likely, the women choosing not to enroll had a higher risk for preterm birth than the women who did enroll in the program. Therefore, the observed "reductions" are probably associated with participant self-selection rather than with the program itself. The randomized trials that would be needed to document whether introduction of prenatal care into a geographic area actually reduces the prematurity rate have often not been undertaken because of the overall impression that prenatal care is beneficial and withholding it would be unethical. At least part of the reluctance to withhold prenatal care is based on reasonably good evidence that prenatal care is associated with a reduction in maternal mortality, stillbirths, and neonatal death of term infants. However, it is not generally associated with a reduction in preterm birth.

Another type of prenatal care study deals with some type of enhanced prenatal care compared to that ordinarily available (Buescher et al., 1991; Olds et al., 1986). On a clinical level, these types of studies are easier to justify, because no woman is deprived of the standard components of prenatal care, while additional care is provided to women in the treatment group. A number of these studies have been conducted as randomized clinical trials. Although other outcomes may have been improved, in the great majority of these studies there has not been a significant reduction in preterm birth. Careful evaluation of these publications reveals some interesting trends. For example, the published results of several of these randomized trials have not emphasized the differences in the preterm delivery rates in the entire population randomized, probably because in most cases, there was not a significant difference in prematurity in the overall population (McLaughlin et al., 1992; Olds et al., 1986). Instead of emphasizing the intent-to-treat analysis of the entire study population, some authors have chosen to emphasize what appears to be a significant reduction in the prematurity or low birth weight rate in some sub-population of the overall study. This type of post-hoc sub-population analysis, while sometimes useful for suggesting additional studies, should never be regarded as providing conclusive proof that a particular intervention is associated with a real improvement in the rate of preterm delivery.

An example of a study of enhanced prenatal care is the March of Dimes Multicenter Prematurity Prevention Trial (Collaborative Group, 1993; Goldenberg et al., 1990a; Herron et al., 1982). In this study, women deemed to be at high risk for preterm birth were randomized to either standard prenatal care or to an intervention that included weekly evaluation for symptoms of preterm labor or cervical change, and more expeditious access to therapy to halt labor (tocolytic therapy) when symptoms arose. Despite evidence from a non-randomized observational study that this intervention held promise in reducing preterm birth (Herron et al., 1982), enhanced prenatal care did not reduce the rate of preterm birth in this randomized trial (Collaborative Group, 1993; Goldenberg et al., 1990a). However, two other studies in which women were randomly assigned to an enhanced type of prenatal care showed reduced preterm birth in the treatment group (Hobel et al., 1994; Meis et al., 1987). Therefore, despite the general finding that enhanced prenatal care has not been associated with a reduction in preterm birth, these two studies suggest that further evaluation of enhanced prenatal care strategies may be warranted.

Risk scoring

One strategy that has been strongly recommended by a number of authors and has been a component of a number of prematurity prevention strategies, is risk-scoring evaluation using a standardized questionnaire to guide the intensity of prenatal care (Alexander and Keirse, 1989; Herron et al., 1982; Main and Gabbe, 1987; Mueller-Heubach and Guznick, 1989; Owen et al., 1990). In most scenarios, women are rated as either being high- or low-risk for preterm birth, and high-risk women then receive an increased level of prenatal care. In general, each of these scoring systems has been able to define a group of women with approximately a two-fold increased risk of preterm birth, based predominantly on the fact that women who have had a previous preterm birth are at significantly increased risk for a repeat preterm birth (Hobel et al., 1994; Main and Gabbe, 1987; Mueller-Heubach and Guznick, 1989; Owen et al., 1990). However, in general, the use of these scoring systems has not been associated with significant reductions in preterm births. The Oxford Group on Effective Care in Pregnancy and Childbirth has voiced the concern that the use of these scoring systems leads to an increase in other interventions that, as will be seen below, have not been demonstrated to be effective (Alexander and Keirse, 1989). Therefore, it is likely that the use of these scoring systems and the resultant increase in surveillance and interventions will be associated with possible harm and increased costs, but not a reduction in the preterm birth rate.

At-risk behavior reduction

A component of prenatal care often advocated and adopted enthusiastically as part of a strategy to reduce preterm births includes smoking, drug, and alcohol cessation programs. As noted above, each of these behavioral characteristics is more closely linked to fetal growth restriction than to preterm birth (Goldenberg et al., 1996c; Wen et al., 1990a). For example, women who smoke have a significant increase in fetal growth restriction and an average reduction in birth weight in term babies of approximately 200 gm. However, smoking is associated with only a very small increase in the risk of spontaneous preterm birth (Cliver et al., 1992; Goldenberg et al., 1996c; Kramer, 1987; Wen et al., 1990b). Because anti-smoking programs, as well as anti-drug and anti-alcohol interventions, all achieve, at best, relatively low quitting rates, and because smoking and alcohol and drug use are only marginally associated with preterm birth, it is not likely that these types of programs are associated with significant reductions in prematurity.

Psychologic interventions

There is a very large literature dealing with the relationship of various psychological characteristics (e.g., perceived stress, anxiety, depression) and preterm birth (Cliver et al., 1992; Copper et al., 1996; Elbourne et al., 1989; Goldenberg et al., 1996c; Goldenberg and Gotlieb, 1991; Graham et al., 1992; Oakley et al., 1990; Rothberg and Lits, 1991; Rowley et al., 1993; Spencer et al., 1989; Villar et al., 1992). In this literature, the association between these psychological characteristics and spontaneous preterm birth is inconsistent, and when a relationship has been discovered, the relative risk of prematurity for those with the specific characteristic is usually not substantially increased (Goldenberg and Gotlieb, 1991). The few intervention studies in which psychosocial support was provided in some sort of randomized fashion did not demonstrate that the support resulted in a reduction in spontaneous preterm birth, although they suggested other benefits to the mother (Elbourne et al., 1989; Oakley et al., 1990; Spencer et al., 1989; Villar et al., 1992). Thus, there is little evidence to support the belief that a significant reduction in preterm birth can be achieved through the systematic provision of psychosocial support.

Early identification of preterm labor

On the premise that labor-inhibiting drugs are most efficacious if administered before fully-established preterm labor, a number of strategies have been used to identify women in early preterm labor. In these strategies, pregnant women are typically educated to detect mild or asymptomatic contractions or other symptoms that may indicate preterm labor. These include pelvic pressure, vaginal discharge, and back pain (Copper et al., 1990; Herron et al., 1982; Iams et al., 1990; Katz et al., 1986). However, although women in early preterm labor are more likely to perceive more contractions and other symptomology suggestive of preterm labor, whether early detection of these findings can be translated into a meaningful reduction in preterm births is unknown. The strategy tested in the

March of Dimes Prematurity Prevention Program included teaching uterine self-palpation and an awareness of symptoms (Herron et al., 1982), but it did not result in a reduction of preterm birth (Collaborative Group, 1993; Goldenberg et al., 1990a).

The methodology currently in use to detect uterine contractions before the onset of preterm labor is called "home uterine activity monitoring," or HUAM (Blondel et al., 1992; Collaborative Home Uterine Monitoring, 1995; Colton et al., 1995; Grimes and Schulz, 1992; Iams et al., 1987, 1988; Morrison et al., 1987; Mou et al., 1991; Nagey et al., 1993; Sachs et al., 1991; USPSTF, 1993; Wapner et al., 1995). This technology involves placing a contraction monitor on the mother's abdomen. The data thus obtained are transferred electronically to a central site for analysis. This intervention, which has been available commercially for approximately 10 years, was approved by the Food and Drug Administration primarily because (1) the device is effective at detecting contractions (Beckmann et al., 1996; Hess et al., 1990); (2) the monitoring results can be transmitted to a central location; and (3) the occurrence of contractions is associated with an increase in the risk of spontaneous preterm birth (Copper et al., 1994). However, the real test of this technology's utility is whether its use results in a reduction in spontaneous preterm birth. Although initial studies were promising (Morrison et al., 1987), nearly all of the subsequent randomized trials have not shown the technology to be efficacious (Blondel et al., 1992; Collaborative Home Uterine Monitoring, 1995; Colton et al., 1995; Grimes and Schulz, 1992; Iams et al., 1987, 1988; Mou et al., 1991; Nagey et al., 1993; Sachs et al., 1991; USPSTF, 1993; Wapner et al., 1995). Several of the studies that failed to show benefit in the overall intent-to-treat analysis have been sub-analyzed with the suggestion of benefit in either earlier detection of preterm labor or a reduction in preterm delivery only in those women who actually experienced preterm labor. However, sub-analyses of this type are subject to many types of biases, some of which have been discussed above. While it remains possible that this technology might ultimately be shown to be beneficial in some specific subgroup of women, based on currently available data, the use of HUAM does not lower the rate of preterm birth.

Strategies employing HUAM have often included daily nurse contact in the women undergoing monitoring, and there are several studies that suggest that daily nursing contact may be associated with a reduction in preterm birth (Dyson et al., 1991, 1997; Hill et al., 1990; Iams et al., 1987, 1988; Knuppel et al., 1990). However, this specific intervention has rarely been compared to routine care in randomized studies. In a recent study, in which high-risk women were randomized to groups receiving home uterine activity monitoring, daily nursing contact, or weekly nursing contact, there were no differences among the groups in the rate of preterm birth (Dyson et al., 1997). The authors of this study believe that the outcomes of each of the three groups were improved when compared to historical rates of prematurity and were better than that reported previously. In fact, however, there is relatively little evidence that daily or weekly nursing contact in high-risk women reduces preterm birth when compared with routine prenatal care (Dyson et al., 1991, 1997; Hill et al., 1990; Iams et al., 1987, 1988; Knuppel et al., 1990). Therefore, although there are some promising initial results, it remains to be proven whether daily or weekly nursing contact should become part of the prenatal care of women at high risk for preterm birth.

Nutrition interventions

The literature dealing with nutrition interventions to reduce preterm birth also is voluminous. In general, nutrition interventions can be divided into four types: (1) nutritional counseling; (2) caloric supplementation; (3) protein supplementation; and (4) vitamin/mineral supplementation. Although it is fairly well established that pregnant women who are starved or consume very low calorie diets are at increased risk for delivering small or growth-restricted infants, it is not clear if they are at increased risk of prematurity (Carmichael and Abrams, 1997; Goldenberg et al., 1993; Goldenberg and Tamura, 1996; Hickey et al., 1997). On the other hand, it seems clear that both low maternal weight or maternal thinness (measured by such criteria as the body mass index) and poor weight gain during pregnancy are associated with an increased risk of preterm birth (Wen et al., 1990a). Whether these associations imply a cause and effect relationship is unknown, because the mediators of this association have not been elucidated. It should be noted that weight gain during pregnancy is not necessarily associated with maternal diet. Weight gain may be a measure of increasing blood volume, increasing amniotic fluid, and a growing fetus, all of which are only loosely correlated with maternal nutritional status (Carmichael and Abrams, 1997). With this in mind, when one examines the literature dealing with specific nutritional interventions, it is not clear whether, in developed countries, any nutritional intervention leads to lowering of the prematurity rate. It should be noted that in underdeveloped countries, when the caloric intake during pregnancy is very low, such as in Gambia during the wet season, nutritional supplementation during pregnancy has been associated with substantial increases in birth weight (Prentice et al., 1983). It is not known whether this increase in birth weight is associated with a reduction in the rate of prematurity.

In developed countries, the evidence for an association between nutritional counseling or supplementation and a reduction in low birth weight or preterm birth is less clear (Kramer, 1993). There is no clear evidence that simply providing advice to pregnant women about their diet actually changes eating behavior, let alone improves pregnancy outcome. Moreover, studies of high-protein supplementation have consistently been associated with worse pregnancy outcomes, to the degree that high protein supplementation during pregnancy actually appears contraindicated (Garner et al., 1992; Rush, 1989; Susser, 1981). We are therefore left with the question of whether, in the U.S. population, caloric supplementation specifically achieves a reduction in the prematurity rate, and whether some type of vitamin/mineral supplementation improves outcome.

In fact, the United States has been involved in a natural experiment of nutritionally supplementing pregnant women in order to improve their pregnancy outcomes: the Special Supplemental Food Program for Women, Infants, and Children (WIC). In this program, pregnant women are provided food vouchers or the food itself in order to achieve a more nutritionally balanced, calorically enriched diet. The results of studies of this program are mixed, but in general, the overall mean increase in birth weight for the infants of WIC mothers has been in the 25–50 gm range and, in all likelihood, much of this birth weight increase has been achieved through improved fetal growth rather than through a prolongation of pregnancy (Kramer, 1993; Metcoff et al., 1985; see also the discussion in Chapter 6). There is no compelling evidence that WIC supplementation is associated with a reduction in preterm birth.

In an excellent paper published in 1993, Kramer evaluated the literature related to nutritional counseling and supplementation and made the following statement: "On the basis of available evidence from randomized trials, clinicians should not expect that energy and protein supplementation, let alone advice to pregnant women to increase their energy and protein intakes, will have a large beneficial impact on the health of mothers or their infants. Similarly, public health policymakers should not place undue expectations on supplementation programs for undernourished pregnant women in their communities. The modest enhancements in fetal growth that can be expected appear to be without important long-term benefits for child growth and development" (Kramer, 1993).

The relationship of vitamin/mineral supplementation to the prematurity rate is a complicated one, and its thorough evaluation would require an in-depth literature review that is beyond the scope of this chapter. Several key vitamins and minerals are discussed here briefly, however. Chapter 3 also addresses these issues.

There is a large literature related to maternal iron status and pregnancy outcome, and there are many studies that suggest that women with "anemia" as defined by low hematocrits or hemoglobins are at increased risk for preterm birth (Blankson et al., 1993; Hemminki and Rimpela, 1991; Klebanoff et al., 1989; Lieberman et al., 1987; Lu et al., 1991; Macgregor, 1963). These findings relate partly to the point in pregnancy when the hematocrit or hemoglobin is evaluated. It has been frequently observed that women in preterm labor tend to have lower hematocrits than do women in term labor. This is readily explained: because of unequal rates of plasma volume and red cell mass expansion during pregnancy, women in the second and early third trimester have lower hematocrits than those at term, resulting in what has been termed a "physiologic anemia." Failure to correct for gestational age thus leads to a misleading association between low hematocrit and prematurity (Lieberman et al., 1987). More appropriate studies, in which the hematocrits or hemoglobins were prospectively evaluated and the timing of the tests were standardized, show little relationship between low hematocrits and preterm birth (Blankson et al., 1993; Klebanoff et al., 1989; Lu et al., 1991). In fact, studies that have been carefully performed demonstrate that it is high hematocrits (probably associated with a failure to expand plasma volume) that are associated with a significant increase in the preterm birth rate, often in association with fetal growth restriction (Blankson et al., 1993). These comments do not necessarily apply to women who have extremely low hematocrits, which in this country are usually due to a hemoglobinopathy and, in underdeveloped countries, to severe iron deficiency or malaria. It is quite possible that severe anemia, as distinct from the more mild anemias seen in developed countries, may represent a significantly increased risk for preterm birth.

A number of studies of iron supplementation during pregnancy have been performed in the United States and other developed countries (Hemminki and Rimpela, 1991). While nearly all show an improvement in the hematocrit or other measures of iron status associated with supplementation, there is no consistent evidence that the preterm birth rate is reduced with iron supplementation, and it may even be increased (Paintin et al., 1966; Simmer et al., 1987).

Low maternal serum levels of folate have been associated with a reduction in infant birth weight (Goldenberg et al., 1992; Tamura et al., 1992). There is also some evidence that high maternal folate serum levels achieved with supplementation are associated with increased infant birth weight. Nevertheless, there is little evidence that folate supplementation itself is associated with a significant reduction in the rate of preterm birth. However, the fact that fetuses of folate-supplemented women have a reduced risk of neural tube defects (spina bifida and anencephaly), coupled with the knowledge that fetal and maternal requirements for folate are increased during pregnancy, have led to a consensus that regardless of its impact on preterm birth, folate supplementation should be given to all pregnant women (Goldenberg and Tamura, 1996).

Maternal zinc status during pregnancy and its relationship to various adverse outcomes is of particular interest (Tamura and Goldenberg, 1996; Neggers et al., 1990). In retrospective studies, low maternal zinc levels have been associated with an increased risk of intrauterine growth restriction and possibly preterm birth as well (Neggers et al., 1990). Several, but not all, randomized trials have shown an increase in birth weight associated with zinc supplementation and some, including our recently published study (Goldenberg et al., 1995b; Simmer et al., 1991), suggested that zinc supplementation may have a positive impact on preterm birth. Our study was conducted in a low-income minority population in the United States, all of whom had moderately low serum zinc values upon enrollment in prenatal care. In contrast, a recently published study from Scandinavia in middle-class white women showed no impact of zinc supplementation on pregnancy outcome (Simmer et al., 1991). In our study, zinc supplementation was associated with an increase in birth weight, half of which resulted from improved fetal growth and half from an increase in the length of gestation. The biggest impact of zinc on birth weight occurred in the study's thinnest women. Further studies on zinc supplementation during pregnancy are therefore indicated. In the United States, because zinc is now a component of the standard vitamin/mineral tablet routinely prescribed to nearly all pregnant women, such studies are not likely to be performed. However, in areas of the world where zinc supplementation is not routinely provided, it still may be reasonable to further evaluate the impact of zinc supplementation on pregnancy outcome.

Whether the entire vitamin/mineral supplement as currently used in many developed countries lowers the risk of prematurity or improves fetal growth has not undergone rigorous evaluation. A recent study by Scholl and colleagues, of an inner city population in Camden, New Jersey, found that women who used a vitamin/mineral supplement had significantly fewer preterm births than those who did not (Scholl et al., 1997). As with many of the studies described above, since this was not a randomized trial, it may be that factors other than the vitamin/mineral supplementation (such as self-selection) accounted for the very large differences in pregnancy outcome observed in that study.

In summary, it appears that women with good nutritional status and a normal body mass index have better pregnancy outcomes than women with poor nutritional status and a low body mass index. However, despite the large number of studies and various institutionalized practices related to nutrition and pregnancy, it remains unclear if any nutritional interventions in developed countries are associated with a reduction in preterm birth.

Tocolytic drugs

Tocolytic drugs literally "break" or stop uterine contractions. There is a very large tocolytic literature, with too many publications to describe individual reports in detail (Canadian Preterm Labor Investigators Group, 1992; Higby et al., 1993; Keirse et al., 1989; King et al., 1988; Menticoglou et al., 1992; Zlatnik, 1992). Some of the tocolytics, such as the betamimetics, have been well evaluated, while drugs such a magnesium sulfate, calcium channel blockers, and non-steroidal anti-inflammatory drugs (NSAIDs) have had less satisfactory evaluations. The effectiveness of each of these drugs is subject to much debate. Nevertheless, certain conclusions can be drawn. First, it is clear that in the short run, many of these drugs are associated with a reduction in uterine contractions. Significant reductions in preterm delivery for 24 or 48 hours are common in clinical trials, and there seems little doubt that at least a few of these drugs are beneficial, if benefit is defined as a delay of delivery for 48 hours. However, if benefit is defined as achieving reductions in preterm delivery overall, or even delaying delivery for more than a week, the impact of tocolytic therapy is minimal.

Because some of these drugs have the potential to delay the delivery for 48 hours or possibly more, the real question is whether that delay confers any benefit to the fetus in terms of reduction in mortality or serious morbidity, and whether the drugs themselves are potentially hazardous to the mother or fetus. The answer to those questions remains unclear, although in the meta-analyses that have been conducted, the use of various tocolytic drugs has not been associated with an improvement in neonatal mortality or a reduction in the most common neonatal morbidity, respiratory distress syndrome. In addition, there is some evidence based on retrospective analyses that betamimetic use is associated with an increased risk of neonatal intraventricular hemorrhage (Groome et al., 1992; Pranikoff et al., 1990). Conversely, there are retrospective data that suggest that magnesium sulfate use for preterm labor is associated with a reduction in neonatal intraventricular hemorrhage, and even in cerebral palsy among children who survive preterm birth (Goldenberg and Rouse, 1997; Nelson and Grether, 1995; Rouse et al., 1996; Schendel et al., 1995). These findings, however, have not been evaluated in prospective randomized studies, which would be difficult to undertake (Rouse et al., 1996).

The relationship between tocolytic drug use and the use of corticosteroids may be of particular importance. Corticosteroid drugs administered to the mother for as few as 12–24 hours before delivery are associated with a significant reduction in neonatal respiratory distress syndrome and intraventricular hemorrhage, as well as a reduction in neonatal mortality (Crowley, 1995; Gardner and Goldenberg, 1995b). Therefore, the combined use of tocolytic drugs and corticosteroids has been advocated as a way of reducing various adverse pregnancy outcomes (Canadian Preterm Labor Investigators Group, 1992). This strategy seems reasonable, and in retrospective analyses seemed to improve various pregnancy outcomes (Atkinson et al., 1995; Piper et al., 1996). The potential benefits of administering prenatal corticosteroids in cases of infants at risk of premature delivery from intrauterine growth restriction is also described in Chapter 7.

The combination of tocolytics and corticosteroid drug use versus placebo treatment has not been tested in a prospective randomized study. However, since the apparent benefit of tocolytic drugs is a delay in delivery for 48 hours, and since that period of time allows for the maximum benefit from corticosteroids, it seems appropriate to suggest that the major indication for the use of tocolytic drugs is to allow appropriate time for the action of corticosteroids. Tocolytic therapy has also been advocated as a means of delaying delivery in order to facilitate transfer of women in preterm labor to a perinatal center. While this strategy seems appropriate, it has not been extensively evaluated.

Bed rest and maternal hydration

The evaluation of some less intensive interventions for the reduction in preterm birth, including bed rest and maternal hydration, is also of particular interest (Freda and DeVore, 1996; Goldenberg et al., 1994; Maloni et al., 1993; Maloni and Kasper, 1991). This relatively small literature can be summarized by saying that there are no convincing data showing a reduction in preterm labor with either treatment, and several studies that suggest there is no benefit. In addition, there are some theoretical and, occasionally, actual negative outcomes associated with each of these interventions (Crowther et al., 1992; Maloni et al., 1993; Maloni and Kasper, 1991). Therefore, while both interventions are commonly used in women at risk for and diagnosed with preterm labor, the evidence supporting their use is minimal at best.

Incompetent cervix and cerclage

An incompetent cervix is diagnosed in 1 in 200 to 1 in 1000 pregnancies, based on a history of spontaneous second trimester abortions or early spontaneous preterm births associated with painless (i.e., without perceived contractions) dilatation of the cervix. The etiology of this condition may be traumatic or structural. The traditional treatment has been the placement of one or several circumferential stitches – termed a cerclage – in the cervix (Grant, 1989). Whether women with a classic history (midtrimester delivery without discernible labor) benefit from cerclage has not been tested prospectively in randomized studies. However, compared to historical controls, it seems likely that benefits accrue to women with classic histories who undergo this procedure. In fact, however, most women do not have a "classic" history, but instead present with a history of preterm delivery in which it is difficult to determine the difference between painless dilatation not related to labor and true, but unrecognized, preterm labor. In a randomized study involving women with non-classic histories, cerclage placement conferred a statistically significant reduction in the rate of preterm birth (defined as birth before 33 weeks), but 25 cerclages were required to prevent one preterm birth (MacNaughton et al., 1993). It therefore seems reasonable to recommend a cerclage for the classic cases of incompetent cervix, but to leave use of cerclage in the non-classic cases to individual judgement.

Progestins

In a number of animal species, there is substantial evidence to indicate that maternal progesterone concentrations decline before labor. There is also some evidence that in human pregnancy declining levels of progesterone are associated with preterm birth. Therefore, several randomized studies have evaluated the effect of administering various types of progesterone supplementation, including weekly injections of 17–alpha-hydroxyprogesterone caproate, a potent progesterone analog, to women at risk of preterm birth (Hartikainen-Sorri et al., 1980; Hauth et al., 1983; Johnson et al., 1975; Keirse, 1990; Yemeni et al., 1985). A meta-analysis by the Oxford Group suggested that progestin supplementation was associated with an approximately 50% reduction in the rate of prematurity (Keirse, 1990). In fact, this intervention is one of the few in which there are sufficient randomized efficacy data to support its use. Nevertheless, because the most widely studied regimen requires a weekly injection, and since identification of appropriate candidates is difficult, progestins are now rarely used to reduce the risk of preterm birth. For these reasons, and because the previous studies were relatively small and had dissimilar study designs, the National Institutes of Health NICHD Maternal–Fetal Medicine Units Network has initiated a randomized prospective trial of this intervention. However, it will be several years before the results of this study are known.

Screening for infection and antibiotic treatment

In recent years, substantial progress has been made in understanding the relationship between maternal infection and spontaneous preterm birth (Andrews et al., 1995; Gibbs et al., 1992). We and a number of other groups have demonstrated that a large proportion (perhaps as many as 80%) of very early preterm births (gestational age < 28 weeks or birth weight < 1000 gm) are associated with an intrauterine infection (Cassell et al., 1993a,b). These infections, involving relatively low virulence organisms such as ureaplasma, mycoplasma, or gardnerella, result from the ascension of organisms from the vagina into the space between the fetal chorion and the maternal endometrium.

The association of intra-amniotic infection and preterm birth has been appreciated since at least the early 1980s. As a result, many antibiotic trials of women in spontaneous preterm labor have been performed in an attempt to reduce intra-amniotic infection-associated prematurity. Although there are a few studies in which a significant reduction in preterm birth seems to have occurred, most have not been associated with a reduction in preterm birth (Gibbs et al., 1992). It is not known whether the failure to reduce the prematurity rate using antibiotics in these symptomatic women is due to the choice of inappropriate antibiotics, the initiation of treatment too late in the cascade leading to spontaneous preterm delivery, or other factors. To date, however, the available literature provides little support for treating women in preterm labor with antibiotics to reduce the risk of preterm delivery.

If treatment with antibiotics in established preterm labor is ineffective, it remains possible that antibiotic therapy might be effective in preventing or forestalling preterm labor in asymptomatic women. Data from the 1960s suggest that women treated with tetracycline for symptomatic urinary tract infections had fewer spontaneous preterm deliveries than those randomized to a control group (Norden and Kass, 1968). However, because tetracycline was observed to adversely affect developing fetal teeth and bones, its use during pregnancy fell into disfavor.

Both symptomatic and asymptomatic urinary tract infections are associated with an increased risk of spontaneous preterm delivery, and there are a number of randomized trials that confirm that treating asymptomatic bacteriuria during pregnancy reduces the risk of maternal pyelonephritis. Several other randomized trials suggest a reduction in the preterm birth rate as well (Andriole and Patterson, 1991; Rouse et al., 1995a). Therefore, in an industrialized country with sufficient resources, it seems reasonable to screen all pregnant women for asymptomatic bacteriuria and treat them appropriately.

Defining which other types of infection may have a causal role in spontaneous preterm birth is the focus of much current research (Goldenberg and Andrews, 1996; Goldenberg et al., 1997). As an example, nearly every sexually transmitted disease has been associated, in one paper or another, with an increase in spontaneous preterm birth. However, women with various sexually transmitted diseases have many other known (and probably unknown) risk factors for preterm birth. These factors have rarely been evaluated as confounding factors in the studies assessing the relationship between sexually transmitted diseases and preterm birth.

Confounding factors aside, maternal infection with syphilis, gonorrhea, and chlamydia has been associated with between a two- and four-fold increase in the risk of spontaneous preterm birth. Screening and treatment for syphilis and gonorrhea is indicated for reasons other than prematurity prevention, and whether the relationship between these two infections and spontaneous preterm birth is causal or simply an association is almost immaterial (Donders et al., 1993). Chlamydia is a known cause of pelvic infection, neonatal ophthalmia, and infant pneumonia, but its role in causing preterm birth is controversial (Harrison et al., 1983; Sweet et al., 1987). In general, the more confounders are adjusted for, the more attenuated the association between chlamydia and preterm birth becomes. As with syphilis and gonorrhea, screening and treatment of chlamydia during pregnancy is recommended for other reasons, but whether this intervention will have an impact on the prematurity rate is unknown.

Maternal vaginal colonization with group B streptococcus (GBS) has been variably associated with spontaneous preterm birth (Regan et al., 1991; White et al., 1984). However, a more consistent relationship has been defined between maternal GBS urinary tract infection and preterm birth. In fact, one treatment trial suggests than a reduction in preterm birth can be achieved by treating GBS urinary tract infection (Regan et al., 1991). It therefore seems reasonable that when pregnant women are diagnosed with a GBS urinary tract infection (or any urinary tract infection for that matter), even if asymptomatic, they should be treated with the intent of preventing preterm birth. Also, during labor, these women should be treated with a penicillin-like drug in order to reduce the rate of vertical transmission of the organism. It does not appear to be reasonable, based on existing data, to screen and treat women early in pregnancy for group B streptococcal genital colonization in order to prevent spontaneous preterm birth.

This leaves us with the question of how, if at all, to prevent spontaneous preterm birth associated with an intrauterine infection. It is known that bacterial vaginosis (BV), either by itself or in association with an intrauterine infection, is associated with between a one-and-a-half- and three-fold increased risk of spontaneous preterm birth (Hay et al., 1994; Hillier et al., 1995a,b; Meis et al., 1995). This association has been confirmed in at least 15 separate studies conducted in a number of different populations and locations. Again, it is not known whether this association is causal and it is not clear whether BV is a marker for an upper tract infection, or whether it is a cause of preterm labor in its own right. Two randomized trials of antibiotic use in women with BV have been associated with reductions in the spontaneous preterm birth rate (Hauth et al., 1995; Morales et al., 1994). Our study, by Hauth and colleagues (1995), enrolled women with BV who were at high risk for spontaneous preterm birth either because of a previous spontaneous preterm birth, or because they were of low maternal weight. We compared a course of metronidazole and erythromycin to placebo. In a similar but smaller study, Morales and colleagues (1994) enrolled women who had BV and a previous preterm birth and treated them with metronidazole alone. Both studies achieved between a 33% and 50% reduction in spontaneous preterm birth. It is not known whether the improvement in outcome in these studies was due to reduction in the number of the vaginal organisms, eradication of organisms in the uterus for which the vaginal organisms were a marker, or some other mechanism.

These two studies suggest that when certain high-risk women with bacterial vaginosis are treated systemically with metronidazole (perhaps in combination with erythromycin) for a week or more, there is a reduction in prematurity. How generalizable these findings are in terms of other antibiotics, to shorter courses of antibiotics, or to lower-risk women remains to be established. Ongoing studies are attempting to answer these and other questions related to the prevention of prematurity in association with various markers for maternal infection. Because so much of the morbidity and mortality in association with prematurity occurs in the early gestational age newborns, and because so much of the early gestational age prematurity seems associated with infection, these types of interventions show great promise in ultimately achieving an improvement in some important outcomes associated with early spontaneous preterm birth. African American women have significantly higher rates of vaginal infections, particularly BV, than do other women (Goldenberg et al., 1996d; Hay et al., 1994). Several studies suggest that approximately 40% of the prematurity in this group, and especially early prematurity, may be associated with BV (Fiscella, 1995b; Goldenberg et al., 1997). The development of effective treatment strategies for BV, therefore, has great potential to lower the high rate of prematurity, especially in African American women.

Strategies related to preterm premature rupture of the membranes (PROM)

Women whose membranes rupture spontaneously are at extremely high risk for subsequent preterm delivery. Although women whose membranes rupture earlier in the preterm period have somewhat longer latency periods (time from PROM to delivery), in the absence of intervention, the vast majority of women whose membranes rupture spontaneously deliver within a week, and only a small minority remain undelivered for more than two weeks. In women with PROM, subsequent infant mortality and morbidity is closely related to the gestational ages at PROM and at delivery. Because these infants almost never remain undelivered until term, strategies used to improve pregnancy outcome in women with PROM rarely have a reduction in the rate of preterm delivery as an endpoint. Instead, endpoints such as an increase in latency or a reduction in specific maternal or combined fetal and neonatal mortality or neonatal morbidity are used. Because the vast majority of infants born at more than 34 weeks gestation do well regardless of treatment strategy, many fewer studies have been done in these women than in those whose membranes have ruptured at less than 34 weeks gestational age.

Until two decades ago, the increased risk of maternal and fetal infection associated with PROM was greatly feared. The management of women with ruptured membranes, therefore, nearly always consisted of delivery, regardless of gestational age. Beginning approximately 20 years ago, with the advent of newborn intensive care and the availability of more potent antibiotics, the management trend, once membranes ruptured at less than 32 or 34 weeks, evolved to a strategy of watchful waiting. Delivery occurred with nearly any sign of infection. This strategy appeared to confer benefit on the infants of mothers who had a spontaneous long latency period, perhaps because infection was less common in these women.

In recent years, several interventions have been tested that have attempted to prolong the latency period. Perhaps the one most studied is the use of antibiotics (Amon et al., 1988; Christmas et al., 1992; Johnston et al., 1990; Lockwood et al., 1993; Mercer et al., 1992, 1997; Morales et al., 1989; Owen et al., 1993). In a number of studies, women with ruptured membranes were randomized to anti-biotics or placebo. The results of these studies are relatively consistent: the use of antibiotics in women with PROM prolongs the latency period. The largest study to date, a recently completed study of PROM at less than 32 weeks by the Maternal–Fetal Medicine Network, confirmed a prolongation of latency and also demon-strated a reduction in maternal chorioamnionitis as well as an improvement in a number of newborn outcomes, including a reduction in respiratory distress syndrome and apparent sepsis (Mercer et al., 1997). However, mortality was not different between the treatment and placebo groups, with survival in both groups approximately 95%.

No study to date has evaluated long-term outcome associated with an antibiotic strategy in the face of PROM, but these data would be important. Theoretically, the greater the gestational age, the lower the rates of maternal and infant infection. The reduced short-term morbidity that has been associated with antibiotic use should result in less long-term infant neurologic morbidity. However, some recent studies, which suggest a worsening of infant neurologic outcomes in association with high levels of intrauterine cytokines, raise the concern that prolonging the pregnancy with antibiotics in some cases of PROM might not be in the ultimate best interest of the neonate. Studies that evaluate long-term neurologic outcomes associated with this strategy are therefore important.

There is also a considerable controversy over whether the use of a strategy involving tocolytic treatment and corticosteroids improves outcome in women with ruptured membranes, or whether corticosteroids themselves will achieve that outcome. In regard to corticosteroids, meta-analyses of the existing studies have produced conflicting results (Crowley, 1995; Ohlsson, 1989). The Consensus Conference on Corticosteroids recommended the use of corticosteroids in the face of PROM at less than 30–32 weeks in order to reduce the risk of intraventricular hemorrhage (NIH, 1994). However, because there have been few randomized trials restricted to women with PROM, the American College of Obstetrics and Gynecology has not made a similar recommendation. A recent small randomized study showed reduced respiratory distress syndrome when corticosteroids were used in conjunction with antibiotics in women with PROM at less than 32 weeks (Lewis et al., 1996). However, until the long-term outcome associated with the use of antibiotics in women with PROM is known, the most appropriate treatment strategy to use with PROM is not clear. The developing consensus is that if a woman with PROM is to be observed in order to achieve the maximum latency period, antibiotic administration is reasonable and likely beneficial. In conjunction with antibiotics, the use of corticosteroids to reduce intraventricular hemorrhage and respiratory distress syndrome in pregnancies that are less than 32 weeks and complicated by PROM also is appropriate. Any benefit of tocolytic use in these women remains to be established.

Conclusion

Given what we know about the effectiveness of the various interventions aimed at reducing preterm birth, it is not surprising that we have had little success in reducing the rate of prematurity in the United States over the past 20 years. Fundamental to achieving greater success is a better understanding of the mechanisms leading to preterm birth, which will allow a more rational approach to intervention. Until then, significant and important reductions in preterm delivery are unlikely to be achieved. In parallel with effects to reduce the risk of prematurity, ongoing efforts should focus on the continued development and refinement of interventions that reduce prematurity-attendant morbidity and mortality.

REFERENCES

Alexander GR, Cornely DA. Prenatal care utilization: its measurement and relationship to pregnancy outcome. American Journal of Preventive Medicine 1987; **3**: 243–53.

Alexander S, Keirse MJNC. Formal risk scoring during pregnancy. In: Chalmers I, Enkin M, Keirse MJNC, eds. Effective care in pregnancy and childbirth. Vol. 1. Pregnancy. New York: Oxford University Press, 1989: 345–65.

Amon E, Lewis SV, Sibai BM, Villar MA, Arheart KL. Ampicillin prophylaxis in preterm premature rupture of the membranes: a prospective randomized study. American Journal of Obstetrics and Gynecology 1988; **159**: 539–43.

Andrews WW, Goldenberg RL, Hauth JC. Preterm labor: emerging role of genital tract infections. Infectious Agents and Disease 1995; **4**: 196–211.

Andriole VT, Patterson TF. Epidemiology, natural history, and management of urinary tract infections in pregnancy. Medical Clinics of North America 1991; **75**: 359–73.

Atkinson MW, Goldenberg RL, Gaudier FL, et al. Maternal corticosteroid and tocolytic treatment and morbidity and mortality in very low birthweight infants. American Journal of Obstetrics and Gynecology 1995; **173**: 299–305.

Beaufils M, Uzan S, Donsimoni R, Colau JC. Prevention of pre-eclampsia by early antiplatelet therapy. Lancet 1985; **I**: 840–2.

Beckmann CA, Beckmann CRB, Stanziano GJ, Bergauer NK, Marth CB. Accuracy of maternal perception of preterm uterine activity. American Journal of Obstetrics and Gynecology 1996; **174**: 672–5.

Belizan JM, Villar J, Gonzalez L, Campodonico L, Bergel E. Calcium supplementation to prevent hypertensive disorders of pregnancy. New England Journal of Medicine 1991; **325**: 1399–405.

Blankson ML, Goldenberg RL, Cutter GR, Cliver SP. The relationship between maternal hematocrit and pregnancy outcome: black–white differences. Journal of the National Medical Association 1993; **85**: 130–4.

Blondel B, Breart G, Berthoux Y, et al. Home uterine activity monitoring in France: a randomized, controlled trial. American Journal of Obstetrics and Gynecology 1992; **167**: 424–9.

Bottoms SF, Paul RH, Iams JD, et al. Obstetric determinants of neonatal survival: influence of willingness to perform cesarean delivery on survival of extremely low-birth-weight infants. American Journal of Obstetrics and Gynecology 1997; **176**: 960–6.

Bucher HC, Guyatt GH, Cook RJ, et al. Effect of calcium supplementation on pregnancy-induced hypertension and preeclampsia. Journal of the American Medical Association 1996; **275**: 1113–17.

Buescher PA, Meis PJ, Ernest JM, Moore ML, Michielutte R, Sharp P. A comparison of women in and out of a prematurity prevention project in a North Carolina perinatal care region. American Journal of Public Health 1988; **78**: 264–7.

Buescher PA, Roth MS, Williams D, Goforth CM. An evaluation of the impact of maternity care coordination on Medicaid birth outcomes in North Carolina. American Journal of Public Health 1991; **81**: 1625–30.

Canadian Preterm Labor Investigators Group. Treatment of preterm labor with the beta-adrenergic agonist ritodrine. New England Journal of Medicine 1992; **327**: 308–12.

Caritis SN. Low dose aspirin does not prevent preeclampsia in high risk women. American Journal of Obstetrics and Gynecology 1997; **176**: S3. SPO abstract.

Carmichael SL, Abrams B. A critical review of the relationship between gestational weight gain and preterm delivery. Obstetrics and Gynecology 1997; **89**: 865–73.

Cassell G, Andrews W, Hauth J, et al. Isolation of microorganisms from the chorioamnion is twice that from amniotic fluid at cesarean delivery in women with intact membranes. American Journal of Obstetrics and Gynecology 1993a; **168**: 424.

Cassell G, Hauth J, Andrews W, Cutter G, Goldenberg R. Chorioamnion colonization: correlation with gestational age in women delivered following spontaneous labor versus indicated delivery. American Journal of Obstetrics and Gynecology 1993b; **168**: 425. Abstract.

Christmas JT, Cox SM, Andrews W, Dax J, Leveno KJ, Gilstrap LC. Expectant management of preterm ruptured membranes: effects of antimicrobial therapy. Obstetrics and Gynecology 1992; **80**: 950–62.

CLASP. A randomised trial of low-dose aspirin for the prevention and treatment of pre-eclampsia among 9364 pregnant women. Lancet 1994; **3443**: 619–29.

Cliver SP, Goldenberg RL, Cutter GR, et al. The relationships among a psychosocial profile, maternal size, and smoking in predicting fetal growth retardation. Obstetrics and Gynecology 1992; **80**: 262–7.

Collaborative Group on Preterm Birth Prevention. Multicenter randomized controlled trial of a preterm birth prevention program. American Journal of Obstetrics and Gynecology 1993; **169**: 352–66.

Collaborative Home Uterine Monitoring Study Group. A multicenter randomized controlled trial of home uterine monitoring: active versus sham device. American Journal of Obstetrics and Gynecology 1995; **173**: 1120–7.

Colton T, Kayne HL, Zhang Y, Heeren T. A metaanalysis of home uterine activity monitoring. American Journal of Obstetrics and Gynecology 1995; **173**: 1499–505.

Copper RL, Goldenberg RL, Creasy RK, et al. A multicenter study of preterm birth weight and gestational age specific neonatal mortality. American Journal of Obstetrics and Gynecology 1993; **168**: 78–84.

Copper RL, Goldenberg RL, Das A, et al. The preterm prediction study: maternal stress is associated with spontaneous preterm birth at less than thirty-five weeks' gestation. American Journal of Obstetrics and Gynecology 1996; **175**: 1286–92.

Copper RL, Goldenberg RL, Davis RO, et al. Warning symptoms, uterine contractions, and cervical examination findings in women at risk of preterm delivery. American Journal of Obstetrics and Gynecology 1990; **162**: 748–54.

Copper RL, Goldenberg RL, DuBard MB, Hauth JC, Cutter GR. Cervical examination and tocodynamometry at 28 weeks gestation: prediction of spontaneous preterm birth. American Journal of Obstetrics and Gynecology 1994; **83**: 609–12.

Creasy RK. Preterm birth prevention: where are we? American Journal of Obstetrics and Gynecology 1993; **168**: 1223–30.

Creasy RK, Gummer BA, Liggins GC. System for predicting spontaneous preterm birth. Obstetrics and Gynecology 1980; **55**: 692–95.

Crowley PA. Antenatal corticosteroid therapy: a meta-analysis of the randomized trials, 1972 to 1995. American Journal of Obstetrics and Gynecology 1995; **173**: 322–34.

Crowther CA, Boumeester AM, Ashurst HM. Does admission to hospital for bed rest prevent disease progression or improve fetal outcome in pregnancy complicated by non-proteinuric hypertension? British Journal of Obstetrics and Gynæcology 1992; **99**: 13–17.

Crowther C, Chalmers I. Bed rest and hospitalization during pregnancy. In: Chalmers I, Enkin M, Keirse MJN, editors. Effective care in pregnancy and childbirth. Vol. 1. Pregnancy. New York: Oxford University Press, 1989: 624–32.

Donaldson PJ, Billy JOG. The impact of prenatal care on birth weight. Evidence from an international data set. Medical Care 1984; **22**: 177–88.

Donders GG, Desmyter J, De Wet DH, Van Assche FA. The association of gonorrhea and syphilis with premature birth and low birthweight. Genitourinary Medicine 1993; **69**: 98–101.

Dyson DC, Crites YM, Ray DA, Armstrong MA. Prevention of preterm birth in high-risk patients: the role of education and provider contact versus home uterine monitoring. American Journal of Obstetrics and Gynecology 1991; **164**: 756–62.

Dyson D, Danbe K, Banber J, et al. A multicenter randomized trial of three levels of surveillance in patients at risk for preterm labor. American Journal of Obstetrics and Gynecology 1997; **176**: S30. Abstract.

ECPPA Collaborative Group. ECPPA: randomised trial of low dose aspirin for the prevention of maternal and fetal complications in high risk pregnant women. British Journal of Obstetrics and Gynæcology 1996; **103**: 39–47.

Elbourne D, Oakley A, Chalmers I. Social and psychological support during pregnancy. In: Chalmers I, Enkin M, Keirse MJNC, eds. Effective care in pregnancy and childbirth. Vol. 1.

Pregnancy. New York: Oxford University Press, 1989: 221–36.

Fink A, Yano EM, Goya D. Prenatal programs: what the literature reveals. Obstetrics and Gynecology 1992; **80**: 867–71.

Fiscella K. Race, perinatal outcome, and amniotic infection. Obstetrics and Gynecological Survey 1995a; **51**: 60–6.

Fiscella K. Does prenatal care improve birth outcomes? A critical review. Obstetrics and Gynecology 1995b; **85**: 468–79.

Floyd RL, Rimer BK, Giovino GA, Mullen PD, Sullivan SE. A review of smoking and pregnancy: interventions, implications, and issues. Annual Review of Public Health 1993; **14**: 379–411.

Freda MC, DeVore N. Should intravenous hydration be the first line of defense with threatened preterm labor? A critical review of the literature. Journal of Perinatology 1996; **16**: 385–9.

Gardner MO, Goldenberg RL. The influence of race and previous pregnancy outcome on outcomes in the current pregnancy. Seminars in Perinatology 1995a; **19**: 191–6.

Gardner MO, Goldenberg RL. The clinical use of antenatal corticosteroids. Clinical Obstetrics and Gynecology 1995b; **38**: 746–54.

Garner PA, Kramer MS, Chalmers I. Might efforts to increase birthweight in undernourished women do more harm than good? Lancet 1992; **79**: 908–12.

Gibbs RS, Romero MD, Hillier SL, Eschenbach DA, Sweet RL. A review of premature birth and subclinical infection. American Journal of Obstetrics and Gynecology 1992; **166**: 1515–28.

Goepfert AR, Goldenberg RL. Prediction of prematurity. Current Opinion in Obstetrics and Gynecology 1996: **8**; 417–27.

Goldenberg RL. The prevention of low birthweight and its sequelae. Preventive Medicine 1994; **23**: 627–31.

Goldenberg RL. Small for gestational age infants. In: Sachs BP, Beard R, Papiernik E, Russell C, eds. Reproductive health care for women and babies. Section V. Impact of adverse infant outcomes. New York: Oxford University Press, 1995: 391–9.

Goldenberg RL, Andrews WW. Editorial. Intrauterine infection and why preterm prevention programs have failed. American Journal of Public Health 1996; **86**: 781–3.

Goldenberg RL, Andrews WW, Yuan A, MacKay T, St. Louis M. Sexually transmitted diseases and adverse outcomes of pregnancy. Clinics in Perinatology 1997; **24**: 23–41.

Goldenberg RL, Bronstein J. Preventing low birth weight. In: Wallace HH, Sweeney PJ, eds. Maternal and child health practices. 4th edn. Oakland (CA): Third Party Publishing Co, 1994: 260–78.

Goldenberg RL, Cliver SP, Bronstein J, Cutter GR, Andrews WW. Bed rest in pregnancy. Obstetrics and Gynecology 1994; **84**: 131–6.

Goldenberg RL, Cliver SP, Mulvihill FX, et al. Medical, psychosocial and behavioral risk factors do not explain the increased risk for low-birth weight in black women. American Journal of Obstetrics and Gynecology 1996a; **175**: 1317–24.

Goldenberg RL, Davis RO, Baker RC, Corliss DK, Andrews J, Carpenter AH. The Alabama preterm birth prevention project. Obstetrics and Gynecology 1990a; 75–93.

Goldenberg RL, Davis RO, Cliver SP, et al. Maternal risk factors and their influence on fetal anthropometric measurements. American Journal of Obstetrics and Gynecology 1993; **168**: 1197–203.

Goldenberg RL, Davis RO, Nelson KG. Intrauterine growth retardation. In: Merkatz IR, Thompson JE, eds. New perspectives on prenatal care. New York: Elsevier Science, 1990b: 461–78.

Goldenberg RL, DuBard MB, Cliver SP, et al. Pregnancy outcome and intelligence at age five years. American Journal of Obstetrics and Gynecology 1996b; **175**: 1511–15.

Goldenberg RL, Gotlieb SJ. Social and psychological factors and pregnancy outcome. In: Merkatz IR, Cherry SH, eds. Rovinsky and Guttmacher's medical complications of pregnancy: medical, surgical, gynecologic, psychosocial, and perinatal. 4th edn. Baltimore (MD): Williams & Wilkins, 1991: 80–96.

Goldenberg RL, Hauth JC, DuBard MB, Copper RL, Cutter GR. Fetal growth in women using low dose aspirin for the prevention of preeclampsia. Journal of Maternal Fetal Medicine 1995a; **4**: 218–24.

Goldenberg RL, Hoffman HJ, Cliver SP. Neurodevelopmental outcome of small-for-gestational-age infants. Paper presented at: IDECG/IUNS Workshop on Causes and Consequences of Intrauterine Growth Retardation, Baton Rouge, Louisiana, November 11–15, 1996c.

Goldenberg RL, Iams JD, Mercer BM, et al. The preterm prediction study: the value of new vs. standard risk factors in predicting early and all spontaneous preterm births. American Journal of Public Health 1998; **88**: 233–8.

Goldenberg RL, Klebanoff MA, Nugent R, et al. Bacterial colonization of the vagina during pregnancy in four ethnic groups. American Journal of Obstetrics and Gynecology 1996d; **174**: 1618–21.

Goldenberg RL, Koski JF, Boyd BW, Cutter GR, Nelson KG. Fetal deaths in Alabama 1974 to 1983 – A birthweight-specific analysis. Obstetrics and Gynecology 1987; **70**: 831.

Goldenberg RL, Rouse DJ. Preterm birth, cerebral palsy and magnesium: where are we? Nature Medicine 1997; **3**: 146–7.

Goldenberg RL, Tamura T. Editorial. Prepregnancy weight and pregnancy outcome. Journal of the American Medical Association 1996; **275**: 1127–8.

Goldenberg RL, Tamura T, Cliver SP, et al. Serum folate and fetal growth retardation: a matter of compliance. Obstetrics and Gynecology 1992; **79**: 719–22.

Goldenberg RL, Tamura T, Neggers Y, et al. The effect of zinc supplementation on pregnancy outcome. Journal of the American Medical Association 1995b; **274**: 463–8.

Graham AV, Frank SH, Zyzanski SJ, Kitson GC, Reeb KG. A clinical trial to reduce the rate of low birth weight in an inner-city black population. Clinical Research Methods 1992; **24**(6): 439–46.

Grant A. Cervical cerclage to prolong pregnancy. In: Chalmers I, Enkin M, and Keirse MJNC, eds. Effective care in pregnancy and childbirth. Vol. 1. Pregnancy. New York: Oxford University Press, 1989: 633–46.

Grimes DA, Schulz KF. Randomized controlled trials of home uterine activity monitoring: a review and critique. Obstetrics and Gynecology 1992; **79**: 137–42.

Groome LJ, Goldenberg RL, Cliver SP, Davis RO, Copper RL, and the March of Dimes Multicenter Study Group. Neonatal periventricular-intraventricular hemorrhage after maternal beta-sympathomimetic tocolysis. American Journal of Obstetrics and Gynecology 1992; **167**: 873–9.

Guinn DA, Goldenberg RL, Hauth JC, Andrews WW, Thom E, Romero R. Risk factors for the development of preterm premature rupture of the membranes after arrest of preterm labor. American Journal of Obstetrics and Gynecology 1995; **173**: 1310–15.

Hack M, Horbar JD, Malloy MH, Tyson JE, Wright E, Wright L. Very low birth weight outcomes of the National Institute of Child Health and Human Development Neonatal Network. Pediatrics 1991; **87**: 587–97.

Harrison HR, Alexander ER, Weinstein L, Lewis M, Nash M, Sim DA. Cervical *Chlamydia trachomatis* and mycoplasmal infections in pregnancy: epidemiology and outcomes. Journal of the American Medical Association 1983; **250**: 1721–7.

Hartikainen-Sorri A-L, Kauppila A, Tuimala R. Inefficacy of 17 alpha-hydroxyprogesterone caproate in the prevention of prematurity in twin pregnancy. Obstetrics and Gynecology 1980; **56**: 692.

Hauth JC, Gilstrap LC, Brekken AL, Hauth JM. The effect of 17 alpha-hydroxyprogesterone caproate on pregnancy outcome in an active-duty military population. American Journal of Obstetrics and Gynecology 1983; **146**: 187–90.

Hauth JC, Goldenberg RL, Andrews WW, DuBard MB, Copper RL. Mid-trimester treatment with metronidazole plus erythromycin reduces preterm birth only in women with bacterial vaginosis. New England Journal of Medicine 1995; **333**: 1732–6.

Hauth JC, Goldenberg RL, Parker CR Jr, et al. Low-dose aspirin therapy to prevent pre-eclampsia. American Journal of Obstetrics and Gynecology 1993; **168**: 1083–93.

Hay PE, Lamont RF, Taylor-Robinson D, Morgan DJ, Ison C, Pearson J. Abnormal bacterial colonisation of the genital tract and subsequent preterm delivery and late miscarriage. British Journal of Medicine 1994; **308**: 295–8.

Hemminki E, Rimpela U. A randomized comparison of routine versus selective iron supplementation during pregnancy. Journal of the American College of Nutrition 1991; **10**: 3–10.

Herron MA, Katz M, Creasy RK. Evaluation of a preterm birth prevention program: preliminary report. Obstetrics and Gynecology 1982; **59**: 452–6.

Hess LW, McCaul JF, Perry KG, Howard PR, Morrison JC. Correlation of uterine activity using the Term Guard monitor versus standard external tocodynamometry compared with the intrauterine pressure catheter. Obstetrics and Gynecology 1990; **76**: 52S–55S.

Hickey CA, Cliver SP, McNeal SF, Goldenberg RL. Low pregravid body mass index as a risk factor for preterm birth: variation by ethnic group. Obstetrics and Gynecology 1997; **89**: 206–12.

Higby K, Xenakis EMJ, Pauerstein CJ. Do tocolytic agents stop preterm labor? A critical and comprehensive review of efficacy and safety. American Journal of Obstetrics and Gynecology 1993; **168**: 1247–59.

Hill WC, Fleming AD, Martin RW, et al. Home uterine activity monitoring is associated with a reduction in preterm birth. Obstetrics and Gynecology 1990; **76**: 13S–18S.

Hillier SL, Krohn MA, Cassen E, Easterling TR, Rabe LK, Eschenbach DA. The role of bacterial vaginosis and vaginal bacteria in amniotic fluid infection in women in preterm labor with intact fetal membranes. Clinical Infectious Diseases 1995a; **20**: S276–8.

Hillier SL, Nugent RP, Eschenbach DA, Krohn MA, Gibbs RS, Martin DH. Association between bacterial vaginosis and preterm delivery of a low-birth-weight infant. New England Journal of

Medicine 1995b; **333**: 1737–42.

Hobel DJ, Ross MG, Benis RL, et al. The West Los Angeles Preterm Birth Project. I. Program impact on high-risk women. American Journal of Obstetrics and Gynecology 1994; **170**: 54–62.

Hulsey TC, Patrick CH, Alexander GR, Ebeling M. Prenatal care and prematurity: is there an association in uncomplicated pregnancies? Birth 1991; **18**: 146–50.

Iams JD, Johnson FF, O'Shaughnessy RW. A prospective random trial of home uterine activity monitoring in pregnancies at increased risk of preterm labor. American Journal of Obstetrics and Gynecology 1987; **157**: 638–43.

Iams JD, Johnson FF, O'Shaughnessy RW. A prospective random trial of home uterine activity monitoring in pregnancies at increased risk of preterm labor. Part II. American Journal of Obstetrics and Gynecology 1988; **159**: 595–603.

Iams JD, Stilson R, Johnson FF, Williams RA, Rice R. Symptoms that precede preterm labor and premature rupture of the membranes. American Journal of Obstetrics and Gynecology 1990; **162**: 486–90.

Johnson JWC, Auston KL, Jones GS, Davis GH, and King TM. Efficacy of 17 alpha-hydroxyprogesterone caproate in the prevention of premature labor. New England Journal of Medicine 1975; **292**: 675–80.

Johnston MM, Sanchez-Ramos L, Vaughn AJ, Todd MW, Benrubi GI. Antibiotic therapy in preterm premature rupture of the membranes: a randomized prospective double-blind trial. American Journal of Obstetrics and Gynecology 1990; **163**: 743–7.

Katz M, Newman RB, Gill PJ. Assessment of uterine activity in ambulatory patients at high risk of preterm labor and delivery. American Journal of Obstetrics and Gynecology 1986; **154**: 44–7.

Keirse MJNC. Progesterone administration in pregnancy may prevent preterm delivery. British Journal of Obstetrics and Gynæcology 1990; **97**: 149–54.

Keirse MNJC, Grant A, King JF. Preterm labour. In: Chalmers I, Enkin M, Keirse MJNC, eds. Effective care in pregnancy and childbirth. Vol. 1. Pregnancy. New York: Oxford University Press, 1989: 694–745.

Kempe A, Wise PH, Barkan SE, et al. Clinical determinants of the racial disparity in very low birth weight. New England Journal of Medicine 1992; **327**: 969–73.

King JF, Grant A, Keirse MJ, Chalmers I. Beta-mimetics in preterm labour: an overview of the randomized controlled trials. British Journal of Obstetrics and Gynæcology 1988; **95**: 211–22.

Klebanoff MA, Shiono PH, Berendes HW, Rhoads GG. Facts and artifacts about anemia and preterm delivery. Journal of the American Medical Association 1989; **262**: 511–15.

Kleinman JC, Kessel SS. Racial difference in low birth weight: trends and risk factors. New England Journal of Medicine 1987; **317**: 749–53.

Knuppel RA, Lake MF, Watson DL, et al. Preventing preterm birth in twin gestation: home uterine activity monitoring and perinatal nursing support. Obstetrics and Gynecology 1990; **76**: 24S–27S.

Kogan MD, Alexander GR, Kotelchuck M, Nagey DA. Relation of the content of prenatal care to the risk of low birth weight. Journal of the American Medical Association 1994; **271**: 1340–5.

Korenbrot CC. Risk reduction in pregnancies of low-income women. Mobius 1984; **4**: 34–43.

Kramer MS. Determinants of low birth weight: methodological assessment and meta-analysis. Bulletin of the World Health Organization 1987; **65**: 663–737.

Kramer MS. Effects of energy and protein intakes on pregnancy outcome: an overview of the research evidence from controlled clinical trials. American Journal of Clinical Nutrition 1993; **58**: 627–35.

Laurin J, Persson P. The effect of bedrest in hospital on fetal outcome in pregnancies complicated by intra-uterine growth retardation. Acta Obstetricia et Gynecologica Scandinavica 1987; **66**: 407–11.

Levine RJ, Esterlitz JR, Raymond EG, et al. The trial of calcium for preeclampsia prevention (CPEP): rationale, design, and methods. Controlled Clinical Trials 1996; **17**: 442–69.

Levine RJ, Hauth JC, Curet LB, et al. The trial of calcium for preeclampsia prevention. New England Journal of Medicine 1997; **337**: 69–76.

Lewis DF, Brody K, Edwards MS, Brouillette RM, Burlison S, London SN. Preterm premature ruptured membranes: a randomized trial of steroids after treatment with antibiotics. Obstetrics and Gynecology 1996; **88**: 801–5.

Lieberman E, Ryan KJ, Monson RR, Schoenbaum SC. Risk factors accounting for racial differences in the rate of premature birth. New England Journal of Medicine 1987; **317**: 743–8.

Lockwood CJ, Costigan KG, Ghidini A, et al. Double-blind placebo-controlled trial of Piperacillin prophylaxis in preterm membrane rupture. American Journal of Obstetrics and Gynecology 1993; **169**: 970–6.

Lu ZM, Goldenberg RL, Cliver SP, Cutter GR. The relationship of maternal hematocrit to intrauterine growth retardation and preterm delivery. Obstetrics and Gynecology 1991; **77**: 190–4.

MacGregor MW. Maternal anaemias as a factor in prematurity and perinatal mortality. Scottish Medical Journal 1963; **8**: 134–40.

MacNaughton MC, Chalmers IG, Dubowitz V, et al. Final report of the Medical Research Council/Royal College of Obstetricians and Gynæcologists multicentre randomised trial of cervical cerclage. British Journal of Obstetrics and Gynæcology 1993; **100**: 516–23.

Main DM, Gabbe SG. Risk scoring for preterm labor: where do we go from here? American Journal of Obstetrics and Gynecology 1987; **157**: 789–93.

Main DM, Gabbe SG, Richardson D, Strong S. Can preterm deliveries be prevented? American Journal of Obstetrics and Gynecology 1985; **151**: 892–8.

Maloni JA, Chance B, Zhang C, Cohen AW, Betts D, Gange SJ. Physical and psychosocial side effects of antepartum hospital bed rest. Nursing Research 1993; **42**: 197–203.

Maloni JA, Kasper CE. Physical and psychosocial effects of antepartum hospital bedrest: a review of the literature. Image 1991; **23**: 187–92.

McCormick MC. The contribution of low birth weight to infant mortality and childhood morbidity. New England Journal of Medicine 1985; **312**: 82–90.

McDuffie RS, Beck A, Bischoff K, Cross J, Orleans M. Effect of frequency of prenatal care visits on perinatal outcome among low-risk women. Journal of the American Medical Association 1996; **275**: 847–51.

McLaughlin FJ, Altemeier WA, Christensen MJ, Sherrod KB, Deitrich MS, Stern DT. Randomized trial of comprehensive prenatal care for low-income women: effect on infant birth weight. Pediatrics 1992; **89**: 129–32.

Meis PJ, Ernest JM, Moore ML, Michielutte R, Sharp PC, Buescher PA. Regional program for prevention of premature birth in northwestern North Carolina. American Journal of Obstetrics and Gynecology 1987; **157**: 550–6.

Meis PJ, Goldenberg RL, Mercer B, et al. The preterm prediction study: significance of vaginal infections. American Journal of Obstetrics and Gynecology 1995; **173**: 1231–5.

Meis PJ, Goldenberg RL, Mercer BM, et al. The preterm prediction study: risk factors for indicated preterm births. American Journal of Obstetrics and Gynecology 1998; **178**: 562–7.

Menticoglou SM, Morrison I, Harman CR, Manning FA, Lange IR. Maximum possible impact of tocolytics in preventing preterm birth: a retrospective assessment. American Journal of Perinatology 1992; **9**: 394–7.

Mercer BM, Goldenberg RL, Das AMS, Moawad AH, Iams JD, Meis PJ. The preterm prediction study: a clinical risk assessment system. American Journal of Obstetrics and Gynecology 1996; **174**: 1885 95.

Mercer BM, Miodovnik M, Thurnau GR, et al. Antibiotic therapy for the reduction of morbidity and mortality after preterm premature rupture of the membranes. Journal of the American Medical Association 1997; **278**: 989–95.

Mercer B, Moretti M, Rogers R, Sibai B. Antibiotic prophylaxis in preterm premature rupture of the membranes: a prospective randomized double-blind trial of 220 patients. American Journal of Obstetrics and Gynecology 1992; **166**: 794–802.

Metcoff J, Costiloe P, Crosby WM, et al. Effect of food supplementation (WIC) during pregnancy on birth weight. American Journal of Clinical Nutrition 1985; **41**: 933–47.

Morales WJ, Angel JL, O'Brien WT, Knuppel RA. Use of ampicillin and corticosteroids in premature rupture of the membranes: a randomized study. Obstetrics and Gynecology 1989; **73**: 721–6.

Morales WJ, Schorr S, Albritton J. Effect of metronidazole in patients with preterm birth in preceding pregnancy and bacterial vaginosis: a placebo-controlled, double-blind study. American Journal of Obstetrics and Gynecology 1994; **171**: 345–9.

Morrison JC, Martin JN Jr., Martin RW, Gookin KS, Wiser WL. Prevention of preterm birth by ambulatory assessment of uterine activity: a randomized study. American Journal of Obstetrics and Gynecology 1987; **156**: 536–43.

Mou SM, Sunderji SG, Gall S, et al. Multicenter randomized clinical trial of home uterine activity monitoring for detection of preterm labor. American Journal of Obstetrics and Gynecology 1991; **165**: 858–66.

Mueller-Heubach E, Guznick DS. Evaluation of risk scoring in a preterm birth prevention study of indigent patients. American Journal of Obstetrics and Gynecology 1989; **160**: 829–37.

Nagey DA, Bailey-Jones C, Herman AA. Randomized comparison of home uterine activity monitoring and routine care in patients discharged after treatment for preterm labor. Obstetrics and Gynecology 1993; **82**: 319–23.

National Institutes of Health (NIH) Consensus Development Conference Statement. Effect of corticosteroids for fetal maturation on perinatal outcomes. American Journal of Obstetrics and Gynecology 1994; **173**: 246–52.

Neggers YH, Cutter GR, Acton RT, et al. A positive association between maternal serum zinc and birth weight. American Journal of Clinical Nutrition 1990; **51**: 678–84.

Nelson KB, Grether JK. Can magnesium sulphate reduce the risk of cerebral palsy in very low birth weight infants? Pediatrics 1995; **95**: 263–9.

Nicolaides KH, Bradley RJ, Soothill PW, Campbell S, Bilardo CM, Gibb D. Maternal oxygen therapy for intrauterine growth retardation. Lancet 1987: 942–5.

Norden CW, Kass EH. Bacteriuria of pregnancy – a critical appraisal. Annual Review of Medicine 1968; **19**: 431–70.

Oakley A, Rajan L, Grant A. Social support and pregnancy outcome. British Journal of Obstetrics and Gynæcology 1990; **97**: 155–62.

Ohlsson A. Treatment of preterm premature rupture of the membranes: a meta-analysis. American Journal of Obstetrics and Gynecology 1989; **160**: 890–906.

Olds DL, Henderson CR Jr., Tatelbaum R, Chamberlin R. Improving the delivery of prenatal care and outcomes of pregnancy: a randomized trial of nurse home visitation. Pediatrics 1986; **77**: 16–28 [published erratum appears in Pediatrics 1986; **78**: 138].

Owen J, Goldenberg RL, Davis RO, Kirk KA, Copper RL. Evaluation of a risk scoring system as a predictor of preterm birth in an indigent population. American Journal of Obstetrics and Gynecology 1990; **163**: 873–9.

Owen J, Groome LJ, Hauth JC. Randomized trial of prophylactic antibiotic therapy after preterm amnion rupture. American Journal of Obstetrics and Gynecology 1993; **169**: 976–81.

Paintin DB, Thomson AM, Hytten FE. Iron and haemoglobin level in pregnancy. Journal of Obstetrics and Gynæcology of the British Commonwealth 1966; **73**: 181–90.

Paul RH, Koh KS, Monfared AH. Obstetric factors influencing outcome in infants weighing from 1001 to 1500 grams. American Journal of Obstetrics and Gynecology 1979; **133**: 503–8.

Piper JM, Atkinson MW, Mitchel EF, Cliver SP, Snowden M, Wilson SC. Improved outcomes for very low birthweight infants associated with the use of combined maternal corticosteroids and tocolytics. Journal of Reproductive Medicine 1996; **41**: 692–8.

Pranikoff J, Helmchen R, Evertson L. Tocolytic therapy and intraventicular hemorrhage in the neonate. American Journal of Obstetrics and Gynecology 1990; **164**: 387. SPO Abstract.

Prentice AM, Whitehead RG, Watkinson M, Lamb WH, Cole TJ. Prenatal dietary supplementation of African women and birthweight. Lancet 1983; **1**: 489–92.

Regan JA, Klebanoff MA, Nugent RP, for the Vaginal Infections and Prematurity Study Group. The epidemiology of group G streptococcal colonization in pregnancy. Obstetrics and Gynecology 1991; **77**: 603–10.

Robertson PA, Sniderman SH, Laros RK, et al. Neonatal morbidity according to gestational age and birth weight from five tertiary care centers in the United States 1983–1986. American Journal of Obstetrics and Gynecology 1992; **166**: 1629–41.

Rothberg AD, Lits B. Psychosocial support for maternal stress during pregnancy: effect on birth weight. American Journal of Obstetrics and Gynecology 1991; **165**: 403–7.

Rouse DJ, Andrews WW, Goldenberg RL, Owen J. Screening and treatment of asymptomatic bacteriuria of pregnancy to prevent pyelonephritis: a cost effectiveness analysis. Obstetrics and Gynecology 1995a; **86**: 119–23.

Rouse DJ, Goldenberg RL, Cliver SP, Cutter GR, Mennemeyer ST, Fargason CA Jr. Strategies for the prevention of early onset neonatal group B streptococcal sepsis: a decision analysis. Obstetrics and Gynecology 1994; **83**: 483–94.

Rouse DJ, Hauth JC, Nelson KG, Goldenberg RL. The feasibility of a randomized clinical perinatal trial: maternal magnesium sulfate for the prevention of cerebral palsy. American Journal of Obstetrics and Gynecology 1996; **175**: 701–5.

Rouse DJ, Owen J, Goldenberg RL, Cliver SP. Determinants of the optimal time in gestation to initiate antenatal fetal testing: a decision-analytic approach. American Journal of Obstetrics and Gynecology 1995b; **173**: 1357–63.

Rowley DL, Hogue CJ, Blackmore CA, et al. Preterm delivery among African-American women: a research strategy. Preventive Medicine 1993; **9**: 1–6.

Rush D. Effects of changes in protein and calorie intake during pregnancy on the growth of the human fetus. In: Chalmers I, Enkin MW, Keirse MJNC, eds. Effective care in pregnancy and childbirth. Vol. 1. Pregnancy. New York: Oxford University Press, 1989: 255–80.

Sachs BP, Hellerstein S, Freeman R, Frigoletto F, Hauth JC. Home monitoring of uterine activity. Does it prevent prematurity? New England Journal of Medicine 1991; **325**: 1374–7.

Savitz DA, Blackmore CA, Thorp JM. Epidemiologic characteristics of preterm delivery: etiologic heterogeneity. American Journal of Obstetrics and Gynecology 1991; **164**: 467–71.

Schendel DE, Berg CJ, Yeargin-Allsopp M, Boyle CA, Decoufle P. Prenatal magnesium sulfate exposure and the risk for cerebral palsy or mental retardation among very low-birth-weight children aged 3 to 5 years. Journal of the American Medical Association 1995; **276**: 1805–10.

Schiff E, Peleg E, Goldenberg M, Rosenthal T, Ruppin E, Tamarkin M. The use of aspirin to prevent pregnancy-induced hypertension and lower the ratio of thromboxane A2 to prostacyclin in relatively high risk pregnancies. New England Journal of Medicine 1989; **321**: 351–6.

Scholl TO, Hediger ML, Bendich A, Schall JI, Smith WK, Krueger PM. Use of multivitamin/mineral prenatal supplements: influence on the outcome of pregnancy. American Journal of Epidemiology 1997; **146**: 134–41.

Scholl TO, Miller LK, Salmon RW, Cofsky MC, Shearer J. Prenatal care adequacy and the outcome of adolescent pregnancy: effects on weight gain, preterm delivery, and birth weight. Obstetrics and Gynecology 1987; **69**: 312–16.

Shiono PH, Klebanoff MA, Graubard BI, Berendes HW, Rhoads GG. Birth weight among women of different ethnic groups. Journal of the American Medical Association 1986; **255**: 48–52.

Sibai BM, Caritis SN, Thom E, et al. Prevention of pre-eclampsia with low-dose aspirin in healthy, nulliparous pregnant women. New England Journal of Medicine 1993; **329**: 1213–18.

Simmer K, James C, Thompson RPH. Are iron-folate supplements harmful? American Journal of Clinical Nutrition 1987; **45**: 122–5.

Simmer K, Lort-Phillips L, James C, Thompson RPH. A double blind trial of zinc supplementation in pregnancy. European Journal of Clinical Nutrition 1991; **45**: 139–44.

Spencer B, Thomas H, Morris J. A randomized controlled trial of the provision of a social support service during pregnancy: the South Manchester Family Worker Project. British Journal of Obstetrics and Gynæcology 1989; **96**: 281–8.

Starfield B, Shapiro S, Weiss J, et al. Race, family income, and low birth weight. American

Journal of Epidemiology 1991; **134**: 1166–74.

Susser M. Prenatal nutrition, birthweight and psychological development: an overview of experiments, quasi-experiments, and natural experiments in the past decade. American Journal of Clinical Nutrition 1981; **34**: 784–803.

Sweet RL, Landers DJ, Walker C, Schachter J. *Chlamydia trachomatis* infection and pregnancy outcome. American Journal of Obstetrics and Gynecology 1987; **156**: 824–33.

Tamura T, Goldenberg RL. Zinc nutriture and pregnancy outcome. Nutrition Research 1996; **16**: 139–81.

Tamura T, Goldenberg RL, Freeberg LE, Cliver SP, Cutter GR, Hoffman HJ. Maternal serum folate and zinc concentrations and their relationship to pregnancy outcome. American Journal of Clinical Nutrition 1992; **56**: 365–70.

Tucker JM, Goldenberg RL, Davis RO, Copper RL, Winkler CL, Hauth JC. Etiologies of preterm birth in an indigent population: is prevention a logical expectation? Obstetrics and Gynecology 1991; **77**: 343–7.

U.S. Preventive Services Task Force (USPSTF). Home uterine activity monitoring for preterm labor: policy statement. Journal of the American Medical Association 1993; **270**: 369–70.

Uzan S, Beaufils M, Breart G, Bazin B, Capitant C, Paris J. Prevention of fetal growth retardation with low-dose aspirin: Findings of the EPREDA trial. Lancet 1991; **337**: 1427–31.

Villar J, Farnot U, Barros F, Victoria C, Langer A, Belizan JM, for the Latin American Network for Perinatal and Reproductive Research. A randomized trial of psychosocial support during high-risk pregnancies. New England Journal of Medicine 1992; **327**: 1266–71.

Wallenburg HCS, Makovitz JW, Dekker GA, Rotmans P. Low-dose aspirin prevents pregnancy-induced hypertension and preeclampsia in angiotensin-sensitive primigravidae. Lancet 1986; **I**: 1–3.

Walsh SW. Preeclampsia: An imbalance in placental prostacyclin and thromboxane production. American Journal of Obstetrics and Gynecology 1985; **152**: 335–40.

Wapner RJ, Cotton DB, Artal R, Librizzi RJ, Ross MG. A randomized multicenter trial assessing a home uterine activity monitoring device used in the absence of daily nursing contact. American Journal of Obstetrics and Gynecology 1995; **172**: 1026–34.

Wen SW, Goldenberg RL, Cutter G, Hoffman H, Cliver SP. Intrauterine growth retardation and preterm delivery: prenatal risk factors in an indigent population. American Journal of Obstetrics and Gynecology 1990a; **162**: 213–18.

Wen SW, Goldenberg RL, Cutter GR, et al. Smoking, maternal age, fetal growth and gestational age at delivery. American Journal of Obstetrics and Gynecology 1990b; **162**: 53–8.

White CP, Wilkins EGL, Roberts C, Davidson DC. Premature delivery and group B streptococcal bacteriuria [letter]. Lancet 1984; **2**: 586.

Yemini M, Borenstein R, Dreazen E, et al. Prevention of premature labor by 17 alpha-hydroxyprogesterone caproate. American Journal of Obstetrics and Gynecology 1985; **151**: 574–7.

Zlatnik FJ. Applicability of tocolytic therapy [editorial; comment]. American Journal of Perinatology 1992; **9**: 494.

5

Long-term outcomes of prematurity

Marie C. McCormick

Introduction

As described in Chapters 3 and 4, medical intervention has not succeeded in preventing a substantial fraction of preterm deliveries in the United States. Instead, recent decreases in neonatal mortality reflect the effectiveness of prenatal and neonatal intensive management in improving the survival of ever smaller, more immature infants. The survival of these infants and the quality of life they are able to enjoy has been a critical concern and one that research is only recently beginning to elucidate.

Concerns about the outcomes of these premature survivors have traditionally focused on neurodevelopmental outcomes. Research has emphasized cognitive development as reflected by developmental or intelligence quotients, and/or neuromotor abnormalities, especially cerebral palsy (CP). More recently, a larger array of outcomes has been reported, as will be illustrated in this chapter. With this expansion of scope of concern, the importance of considering a broad array of potential confounders in the relationship between prematurity and various outcomes has been underscored. For example, it cannot be assumed that the factors other than prematurity that may contribute to the risk of poor cognitive development are the same as those that influence social–emotional development.

This chapter discusses the impact of prematurity on physical and developmental outcomes and proposes several options for using current technology to improve the outcomes of premature infants.

Any overview of this outcomes literature should be prefaced by a few caveats. Although the outcomes literature appears at first blush to be extensive, it is plagued with recurring flaws (Aylward et al., 1989; Escobar et al., 1991; Hack et al., 1995; Kitchen et al., 1982; McCormick, 1989, 1993, 1997). These include:

- a lack of standard definitions of outcomes across studies and a reliance on broad characterization of the child's state;
- a lack of documented valid and reliable measures of outcomes;

- a lack of appropriate comparison groups or statistical adjustments for other factors that might affect outcomes;
- a lack of adequate description of cohort definition and attrition;
- a preponderance of single-site studies with limitations in sociodemographic heterogeneity;
- an inability to tease out variations in neonatal intensive care unit (NICU) practices as contributors to outcomes; and
- a failure to incorporate relevant pathogenic or theoretic perspectives.

Another methodologic limitation of the literature is a tendency to characterize the study population of interest solely in terms of birth weight (e.g., < 500 gm, < 1000 gm). While such tiny infants are assuredly prematurely born, they may also be small-for-gestational-age, because a survival advantage accrues to infants who are biologically more mature than their birth weight suggests. As later chapters show, intrauterine growth restriction may confer a separate hazard. These methodologic problems make this literature difficult to summarize into a clear picture of the outcomes of these infants. For example, most studies would probably agree on the types of morbidity that lead to severe impairment, and the proportions of children considered severely affected are generally consistent across most reports. However, the patterns of less severe conditions and their effect on functioning are much more variably described and categorized. These less severe conditions include the cognitive and behavioral impairments underlying much of the need for special education and health services for these children.

Developmental processes

The morbidity incurred by premature infants reflects disruption of developmental processes that occur normally in utero and the potential for further compensatory growth and development. By the second half of pregnancy, most organ systems have developed, but substantial maturation of function continues to occur in preparation for extra-uterine life. For example, while the structures of immune and endocrine systems may be present, they may not be fully functional, and the infant may not adapt well to the stress of birth or be able to fight off infection readily. In the brain, cells are migrating into position, a process that continues into the first year of life. If disruption is severe, this migration may not occur, thus precluding the activities associated with the disrupted cells. Later migration may compensate for these minor disruptions, however. In the lung, the alveoli or air sacs where gasses are exchanged are present but lack a chemical, surfactant, to keep them distended. The premature infant requires artificial surfactant, and may require mechanical ventilation to breathe, with the latter sometimes contributing to injury to the lung. However, because lung development continues into early childhood, improvement in pulmonary function may be seen beyond infancy.

The immaturity of the various organ systems is reflected in the neonatal complications familiar to any neonatologist. For example, hyaline membrane disease, also known as respiratory distress syndrome (RDS), is a result of pulmonary immaturity and is a major cause of death among premature infants. Oxygendependence at 28 days, formerly called bronchopulmonary dysplasia but now more often called chronic lung disease, reflects both immaturity of the lung and damage from the mechanical ventilation needed to keep the baby alive. Patent ductus arteriosus is the failure to close of a blood vessel needed in utero but not after birth, and occurs largely in the context of RDS. Necrotizing enterocolitis reflects immaturity of the gut in digestive as well as immune functions. Intraventricular hemorrhage occurs because the cells lining the ventricles of the brain are immature and therefore unable to regulate intracranial blood pressure. Intraventricular hemorrhage is associated with relatively severe neurodevelopmental outcomes.

The incidence and prevalence of these outcomes vary substantially across neonatal intensive care units (Avery et al., 1987; Hack et al., 1991; Horbar et al., 1988). This variation is probably a function of some combination of the severity of illness of the infant on admission (Richardson et al., 1993) and management of practices within individual NICUs. To the extent that these complications affect the risk of later outcomes, such variations may reflect an opportunity to improve outcomes with current technology.

This consideration raises a larger issue of causality. The literature generally is written as though prematurity "causes" the outcomes being assessed. However, as noted in Chapter 3, multiple causal pathways are possible and should be considered when assessing the potential effect of interventions to improve survival or reduce prematurity. For example, factors known in epidemiology as "confounders" may lead to premature delivery and to the outcomes independently. Crack cocaine, which can cause premature labor, also may cause brain lesions. Bacterial vaginosis may lead to preterm labor and to the brain lesions seen in CP. Poverty increases the risk of prematurity and poor cognitive development. It is thus important to consider whether it is prematurity or the environmental insult that is responsible for the adverse health outcome.

Adverse outcomes may occur in some, but not all, preterm infants who have a particular developmental vulnerability to the stresses of preterm delivery. An argument supporting this assertion may be derived from the literature on variations in admission severity, and on the prepartum interventions to reduce this vulnerability. For example, not all infants of the same birth weight and gestational age are equally "sick" on admission to the intensive care unit, and these differences in severity account for differences in mortality among infants (Richardson et al., 1993).

Another possible causal pathway for the complications associated with premature delivery described previously is the NICU environment, which may ameliorate or exacerbate these complications. Factors that can influence health outcomes include the medical management of the infants, their exposure to environmental stimuli (e.g., light, noise) and pathogens, and the developmental interventions within the unit (Als et al., 1996; Gilkerson et al., 1990; Parker et al., 1992; Resnick et al., 1988).

Finally, observed outcomes may reflect the post-discharge environment of the infant either entirely, or in association with developmental vulnerability. For example, the temperamental difficulties encountered in many premature infants with certain neonatal complications (Ross, 1987) can lead to alterations in how their mothers interact with them (Davis and Thomas, 1988; Macey et al., 1987; McCormick, 1985).

Outcomes

At least two meta-analyses (Aylward et al., 1989; Escobar et al., 1991) and several previous reports (Hack et al., 1995; Kitchen et al., 1982; McCormick, 1989, 1993, 1997) have reviewed the literature on long-term outcomes of premature birth. To the extent possible, this chapter relies on these reports and summarizes outcomes in categories, as they do. However, these categories may be overlapping, and some of the specific conditions within categories may encompass a broad range of severity. It should be recognized that many preterm infants survive without any sequelae, and others may have varying combinations of outcomes.

Assessing the functional impact of individual conditions or combinations of conditions is a relatively recent phenomenon, and only recently has a significant body of literature emerged on the outcomes of children at early school age. Very little, if any, information deals with outcomes in adolescence and adulthood. Data in more recent reports are presented as population averages or percentages. This more recent literature contrasts with previously published work, which is characterized by the use of broad, non-comparable clinical assessments. The more recent literature on outcomes is described below and summarized in Tables 5.1 and 5.2.

Specific conditions and diagnoses

Several health problems appear to occur more frequently in premature infants. They are at increased risk for congenital malformations (McCormick, 1985; Mili et al., 1991), which contribute to their higher risk of mortality (Thompson et al., 1997) and to their use of health care services after discharge from the NICU

Table 5.1. Specific conditions and diagnoses: risk among premature infants relative to term infants

Condition	Relative risk
Congenital malformations	2–5
Neurodevelopmental disorders	
Cerebral palsy	4–30
Hydrocephalus	4–8
Seizures	3
Visual defects	
Blindness	1–2
Retractive errors/Strabismus	7–20
Hearing defects/deafness	
Loss of hearing	Variable
Asthma/Reactive airway disease	2

Sources: Escobar et al., 1991; Grogaard, 1988; McCormick, 1985;
McCormick and Peckham, 1992; McCormick et al., 1995; Mili et
al., 1991.

Table 5.2. Developmental abnormalities: risk among premature infants relative to term
infants

	Birth weight (gm)	Relative risk
Cognitive development		
IQ < 70	< 1000	4–13
	< 1500	3
IQ 70–84	< 1000	2–6
	< 1500	1.7
Physical growth		
Weight < 2 SD for age	< 1000	8
	1001–1500	3
Height < 2 SD for age	< 1000	8
	1001–1500	6
Head circumference < 2 SD for age	< 1000	13
	1001 – 1501	3
Social/emotional development		
Behavior problems		2–3
Lack of social competence		2

Sources: Aylward et al., 1989; Binkin et al., 1988; Casey et al., 1991; Hack et al., 1995;
McCormick and Peckham, 1992; McCormick et al., 1995, 1996.

(McCormick et al., 1980). Premature infants also are at increased risk of cerebral palsy (Escobar et al., 1991) as a result of higher rates of intracranial bleeding and the vulnerability of their cortical white matter to injury (Kuban and Leviton, 1994). An increased risk of seizures and hydrocephalus is associated with these types of injuries (McCormick and Peckham, 1992).

The increased number of visual defects that occur in these infants further underscores the vulnerability of the central nervous system to premature birth. Almost half the infants born weighing 1250 gm or less develop retinopathy of prematurity (ROP). Even if this problem resolves uneventfully, the development of ROP is associated with increased risk of myopia, astigmatism, anisometropia, and strabismus (McCormick et al., 1995). Fortunately, complete blindness is rare, as is deafness (Grogaard, 1988). However, less severe auditory problems are relatively common. In addition to these problems, premature children are more likely to report having asthma or reactive airway disease (McCormick et al., 1992), and to have other pulmonary symptoms and abnormalities of pulmonary function than are full-term children (Yerksel and Greenough, 1991).

Developmental abnormalities

Premature infants are at increased risk of difficulties in cognitive, physical growth, and social–emotional development.

Cognitive development

On average, premature children score only slightly lower on IQ tests than term children (Aylward et al., 1989; Hack et al., 1995). However, this average obscures the fact that a substantial percentage may have difficulties in specific areas, especially expressive language and visual-motor activities (McCormick, 1989). They also are disproportionately more likely to have IQs in the subnormal and borderline range. About 8–18% of children born weighing less than 1000 gm have IQs less than 70, and another 25–30% will be in the range of 70–84 (Table 5.2) (Hack et al., 1995).

Physical growth

On average, premature children do not achieve the 50th percentile in height or weight (Binkin et al., 1988; Casey et al., 1991). In addition, premature infants are disproportionately more likely to be in the very small range (i.e., 3–8 times more likely to be two standard deviations below the mean for their age in height and weight), and 3–13 times more likely to have microcephaly (McCormick and Peckham, 1992). This high rate of head growth failure, however, may reflect the contribution of intrauterine growth restriction, and poor head growth is also associated with other neurodevelopmental problems.

Social–emotional development

Social–emotional development reflects emotional health, behavioral competence, and self-esteem. Unfortunately, most of the measures in this domain focus on problems, and the literature is dominated by information on behavior problems. Premature children are twice as likely to experience clinically significant behavior problems as are term infants (McCormick et al., 1996). A particular area of concern is attention deficits and easy distractibility (Hack et al., 1995). Differences in affective symptoms (depression, anxiety, or emotional well-being) have not been documented, but their parents and teachers rate the children as less socially competent (McCormick et al., 1996). The latter rating reflects almost all aspects of social competence except in physical appearance (Aylward et al., 1989). As with behavior problems, premature children are twice as likely to be rated as less socially competent as normal birth weight children (McCormick et al., 1995).

Impact of morbidity

Functional limitations

As noted above, the use of valid, standard measures of the effect of various health problems on a child's ability to perform the usual activities of daily living is relatively recent. However, assessments of severe impairment have been reported in a relatively comparable fashion for some time. Overall, about 10% of children who weigh less than 1500 gm at birth, and 10% of those who weigh less than 1000 gm are characterized as severely impaired, and this proportion has not changed with increases in survival (McCormick, 1993; OTA, 1987). For the very tiniest infants, the rate goes up to 20–25% (Hack et al., 1994; LaPine et al., 1995; Msall et al., 1991).

Less severe limitations are more frequently encountered, with 46% of those weighing less than 1000 gm and 34% of those weighing 1001–1500 gm having at least one activity of daily living affected by a health problem (McCormick et al., 1992). In addition, premature children experience a variety of motor and coordination problems (Gorga et al., 1991), which generate an overall impression of clumsiness (Marlow et al., 1989; Scottish Low Birth Weight Study Group, 1992).

Educational resources

Not surprisingly, in view of the cognitive and behavioral difficulties experienced by premature children, they have higher rates of school difficulties than do children born at term. Almost half of children born weighing 1000 gm or less have repeated a grade or been classified for special education early in their schooling (Klebanov et al., 1994). Even among those in an age-appropriate grade, achievement scores are lower, suggesting the potential for further difficulty (Klebanov et al., 1994).

Use of health services

Premature children use more health services than do term children. The higher rates of hospitalization in infancy have been well documented (Hack et al., 1983; McCormick et al., 1980) and more recent evidence has shown that the increased rates of morbidity seen in school-aged children who were born prematurely continues to lead to hospital use (Hack et al., 1995; McCormick et al., 1993b).

Family effects

The birth of a premature child also has broad effects on the family, one of the most important of which is financial. The increased morbidity and use of health services early in infancy as well as in succeeding years has clear financial implications for the family (Escobar et al., 1991; Lewit et al., 1995; McCormick et al., 1991; Shankaran et al., 1988). While some of these costs have been estimated (Lewit et al., 1995), how much is directly borne by the family and how much is covered by insurance is not known. Other effects, which have not been examined in detail, include the time burden of taking children for medical care and of advocacy for educational services. In addition, early in infancy, parents may restrict their social networks and may have fewer resources for social support and respite (McCormick et al., 1991). Whether this effect persists has not been investigated.

Only recently has it been possible to ask the child directly about his or her assessment of the quality of life. Saigal et al. (1996) have reported on a cohort of children born weighing 1000 gm or less. At age 13, the youth clearly recognize that they have more functional limitations due to health problems than their normal birthweight peers, but actually rate their quality of life as higher.

In summary, the older, simpler paradigm of outcomes focused on neuro-development is inadequate to describe the varied outcomes seen among premature infants. Such infants appear to have two to four times the risk of term infants of a variety of health problems. However, none of these problems is unique to premature infants, but occur in children born at term as well. A small proportion are severely impaired by the sequelae of prematurity or its management. A larger proportion have less severe problems, which may consist of some combination of mild cognitive delay or difficulties with specific aspects of cognition, attention deficits, and chronic health problems such as reactive airway disease (asthma). Moreover, because very premature children represent only a small fraction of newborns, most of the children with these problems will have been born at term. This observation is not meant to dismiss the difficulties of some families with premature children, but to underscore the relatively good outcomes of many, and to refute the notion that the increased survival of these children is overwhelming the health care system. Furthermore, some of the health problems that these children experience may not be the inevitable consequences of being born premature, but reflect the environments to which the children are exposed. This consideration, in turn, offers potential to improve outcomes.

Conclusion

As noted earlier in this chapter, much of the literature posits a rather static model that assumes that the outcomes observed are a consequence of prematurity. Different or more complex causal models may be needed. If, as Chapter 4 suggests, decreases in prematurity rates through prenatal interventions may not be a near-term achievement, then the following may serve as options for improving outcomes through the use of current technology:

- *Appropriate prenatal and peripartum management:* An underappreciated component of prenatal care is the opportunity for routine and regular risk assessment and referral to appropriate centers for delivery. Evidence supports the effectiveness of regionalized prenatal care in reducing mortality among premature infants (McCormick and Richardson, 1995). A recent analysis of improvements in severity-adjusted mortality in seven NICUs (Richardson et al., 1996) attributed a third of the change to the improved condition of the infant on admission, which had resulted from better obstetric management.
- *Decreasing variations in neonatal complications:* We have previously commented on the variability among NICUs of the major neonatal complications that may predispose infants to later morbidity and slower development. Efforts by each NICU to reduce these complications to the lowest possible rate may also reduce the later burden of ill health among premature infants.
- *Post-discharge interventions:* Chapter 3 notes the role of poverty in increasing the risk of preterm delivery. Poverty has an equally negative effect on child development. Data from a large, multi-site randomized trial of intensive early educational intervention in the first three years of life showed that such interventions can lead to improved cognitive and social–emotional development even among very tiny infants (McCormick et al., 1993a). However, the effect of intervention may not be sustained in smaller infants without continued support (Brooks-Gunn et al., 1994; McCarton et al., 1997). For this reason, early and continued intervention, particularly for families who lack resources, is critical for improving health outcomes for premature infants.
- *Maternal health care:* Finally, as later chapters in this book will argue, we have only begun to think through the potential for improving outcomes in subsequent pregnancies. That the risk of prematurity persists is well documented (Wang et al., 1995). Perhaps greater attention to the health of women already known to have a risk of adverse outcomes will help in reducing the prevalence of prematurity.

REFERENCES

Als H, Duffy FH, McAnulty GGB. Effectiveness of individualized neurodevelopmental care in the newborn intensive care unit (NICU). Acta Pædiatrica. Supplement 1996; **116**: 21–30.

Avery ME, Tooley WH, Keller JB, et al. Is chronic lung disease in low birth weight infants preventable? A survey of eight centers. Pediatrics 1987; **79**: 26–30.

Aylward GP, Pfeiffer SI, Wright A, Verhulst SJ. Outcomes studies of low birth weight infants published in the last decade: a meta-analysis. The Journal of Pediatrics 1989; **115**: 515–20.

Binkin NJ, Yip R, Fleshood L, Trowbridge FL. Birth weight and childhood growth. Pediatrics 1988; **82**: 828–34.

Brooks-Gunn J, McCarton CM, Casey PH, et al. Early intervention in low-birth-weight premature infants: results through age 5 years from the Infant Health and Development Program. Journal of the American Medical Association 1994; **272**: 1257–62.

Casey PH, Kraemer HC, Bernbaum J, et al. Growth status and growth rates of a varied sample of low birth weight, preterm infants: a longitudinal cohort from birth to three years of age. The Journal of Pediatrics 1991; **119**: 599–605.

Davis DH, Thomas EB. The early social environment of premature and full term infants. Early Human Development 1988; **17**: 221–32.

Escobar GJ, Littenberg B, Pettiti DB. Outcome among surviving very low birth weight infants: a meta-analysis. Archives of Disease in Childhood 1991; **66**: 204–11.

Gilkerson L, Gorski P, Panitz P. Hospital-based intervention for preterm infants and their families. In: Meisels SJ, Shenkoff JP, eds. Handbook of early childhood intervention. Cambridge: Cambridge University Press, 1990.

Gorga D, Stern FM, Ross G, Nagler W. The neuromotor behavior of preterm and full-term children by three years of age: equality of movement and variability. Journal of Developmental and Behavioral Pediatrics 1991; **12**: 102–7.

Grogaard J. High risk neonates and long-term outcomes. In Bess FD, ed. Hearing impairment in children. Parkton (MD): York Press, Inc., 1988.

Hack M, Horbar JD, Malloy MH, Tyson JE, Albright E, Wright L. Very low birth weight outcomes of the National Institute Child Health and Human Development neonatal network. Pediatrics 1991; **87**: 587–97.

Hack MD, Klein NK, Taylor HG. Long-term developmental outcomes of low birth weight infants. The Future of Children 1995; **5**(1): 176–96.

Hack M, Rivera A, Fanaroff AA. The very low birth weight infant: the broader spectrum of morbidity during infancy and childhood. Journal of Developmental and Behavioral Pediatrics 1983; **4**: 43–9.

Hack M, Taylor HG, Klein N, Eiben R, Schatschneider C, Mecuri-Minick N. School-age outcomes in children with birth weights under 750 g. New England Journal of Medicine 1994; **331**: 753–9.

Horbar JD, McGuiliffe TL, Adler SM. Variability in 28–day outcomes for very low birth weight infants in 11 neonatal intensive care units. Pediatrics 1988; **82**: 554–9.

Kitchen WH, Ryan MM, Richards A, et al. Changing outcomes over 13 years of very low birth weight infants. Seminars in Perinatology 1982; **4**: 373–89.

Klebanov PK, Brooks-Gunn J, McCormick MC. School achievement and failure in very low birth weight children. Journal of Developmental and Behavioral Pediatrics 1994; **15**: 248–56.

Kuban KCK, Leviton A. Cerebral palsy. New England Journal of Medicine 1994; **330**: 188–95.

LaPine TR, Jackson JC, Bennett FC. Outcome of infants weighing less than 800 grams at birth: 15 years' experience. Pediatrics 1995; **96**: 479–83.

Lewit EM, Baker ES, Corman H, Shiono PH. The direct cost of low birth weight. The Future of Children 1995; **5**(1): 35–56.

Macey TJ, Harmon RJ, Easterbrooks MA. Impact of premature birth on development of the infant in the family. Journal of Consulting and Clinical Psychology 1987; **55**: 846–52.

Marlow N, Roberts BL, Cooke RWI. Motor skills of extremely low birth weight children at 6 years. Archives of Disease in Childhood 1989; **64**: 839–47.

McCarton CM, Brooks-Gunn J, Wallace IF, et al. Results at age 8 years of early intervention for low-birth-weight premature infants: the Infant Health and Development Program. Journal of the American Medical Association 1997; **277**: 126–32.

McCormick MC. The outcomes of very low birth weight infants: are we asking the right questions? Pediatrics 1997; **99**: 869–76.

McCormick MC. Has the prevalence of handicapped infants increased with improved survival of very low birth infants? Clinics in Perinatology 1993; **20**: 263–77.

McCormick MC. The contribution of low birthweight to infant mortality and childhood morbidity. New England Journal of Medicine 1985; **312**: 82–90.

McCormick MC. Long-term follow-up of infants discharged from neonatal intensive care units. Journal of the American Medical Association 1989; **261**: 1767–72.

McCormick MC, Bernbaum JC, Eisenberg JM, Kurstra SL, Finnegan E. Costs incurred by parents of very low birth weight infants after the initial neonatal hospitalization. Pediatrics 1991; **88**: 533–41.

McCormick MC, Brooks-Gunn J, Workman-Daniels K, Turner J, Peckham GJ. The health and developmental status of very low birth weight children at school age. Journal of the American Medical Association 1992; **267**: 2204–8.

McCormick MC, McCarton C, Tonascia J, Brooks-Gunn J. Early educational intervention for very low birth weight infants: results from the infant health and development program. The Journal of Pediatrics 1993a; **123**: 527–53.

McCormick MC, Peckham GJ. Final report of the study of long-term outcomes of very low birth weight infants. Boston: Harvard School of Public Health, 1992.

McCormick MC, Richardson DK. Access to neonatal intensive care. The Future of Children 1995; **5**(1): 162–75.

McCormick MC, Shapiro S, Starfield BH. Rehospitalization in the first year of life for high risk survivors. Pediatrics 1980; **66**: 991–9.

McCormick MC, Stewart JE, Cohen R, Joselow M, Osborne PS, Ware J. Follow-up of NICU graduates: why, what and by whom. Journal of Intensive Care Medicine 1995; **10**: 213–55.

McCormick MC, Workman-Daniels K, Brooks-Gunn J. The behavioral and emotional well-being of school-age children with different birth weights. Pediatrics 1996; **97**: 18–25.

McCormick MC, Workman-Daniels K, Brooks-Gunn J, Peckham GJ. Hospitalization of very low birth weight children at school age. The Journal of Pediatrics 1993b; **122**: 360–5.

Mili F, Edwards LD, Khoury MJ, McClearn AB. Prevalence of birth defects among low birth-weight infants. A population study. American Journal of Diseases of Children 1991; **145**: 1313–18.

Msall ME, Buck GE, Rogers BT, Merke D, Catanzaro NC, Zorn WA. Risk factors for major neurodevelopmental impairments and need for special education resources in extremely premature infants. The Journal of Pediatrics 1991; **119**: 606–14.

Office of Technology Assessment (OTA). Neonatal intensive care for low birth weight infants: cost and effectiveness. Health Technology Case Study 38. Washington DC: Office of Technology Assessment. Office of Technology Assessment – Health Technology Case Study 38, 1987.

Parker SJ, Zahr LK, Cole JG, Brecht M. Outcome after developmental intervention in the neonatal intensive care unit for mothers of preterm infants with low socio-economic status. The Journal of Pediatrics 1992; **120**: 780–5.

Resnick MB, Armstrong S, Carter RL. Developmental intervention program for high-risk premature infants: effects on development and parent–infant interactions. Journal of Developmental and Behavioral Pediatrics 1988; **9**: 73–8.

Richardson DK, Gray JE, Gortmaker S, Goldmann DA, McCormick MC, and the SNAP-II Study Group. Evidence of improving NICU care: declining SNAP-adjusted mortality. Pediatric Research 1996; **39**: 276A.

Richardson DK, Phibbs CS, Gray JE, McCormick MC, Workman-Daniels K, Goldmann DA. Birth weight and illness severity: independent predictors of neonatal mortality. Pediatrics 1993; **91**: 969–75.

Ross G. Temperament of preterm infants: its relationship to perinatal factors and one-year outcome. Journal of Developmental and Behavioral Pediatrics 1987; **8**: 106–10.

Saigal S, Feeny D, Rosenbaum P, Furlong W, Burrows E, Stoskopf B. Self perceived health status and health related quality of life of extremely low-birth-weight infants at adolescence. Journal of the American Medical Association 1996; **276**: 453–9.

Scottish Low Birth Weight Study Group. The Scottish low birth weight study: I. Survival, neuromotor and sensory impairment. Archives of Disease in Childhood 1992; **67**: 675–81.

Shankaran S, Cohen SN, Linver M, Zonia S. Medical care costs of high-risk infants after neonatal intensive care. Pediatrics 1988; **81**: 372–8.

Thompson M, Richardson D, Stark AR, Weisberger S, Bednark F, McCormick MC, and the SNAP-II Study Group. Impact of congenital anomalies on inter-NICU comparisons of VLBW outcomes. Pediatric Research 1997; **41**: 221A.

Wang X, Zuckerman B, Coffman GA, Corwin MJ. Familial aggregation of low birth weight among whites and blacks in the United States. New England Journal of Medicine 1995; **333**: 1744–9.

Yerksel B, Greenough A. Relationship of symptoms to lung function abnormalities in preterm infants at follow-up. Pediatric Pulmonology 1991; **11**: 202–6.

Part III

New Findings and Long-term Evidence on Intrauterine Growth Restriction

6

Causes of intrauterine growth restriction

Kathleen Maher Rasmussen

Introduction

Although intrauterine growth restriction (IUGR) has only recently been consistently distinguished from low birth weight (LBW) and prematurity, this distinction has been crucial in our understanding of the causes and consequences of small size at birth and of interventions that might be successful in reducing the incidence and severity of this condition. To provide background information for subsequent chapters, concepts about the etiology of IUGR will be discussed here. The causes of IUGR in diverse circumstances will be presented, along with implications for preventing this condition in American population groups. This chapter focuses primarily on nutritional and behavioral factors, such as smoking, related to IUGR. Other factors related to IUGR are considered in Chapter 7.

Infants who are small at birth also have been described as "small-for-date" or as "small-for-gestational-age." Most recently, they have been described as having "fetal growth restriction." In this paper, the term IUGR will be used synonymously with these other terms, although – strictly speaking – this is not correct (Altman and Hytten, 1989).

Definition of intrauterine growth restriction

In classifying infants as having IUGR, we are trying to identify those individuals whose growth, in the simplest terms, is less than their genetic potential. This is not easy to do because it is difficult to know a particular individual's genetic potential for growth. Researchers recently have devised workable approaches, such as the "individualized birthweight ratio" (Wilcox et al., 1993) or customized fetal growth standards (Mongelli and Gardosi, 1996), which account for known predictors of size at birth. However, these approaches have not yet been widely applied.

As a result of these challenges, most investigators have resorted to using a statistical definition of IUGR: weight at birth below a specific cut-off value

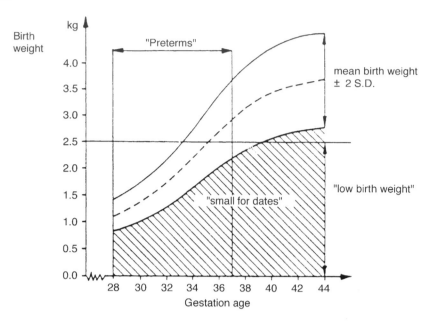

Figure 6.1   The distribution of birth weight by gestational age, Sweden 1958–59. This figure illustrates the fact that an infant can weigh more than 2500 gm and still be growth retarded (Pettersson et al., 1978).

(usually the 10th percentile) on a distribution of birth-weight-for-gestational-age (WHO, 1995) (Figure 6.1). Thus, IUGR does not have a single value for weight; it varies with gestational age (Pettersson et al., 1978). Many IUGR infants are also LBW (i.e., weighing < 2500 gm at birth). In addition, many IUGR infants are premature (i.e., < 37 weeks gestational age at birth). As is evident from Figure 6.1, an infant born at term who weighs more than 2500 gm can still have IUGR. For these infants, the IUGR cut-off point is usually less than the 10th percentile on a standard weight-for-gestational age chart. In fact, because more infants are born at these gestational ages and weights, they comprise the largest fraction of IUGR infants. In some populations, three-fourths of the growth-restricted infants weigh > 2500 gm at birth (Lang et al., 1996). Finally, the weight at any gestational age at which an infant is determined to be IUGR depends on the reference birth weight distribution that is used (Alexander et al., 1996; Goldenberg et al., 1989b) as well as whether the pregnancy was dated by last menstrual period or ultrasonography (Goldenberg et al., 1989a).

As is the case whenever a cut-off point is used, the potential for misclassification exists because a cut-off is often an imperfect proxy for the underlying concept. For example, in any population, it is expected that 10% of individuals will have a birth weight below the 10th percentile of their weight-for-gestational-age. However, some of these individuals are genetically small and healthy. Others are smaller than

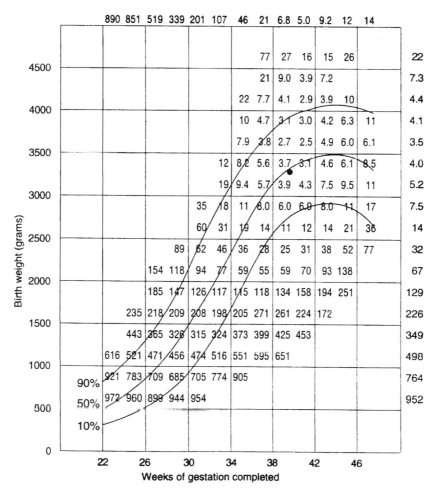

Figure 6.2 Birth weight percentiles and perinatal mortality rates (per 1000) for singleton female births (WHO, 1995).

expected, and it is these individuals whose small size is potentially of concern. It has been estimated that only about 60% of infants classified as IUGR using a traditional birth-weight-for-gestational-age chart would be identified as growth-restricted using a reference that accounted for individuals who were genetically small (Mongelli and Gardosi, 1996; Wilcox et al., 1993). Similarly, some individuals whose weight-for-gestational-age is above the chosen cut-off value will also be smaller than expected. These individuals are also growth-restricted, but are not classified as such. It is difficult to estimate the number of individuals who are misclassified in this way, but it could be large (Chard et al., 1993). In theory, growth restriction can occur at any birth weight. The consequences of growth restriction at higher birth weights have not been investigated.

Table 6.1. Conditions associated with human fetal growth restriction

Intrinsic	Extrinsic
Fetal factors:	Environmental factors:
Intrauterine infection	High altitude, food availability, pollution, hyperthermia, irradiation
Chromosomal mosaicism	
Chromosomal anomalies	Maternal factors:
Congenital malformations	Undernutrition, young age, low weight gain, drug use, low SES, medical complications
Inborn errors of metabolism	
Anemia (Rh disease)	Placental factors:
	Abnormalities, abnormal placentation
	Other factors:
	Reproductive technologies

Source: Adapted from Owens et al., 1995.

At any given gestational age, the more severe the growth restriction, the higher the infant's risk of perinatal death (WHO, 1995) (Figure 6.2). In fact, the perinatal mortality rate is substantially higher for growth-restricted babies than it is for equally preterm babies who are normally grown (WHO, 1995) (Figure 6.2). Growth-restricted infants who are part of a multiple pregnancy are not at increased risk of perinatal mortality above that associated with the earlier-than-normal delivery of multifetal gestations (WHO, 1995).

Common pathways to IUGR

IUGR is not a single entity. Rather, poor fetal growth reflects the presence of one or more adverse events or processes occurring in utero. These events or processes can act on the mother, the placenta, and/or the fetus (Tables 6.1 and 6.2). These result in the reduced delivery of nutrients (including oxygen) to the placenta; altered placental development; reduced placental volume, weight, or surface area for exchange; reduced uterine or umbilical blood flow; and/or reduced substrate acquisition by the fetus (Owens et al., 1995). Immediate predictors of the un-availability of substrates for adequate growth include maternal nutrient deficiencies, defective placentation, placental damage, fetal chromosomal mosaicism, reduced cell proliferation or cardiac output, and absence of the organs or glands that direct growth (Owens et al., 1995).

Table 6.2. Causes of human fetal growth restriction and consequences for the fetus and placenta

Initiating causes	Consequences for the placenta	Consequences for the fetus
Maternal or placental:		
Reduced substrate availability (oxygen and nutrients)	Reduced delivery of substrates, altered placental development	*In utero*: Hypoxemia, hypercapnia, hypoglycemia, acidosis, low concentration of essential amino acids; increased blood alanine, lactate, triglycerides; reduced plasma insulin, thyroid hormones, IGF-1, ACTH; increased plasma cortisol, IGFBP-1 *Perinatal*: Asphyxia, acidosis, hypoglycemia, normal or low birthweight, low ponderal index, soft tissue wasting
Defective placentation, placental damage	Reduced placental volume, weight, surface area; reduced uterine and/or umbilical blood flow; early maturation or slowing of growth; failure of normal ontogenic changes	
Fetal:		
Chromosomal mosaicism, reduced cell proliferation, absence of glands directing growth	Reduced substrate acquisition and delivery to tissues	Low growth velocity, low birth weight, reduced cell number in tissues, normal ponderal index

Source: Adapted from Owens et al., 1995.

The placenta affects fetal growth from the beginning of pregnancy by physiologic (Duvekot et al., 1995), metabolic, and endocrine mechanisms (Aldoretta and Hay, 1995; Garnica and Chan, 1996; Robinson et al., 1995). When the availability of substrates for growth is limited, the fetus must alter its metabolism and endocrine milieu to survive, and reducing its rate of growth is one possible adaptation (Harding, 1995). In fact, it has long been debated whether small size at birth represents a successful adaptation or a pathological finding (Warshaw,

1985). However, the excess mortality associated with IUGR is, alone, sufficient reason to try to prevent it.

It is noteworthy that even with the extensive ontogenic changes in the placenta during the latter half of pregnancy, which increase its transport capacity, fetal growth can still outstrip placental capacity for nutrient transfer (Schneider, 1996). Thus, even with normal growth of the placenta, there may be some fetal growth restriction in healthy pregnancies.

As expected from the pathways that result in IUGR, many factors could activate the mechanisms that produce fetal growth restriction. Established determinants of IUGR include infant sex, racial/ethnic origin, maternal and paternal height, obstetric history, previous LBW (either of the mother herself at her own birth or of an earlier infant), or IUGR (Klebanoff et al., 1997; Lumey, 1992) of the mother herself, prepregnant weight and weight gain during pregnancy, caloric intake during pregnancy, various morbidities, and use of tobacco and alcohol (Kramer, 1998). The relative importance of these factors in various settings is discussed below. A cautionary note: in spite of this well-developed list of risk factors for fetal growth restriction, it has been estimated that more than one-half of the infants with IUGR are not diagnosed until after birth (Langer et al., 1986). This statistic comes from research published before the widespread use of ultrasound, but the general concept that our ability to predict IUGR prenatally is imperfect remains valid.

The incidence of IUGR

By the latest estimates (de Onis et al., 1998), at least 13.7 million babies in developing countries are IUGR-LBW at birth, representing approximately 11% of the newborns in these countries. This contrasts with the rate of 2% for IUGR-LBW for developed countries. Of course, these figures underestimate the total number of growth-restricted babies born each year because they exclude those who are growth-restricted and have a birth weight above the 10th percentile for their gestational age.

The meaning of IUGR

Inasmuch as the statistical definition of IUGR creates the possibility of misclassification, investigators have sought additional ways of identifying those infants who are both small at birth and at risk of poor health or development. One approach has been to characterize IUGR as primary or secondary (Fay and Ellwood, 1993). Primary IUGR is a birth weight below the 10th percentile for gestational age with a normal ponderal index (a measure of adiposity relatively independent of length, defined as weight (g)/[length(cm)]$^3 \times 100$), also known as symmetrical growth restriction (Rosso and Winick, 1974; Villar and Belizán, 1982a). Secondary IUGR is a birth weight below the 10th percentile for gestational age with a low ponderal index, also known as asymmetrical growth restriction (Rosso and Winick, 1974; Villar and Belizán, 1982a). However, it is possible that these are merely the extremes of a continuum, with progressively increasing disproportionality occurring as the severity of growth restriction increases (Kramer et al., 1989, 1990b).

Research carried out in developed (Fay et al., 1991) and various developing countries (Adair and Popkin, 1988; Caulfield et al., 1991; Haas et al., 1987; Villar et al., 1982, 1984, 1990) suggests that the causes and consequences of these two types of IUGR differ. However, Kramer and colleagues (1990a), working in a developed-country setting with more accurate estimates of gestational age, have not found this to be the case. Using data from the National Collaborative Perinatal Project, Conlisk and colleagues (submitted for publication) have recently used body proportionality to explain the paradox of the lower neonatal mortality of African American than white infants at birth weights less than 2800 gm. Others (Chard et al., 1993) have questioned the validity of subtyping IUGR at all. Thus, although associations between body proportionality and short- and long-term outcomes among IUGR infants remain intriguing, further research is needed to clarify whether this classification is valid and useful. This issue is discussed in greater detail in Chapter 8.

We outlined another way of thinking about the meaning of small size at birth a number of years ago (Rasmussen et al., 1985), and these concepts are fundamental to this discussion. IUGR is most likely to be biologically important if it is in the causal pathway from some determinant of poor fetal growth to an adverse consequence of that poor fetal growth (Figure 6.3). An example of such a determinant of IUGR is pregnancy-induced hypertension; it causes both IUGR and preterm birth with predictable consequences for mortality. Similarly, IUGR may be in the causal pathway from a determinant of restricted fetal growth, but there may be no adverse consequence of this seemingly poor fetal growth. An example of such a determinant of IUGR is female sex of the fetus. Other examples include low maternal height or intergenerational IUGR among women of high socioeconomic status.

Other possibilities are important to consider because they are quite common. IUGR may appear to be in the causal pathway from a determinant to an adverse consequence, but the determinant of IUGR may also be the determinant of the adverse consequence. In this case, IUGR is a proxy for the determinant, and is not the only or necessarily even the most important cause of the infant's poor outcome. An example of this situation is poverty, which can be the cause of small maternal size, poor diet and poor weight gain during pregnancy, and other

Causal inference and IUGR

*IUGR is the causal pathway from determinant to an
adverse outcome*

PIH ⟶ IUGR ⟶ Excess mortality

*IUGR is the causal pathway from determinant to an
outcome without adverse consequences*

Female sex of fetus ⟶ IUGR

*IUGR is the causal pathway from determinant to
adverse outcome, but is a proxy for a factor that causes
both the determinant and the outcome*

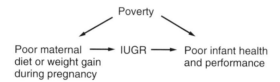

Figure 6.3   Diagram of the various ways IUGR may function between determinants and consequences.

outcomes. These are the proximal causes of the infant's small size at birth, but it may be the conditions of poverty into which that child is born that are responsible for his or her later poor health and development.

Lastly, IUGR may occur without identifiable antecedent determinants or any known adverse consequences. In fact, about one-third of IUGR births occur in the absence of any of the known risk factors for this condition (Galbraith et al., 1979). This proportion of IUGR infants accounts for most of the misclassification rate described above (i.e., those who are have grown to their full biological potential and are genetically small).

Thus, being small at birth is not necessarily a problem that needs a solution. What requires our action, however, is that proportion of fetal growth restriction that both has adverse consequences and is preventable. This preventable proportion of IUGR is strongly related to maternal nutritional status and, more generally, to poor living conditions.

Determinants of IUGR in various settings

Unlike the prematurity rate, which varies by a factor of two between developed and developing countries, the IUGR rate varies more than six-fold (Villar and Belizán, 1982b). In developing-country settings, IUGR accounts for a far higher proportion of LBW infants than does premature birth (Villar and Belizán, 1982b). In his exhaustive and informative review of the literature on IUGR and preterm birth, Kramer (1987) showed that the relative importance (etiologic fraction or population attributable risk) of the determinants of IUGR was different in the resource-poor conditions that characterize developing countries than in developed-country settings.

Many of the causes of fetal growth restriction in poor environments are amenable to intervention, but only a subset of these causes are amenable to interventions begun during pregnancy. For example, to correct short maternal (or paternal) stature, intervention would have to begin in childhood; to correct low prepregnant weight, intervention would have to begin before conception. However, other causes respond to interventions after conception. These include low caloric intake during pregnancy, poor maternal weight gain, and malaria. Other factors, such as female sex of the fetus, maternal non-white race, and obstetric history (parity and prior history of LBW), are not changeable.

Kramer's (1987) analysis revealed that most of the same factors cause IUGR in industrialized and developing countries. However, their relative importance is often different. For example, the etiologic fraction of IUGR that is attributable to non-white race is much smaller in an industrialized setting. Short stature, low pre-pregnant weight, and low caloric intake or weight gain also account for somewhat smaller etiologic fractions of IUGR. In an industrialized setting, malaria as a cause is eliminated, but cigarette smoking appears and is the single largest contributor to IUGR. In a recent update of this analysis, Kramer (1998) showed that, in addition, alcohol/drug use and pre-eclampsia cause a substantial proportion of the IUGR in industrialized countries.

Nutrition-related causes of IUGR

Nutrition-related conditions seem most amenable to change once pregnancy has begun, and effects of nutrition interventions are likely to be detectable in developing-country settings. Interventions designed to raise birth weight by increasing low dietary intake during pregnancy have had variable success. For example, in a four-village study in highland Guatemala conducted during the 1970s, the effect of food supplementation on birth weight was estimated as 25 gm/10 000 additional kcal consumed during pregnancy (Lechtig et al., 1975). Supplementation studies conducted in other locations also have reported effect sizes of this or higher magnitude (Lechtig and Klein, 1981). Other analyses of the data from Guatemala suggest that the improvement in birth weight resulted from an increase in the length of gestation (Delgado et al., 1982) rather than a reduction in IUGR (Villar et al., 1986), but these findings require cautious interpretation. Few other investigations have considered IUGR separately from preterm birth, much less IUGR separately from LBW, so little information on the amelioration of IUGR per se by nutritional supplementation is actually available.

Two supplementation trials provide data with which to evaluate the usefulness of improving maternal nutritional status before conception. In one, which was carried out in Taiwan during the 1960s, supplementation began after one birth and continued until the next. This dietary treatment did not increase the birth weight of the second compared to the first sibling (Adair and Pollitt, 1985). In the Guatemalan study described above, however, women with consistently high intakes of a food supplement during a first study pregnancy, during lactation, and also during the next study pregnancy, had babies whose birth weights were 301 gm higher than women whose intake of the food supplement was low during all three of these periods (Villar and Rivera, 1988). It is not known whether the supplement acted by increasing maternal weight or whether it prevented preterm birth or reduced IUGR.

In developed countries, evidence that interventions during pregnancy can eliminate the IUGR attributable to low pre-pregnant weight (or low body mass index) and poor weight gain during pregnancy is more difficult to obtain. Supplementation trials specifically designed to improve weight gain during pregnancy and birth weight have not been especially successful in the United States (Adams et al., 1978; Paige et al., 1981; Rush et al., 1980) or the United Kingdom (Atton and Watney, 1990; Doyle et al., 1992; Viegas et al., 1982a,b).

In the United States, nutrition supplementation during pregnancy has been evaluated in the context of a major food supplementation program. Rush and colleagues showed that participation in the Special Supplemental Food Program for Women, Infants and Children (WIC) had a small (but statistically significant) effect on birth weight (Rush et al., 1988a,b) and also had a positive effect on another measure of IUGR, head circumference (Rush et al., 1988b). Increases in birth weight were larger among less educated white women than among the sample as a whole (Rush et al., 1988a).

In addition, there is evidence among adolescents for an improvement in birth weight in response to more adequate levels of prenatal care, primarily through adequate weight gain. However, this effect seems to result primarily from a reduction in preterm delivery, not IUGR (Scholl et al., 1987). These same researchers have shown that the attributable risk for a small-for-gestational-age birth was 12.3% with inadequate total weight gain and more than double this when weight gain was inadequate early or late or during both periods of gestation (Hediger et al., 1989). This finding suggests that interventions, including prenatal care, that are successful in increasing weight gain should be successful in reducing small-for-gestational-age births.

Although Kramer's analysis (1987) of the etiologic fraction of IUGR attributable to various causes has been helpful in focusing attention on those causes that could be ameliorated by interventions at various stages during a woman's lifetime, it is important to note that this analysis included only the most *immediate* causes of IUGR. More distal determinants of IUGR, such as socioeconomic status, were not explicitly included because they are associated with more than one of the more immediate causes of IUGR. Nonetheless, disparities in socioeconomic status between population groups in industrialized countries remain a concern. In his recent analysis, Kramer (1998) proposed that an important portion of the observed socioeconomic gradient in IUGR in developed countries is primarily attributable to cigarette smoking, low gestational weight gain, and short stature. Alcohol, drug abuse, and maternal work and physical activity may explain an additional, small portion of this socioeconomic gradient. In a recent exploratory analysis, Roberts (1997) showed that community-level characteristics associated with poverty are negatively associated with birth weight and contended that such economic and structural factors limit the ability of individual women to optimize birth weight.

Non-nutritional causes of IUGR

The non-nutritional causes of IUGR with the highest etiologic fraction are cigarette smoking, pregnancy-induced hypertension, and use of alcohol and other drugs. The major drugs of abuse during pregnancy (nicotine, morphine, and cocaine) cause fetal growth restriction by depressing active uptake of amino acids by the placenta and their transplacental transport (Rama Sastry, 1991). Carbon monoxide and other tobacco gases induce placental hypoxia and depress energy-dependent processes in the placenta and fetus (Rama Sastry, 1991). Cigarette smoking has the highest population attributable risk of IUGR of any factor in developed countries (Kramer, 1998). The etiologic fraction of IUGR that is attributable to the use of alcohol or other drugs is much lower than that for smoking (Kramer, 1998). For more than two decades, ethanol has been recognized as an inhibitor of fetal growth, particularly in weight and head circumference. An overall decline in ethanol consumption by pregnant women (down from 32% in 1985 to 20% in 1988) has been reported (Serdula et al., 1991). The most recent data show that alcohol consumption among pregnant women reached a nadir of 12% in 1991, but by 1995 had begun to increase again, reaching 16% (CDC, 1997). Use of alcohol has remained highest among smokers (37%) and the unmarried (28%) women who are already at high risk of bearing growth-restricted fetuses (Serdula et al., 1991). Smoking and the use of alcohol and other drugs during pregnancy are also discussed in several other chapters, particularly Chapter 2.

Smoking

Despite its widely known adverse effects on fetal growth and pregnancy outcome, 25–30% of American women still smoke during pregnancy (Floyd et al., 1993). Both smoking cessation and improved maternal food intake have been examined as ways to prevent the IUGR associated with maternal smoking during pregnancy. Smoking cessation is the more important of these approaches because it eliminates both the nutritional and non-nutritional routes by which smoking causes fetal growth restriction.

Unfortunately, in a national sample only 27% of smokers quit spontaneously when they found out they were pregnant, and only another 12% later during pregnancy (Fingerhut et al., 1990). Even the best smoking cessation programs report only a 50% increase over the spontaneous quit rate (Floyd et al., 1993). In addition, more than 20% of those who quit start smoking again later in gestation (Quinn et al., 1991). In view of the fact that about one-third of women receive no guidance from their health care providers about the importance of not smoking during pregnancy (Kogan et al., 1994), the vast majority of women who smoke at conception are still smoking at delivery (Floyd et al., 1993). In a study conducted in Sweden, factors that were associated with continuing to smoke during pregnancy included high parity, not living with the infant's father, having been a heavy smoker, and daily passive smoking at home (Cnattingius et al., 1992).

In a meta-analysis of the randomized trials of prenatal smoking cessation, Dolan-Mullen and colleagues (1994) concluded that such programs do increase the rate of smoking cessation and simultaneously reduce the rate of LBW. Quitting at any time during pregnancy appears to increase birth weight, but quitting early produces the largest improvement in birth weight compared to continuing to smoke (Macarthur and Knox, 1988). Women who smoke during the second and third trimester of pregnancy have about the same elevation in risk of delivering a small-for-gestational-age baby as those who smoke throughout pregnancy (Lieberman et al., 1994). The risk of having a small baby increases with the number of cigarettes smoked in the last trimester (Lieberman et al., 1994).

The interaction of maternal nutritional status, dietary intake, and smoking on IUGR is not straightforward. Women who smoke tend to be thinner before conception and to gain less weight during pregnancy than those who do not smoke. They also consume a less nutritious diet (IOM, 1991). Being obese before conception (Hellerstedt et al., 1997) or increasing energy intake (Muscati et al., 1996) or weight gain (Hellerstedt et al., 1997) during pregnancy reduces, but does not eliminate, growth-restricting effects of cigarette smoking.

Taken together, these findings argue that reduction of the IUGR attributable to smoking during pregnancy will require including both nutritional counseling and smoking cessation programs as part of prenatal care (Rasmussen and Abrams, 1997).

Pregnancy-induced hypertension

Recent research demonstrates a continuous inverse association between fetal growth and maternal blood pressure throughout the range of blood pressures observed in normal pregnancies (Churchill et al., 1997). It has long been thought that blood pressures within the hypertensive range were associated with fetal growth restriction (Naeye, 1981). However, a recent review of this literature identified substantial variability between studies in the relationship between hypertension during pregnancy and fetal growth restriction (Misra, 1996). Although its name has changed over the last several decades from toxemia to pre-eclampsia/eclampsia and now to pregnancy-induced hypertension, this condition remains "the disease of theories." Zuspan (1991) even contends that pre-eclampsia "more likely than not, is a birth defect acquired at the time of implantation, and hence, it is not preventable." In fact, it has proved difficult to prevent pregnancy-induced hypertension and the fetal growth restriction that is so strongly associated with it. This condition is six to eight times more frequent among nulliparas than among parous women, and five times more frequent among twin pregnancies than among those with singleton pregnancies (NHBPEP, 1997). Maternal age under 20 years is also an important predictor of the development of pre-eclampsia (Saftlas et al., 1990). Other risk factors include high body mass and African American race (but only among nulliparas) (Eskenazi et al., 1991). A more detailed discussion of pregnancy-induced hypertension can be found in Chapter 1.

Many possible etiologies have been proposed, and therapies as diverse as supplementation with calcium or the use of low-dose aspirin have been tried recently. Calcium lowers blood pressure (Hamet, 1995), supplemental calcium lowers blood pressure in pregnant women (Repke and Villar, 1991), and supplemental calcium prevents hypertensive disorders of pregnancy without changing birth weight or the rate of preterm delivery (Belizán et al., 1991; Carroli et al., 1994). As noted in Chapter 4, low-dose aspirin has not been uniformly successful in preventing pregnancy-induced hypertension. An early meta-analysis concluded that this treatment reduced the risk of pregnancy-induced hypertension and very low birth weight (Imperiale and Petrulis, 1991), but a more recent study of the data is less supportive of this therapy, particularly for women at low risk of the disease (Italian Study, 1993; Villar and Bergsjo, 1996).

Cocaine

The mechanisms by which cocaine causes fetal growth restriction are well understood (Dicke et al., 1993; Rama Sastry, 1991). This drug is a potent predictor of fetal growth restriction (as well as of prematurity and other complications of pregnancy). However, despite the seeming epidemic of cocaine use in inner-city populations, where up to 15% of women may admit to cocaine use during pregnancy (Streissguth et al., 1991), the etiologic fraction remains small because population-based surveys identify a low proportion (1% or less) of affected mother–infant dyads (Weathers et al., 1993). Most cocaine use in pregnancy is identified by a positive drug screen of the mother (often late in pregnancy or at delivery because drug-abusing women often participate poorly or not at all in prenatal care) or of her newborn infant. Thus, prevention of the fetal growth restriction that results from the use of cocaine is difficult indeed.

Targeting nutritional interventions to prevent IUGR

Targeting of nutritional interventions for optimal performance in the prevention of fetal growth restriction requires consideration of three factors: what is to be given, when it is to be given, and to whom. It is axiomatic that women should be provided with an intervention that is relevant to their condition (e.g., a food supplement containing those nutrients that are thought to be lacking in their diets).

Timing of interventions also may be an important factor in their success. In distinguishing between symmetrical and asymmetrical growth restriction, Villar and Belizán (1982a) developed the "timing hypothesis," in which they proposed that insults that occur at a particular period during pregnancy were more likely to result in one or the other form of IUGR. This hypothesis led to the concept that maternal supplementation during the last trimester of pregnancy (when fetal fat gain is the fastest) would be more effective in raising birth weight than supplementation earlier in pregnancy (when maternal fat gain is the fastest). Supplementation trials have therefore focused on increasing maternal intake in the third trimester of pregnancy, although the effects on birth weight have often been disappointing.

More recent research suggests that the maternal gain of fat or weight earlier in pregnancy is an even more important determinant of birth weight than that later in pregnancy. For example, healthy Guatemalan women who gained more fat early in pregnancy had larger infants than those who gained less fat during this period (Villar et al., 1992). Among low-income, pregnant teenagers in New Jersey, those whose early weight gain was inadequate were more likely to have an IUGR infant than those whose early weight gain was adequate (Hediger et al., 1989). Finally, using data from the supplementation trial carried out among undernourished Guatemalan women, Li and colleagues (1997) have recently shown that each kilogram of maternal weight gain during the second trimester of pregnancy produces almost a three-fold larger increase in birth weight than does a similar

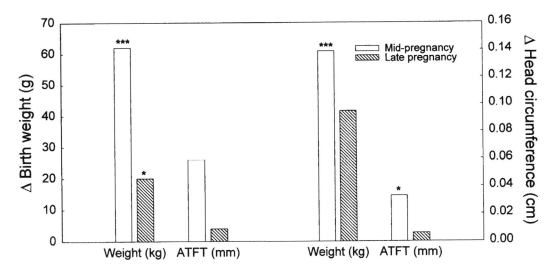

Change in maternal anthropometric measure

Figure 6.4   Association of change during mid- or late pregnancy in maternal weight or anterior thigh fatfold thickness (ATFT) with change in birth weight (left) and head circumference (right). Partial regression coefficients are graphed; * $P < 0.05$, *** $P < 0.001$ (Li et al., 1997).

maternal weight gain in the third trimester (62 gm compared to 26 gm, respectively) (Figure 6.4). The difference between trimesters in birth weight was even more extreme for changes in fatfold thickness of the maternal thigh. This concept, that the timing of the insult or the intervention to correct it matters, has proved valuable, and suggests that future supplementation of women should begin earlier in pregnancy if it is to have the maximum positive impact on birth weight.

Although much of the available literature has concentrated on who is at risk of delivering a small infant, a more useful approach for targeting scarce resources is to consider who will benefit from an intervention. Our analysis of the supplementation study in Guatemala showed that supplemental energy had a greater effect on birth weight among women who had lower skinfold thicknesses, greater knee breadths, and a lower proportion of prior fetal deaths; who were literate; and who were not lactating at the time of conception (Olson, 1994). Unfortunately, this analysis did not distinguish whether the higher birth weight resulted from a longer period of gestation or a reduction in fetal growth restriction. Analyses of data from other supplementation trials reveal that birth weight increased more among women of lower as compared to higher initial weight-for-height [urban setting, Bogotá, Colombia (Herrera et al., 1980)] and among women who delivered in the wet as compared to the dry season [rural setting, Keneba, The Gambia (Prentice et al., 1987)].

The women who participated in the trials in developed countries were selected because they met one or more criteria for risk of having a LBW infant. The results of these studies confirmed that women who are at risk of having a bad outcome of pregnancy are not necessarily those who will benefit most from the intervention. Those who benefited the most included those under 16 years of age (Paige et al., 1981), those whose triceps skinfold thickness increased the most at mid-pregnancy (Viegas et al., 1987; Viegas et al., 1982a), smokers (Rush et al., 1980), and paradoxically, non-smokers (Paige et al., 1981).

Our research in laboratory rats (Fellows, 1985) and secondary data analysis using data from the Guatemala trial (Olson, 1994; Winkvist, 1992) suggest that nutrient partitioning between mother and infant changes with maternal nutritional status. In particular, individuals who were more malnourished will respond to food supplements with increased birth weight, whereas those who are better nourished will gain more themselves without much change in the birth weight of their infants. For example, data from the Olson study (1994) showed that increasing the level of supplement intake from low to high among women in the lowest quartile of subscapular skinfold thickness resulted in an 380 gm increase in their infant's birth weight, but a 300 gm loss in their own weight. In contrast, increasing the level of supplement intake from low to high among women in the highest quartile of subscapular skinfold thickness resulted in only an 80 gm increase in their infant's birth weight, but a 301 gm gain in their own weight.

It is possible, therefore, that some of the lack of effect of the trials in industrialized countries results from the fact that the supplemented women, while undernourished in comparison to others in their community, were not so undernourished that fetal growth restriction was a likely outcome.

Conclusion

Studies of the causes and consequences of small size at birth remain plagued by the inadequacies of the statistical approach to defining IUGR. Eliminating this misclassification would remove infants who are not actually growth restricted (i.e., they are genetically small and healthy) and would also identify those infants who are actually growth restricted but whose birth weight is above the 10th percentile for their gestational age. Some tools are now available for identifying the former but not the latter group, which remains essentially unstudied.

This chapter has focused on the most immediate determinants of IUGR in a range of settings. There is a discrepancy between our knowledge of the physiology of how fetal growth restriction is produced and how to prevent its occurrence. A high proportion of the preventable etiologic fraction of IUGR in developing country settings is related to maternal nutrition, and supplementation trials in this setting reveal an increase in birth weight. A smaller proportion of the preventable etiologic fraction of IUGR in developed country settings is related to maternal nutrition, and supplementation trials in this setting reveal negligible improvement in birth weight. When interventions are scaled up from a research trial to a public health program (e.g., WIC), it remains, not surprisingly, difficult to demonstrate a reduction in fetal growth restriction. Part of the explanation for these disparate findings may lie in differential partitioning of nutrients between mother and fetus as maternal nutritional status improves.

The largest proportion of the preventable etiologic fraction of IUGR in developed country settings is non-nutritional. Unfortunately, we lack information about how to prevent the growth restriction that results from pregnancy-induced hypertension and how to reduce smoking and drug and alcohol use/abuse effectively during pregnancy. Smoking cessation programs and nutritional counseling remain important to include in prenatal care.

Acknowledgment

The author is indebted to Dr. Jean-Pierre Habicht for constructive criticism of an earlier draft of this document.

REFERENCES

Adair LS, Pollitt E. Outcome of maternal nutritional supplementation: a comprehensive review of the Bacon Chow study. American Journal of Clinical Nutrition 1985; **41**: 948–78.

Adair LS, Popkin BM. Birth weight, maturity and proportionality in Filipino infants. Human Biology 1988; **60**: 319–39.

Adams SO, Barr GD, Huenemann RL. Effect of nutritional supplementation in pregnancy. I. Outcome of pregnancy. Journal of the American Dietetic Association 1978; **72**: 144–7.

Aldoretta PW, Hay WW Jr. Metabolic substrates for fetal energy metabolism and growth. Clinics in Perinatology 1995; **22**: 15–36.

Alexander GR, Himes JH, Kaufman RB, Mor J, Kogan M. A United States national reference for fetal growth. Obstetrics and Gynecology 1996; **87**: 163–8.

Altman DG, Hytten FE. Intrauterine growth retardation: let's be clear about it. British Journal of Obstetrics and Gynæcology 1989; **96**: 1127–32.

Atton C, Watney PJM. Selective supplementation in pregnancy: effect on birth weight. Journal of Human Nutrition and Dietetics 1990; **3**: 381–92.

Belizán J, Villar J, Gonzalez L, Campodonico L, Bergel E. Calcium supplementation to prevent hypertensive disorders of pregnancy. New England Journal of Medicine 1991; **325**: 1399–405.

Carroli G, Duley L, Belizan J, Villar J. Calcium supplementation during pregnancy: a systematic review of randomised controlled trials. British Journal of Obstetrics and Gynaecology 1994; **101**: 753–8.

Caulfield LE, Haas JD, Belizán J, Rasmussen KM, Edmonston B. Differences in early postnatal morbidity risk by pattern of fetal growth in Argentina. Pædiatric and Perinatal Epidemiology 1991; **5**: 263–75.

Centers for Disease Control and Prevention (CDC). Alcohol consumption among pregnant and childbearing-aged women – United States, 1991 and 1995. Morbidity and Mortality Weekly Report 1997; **46**(16): 346–50.

Chard T, Young A, Macintosh M. The myth of fetal growth retardation at term. British Journal of Obstetrics and Gynæcology 1993; **100**: 1076–81.

Churchill D, Perry IJ, Beevers DC. Ambulatory blood pressure in pregnancy and fetal growth. Lancet 1997; **349**: 7–10.

Cnattingius S, Lindmark G, Meirik O. Who continues to smoke while pregnant? Journal of Epidemiology and Community Health 1992; **46**: 218–21.

Conlisk EA, Haas JD, Habicht J-P. Body proportionality and the paradox of black–white differences in birthweight-specific neonatal mortality. Submitted for publication.

de Onis M, Bolanos F, Villar J. Levels and patterns of intrauterine growth retardation in developing countries. European Journal of Clinical Nutrition 1998; **52**(S1): S5–S15.

Delgado H, Martorell R, Brineman E, Klein RE. Nutrition and length of gestation. Nutrition Research 1982; **2**: 117–26.

Dicke JM, Verges DK, Polakoski KL. Cocaine inhibits alanine uptake by human placenta microvillus membrane vesicles. American Journal of Obstetrics and Gynecology 1993; **169**: 515–21.

Dolan-Mullen P, Ramírez G, Groff JY. A meta-analysis of randomized trials of prenatal smoking cessation interventions. American Journal of Obstetrics and Gynecology 1994; **171**: 1328–34.

Doyle W, Wynn AHA, Crawford MA, Wynn SW. Nutritional counselling and supplementation in the second and third trimester of pregnancy, a study in a London population. Journal of Nutritional Medicine 1992; **3**: 249–56.

Duvekot JJ, Cheriex EC, Pieters FAA, Menheere PPCA, Schouten HJA, Peeters LLH. Maternal volume homeostasis in early pregnancy in relation to fetal growth restriction. Obstetrics and Gynecology 1995; **85**: 361–7.

Eskenazi B, Fenster L, Sidney S. A multivariate analysis of risk factors for preeclampsia. Journal of the American Medical Association 1991; **266**: 237–41.

Fay RA, Dey PL, Saadie CMJ, Buhl JA, Gebski VJ. Ponderal index: a better definition of the "at risk" group with intrauterine growth problems than birth-weight for gestational age in term infants. Australian and New Zealand Journal of Obstetrics and Gynæcology 1991; **31**: 17–19.

Fay RA, Ellwood DA. Categories of intrauterine growth retardation. Fetal–Maternal Medicine Review 1993; **5**: 203–12.

Fellows WD. Partition of nutrients between dam and fetuses in rats underfed acutely and chronically. M.S. thesis. Ithaca (NY): Cornell University, 1985.

Fingerhut LA, Kleinman JC, Kendrick JS. Smoking before, during, and after pregnancy. American Journal of Public Health 1990; **80**: 541–4.

Floyd RL, Rimer BK, Giovino GA, Mullen PD, Sullivan SE. A review of smoking in pregnancy: effects on pregnancy outcomes and cessation efforts. Annual Review of Public Health 1993; **14**: 379–411.

Galbraith RS, Karchman EJ, Piercy WN, Low JA. The clinical prediction of intrauterine growth retardation. American Journal of Obstetrics and Gynecology 1979; **133**: 281–6.

Garnica AD, Chan W. The role of the placenta in fetal nutrition and growth. Journal of the American College of Nutrition 1996; **15**: 206–22.

Goldenberg RL, Davis RO, Cutter GR, Hoffman HJ, Brumfield CG, Foster JM. Prematurity, postdates, and growth retardation: the influence of use of ultrasonography on reported gestational age. American Journal of Obstetrics and Gynecology 1989a; **160**: 462–70.

Goldenberg RL, Cutter GR, Hoffman HJ, Foster JM, Nelson KG, Hauth JC. Intrauterine growth retardation: standards for diagnosis. American Journal of Obstetrics and Gynecology 1989b; **161**: 271–7.

Haas JD, Balcazar H, Caulfield LE. Variation in early neonatal mortality for different types of fetal growth retardation. American Journal of Physical Anthropology 1987; **73**: 467–73.

Hamet P. The evaluation of the scientific evidence for a relationship between calcium and hypertension. Journal of Nutrition 1995; **125**: 311S–400S.

Harding JE, Johnston BM. Nutrition and fetal growth. Reproduction, Fertility, and Development 1995; **7**: 539–47.

Hediger ML, Scholl TO, Belsky DH, Ances IG, Salmon RW. Patterns of weight gain in adolescent pregnancy: effects on birth weight and preterm delivery. Obstetrics and Gynecology 1989; **74**: 6–12.

Hellerstedt WL, Himes JH, Story M, Alton IR, Edwards LE. Effects of cigarette smoking and gestational weight gain on birth outcomes in obese and normal-weight women. American Journal of Public Health 1997; **87**: 591–6.

Herrera MG, Mora JO, de Paredes B, Wagner M. Maternal weight/height and the effect of food supplementation during pregnancy and lactation. In: Aebi H, Whitehead R, eds. Maternal Nutrition During Pregnancy and Lactation. Bern: Hans Huber Publishers, 1980: 252–3.

Imperiale TF, Petrulis AS. A meta-analysis of low-dose aspirin for the prevention of pregnancy-induced hypertensive disease. Journal of the American Medical Association 991; **266**: 261–5.

Institute of Medicine (IOM), Subcommittee on Nutrition During Lactation, Committee on Nutrition During Pregnancy and Lacation, Food and Nutrition Board. Washington, DC: National Academy Press, 1991.

Italian Study of Aspirin in Pregnancy. Low-dose aspirin in prevention and treatment of intrauterine growth retardation and pregnancy-induced hypertension. Lancet 1993; **341**: 396–400.

Klebanoff MA, Schulsinger C, Mednick BR, Secher NJ. Preterm and small-for-gestational-age birth across generations. American Journal of Obstetrics and Gynecology 1997; **176**: 521–36.

Kogan MD, Kotelchuck M, Alexander GR, Johnson WE. Racial disparities in reported prenatal care advice from health care providers. American Journal of Public Health 1994; **84**: 82–8.

Kramer MS. Intrauterine growth and gestational duration determinants. Pediatrics 1987; **80**: 502–11.

Kramer MS. Socioeconomic determinants of intrauterine growth retardation. European Journal of Clinical Nutrition 1998; **52**(S1): S29–S33.

Kramer MS, McLean FH, Olivier M, Willis DM, Usher RH. Body proportionality and head and length "sparing" in growth-retarded neonates: a critical reappraisal. Pediatrics 1989; **84**: 717–23.

Kramer MS, Olivier M, McLean FH, Dougherty GE, Willis DM, Usher RH. Determinants of fetal growth and body proportionality. Pediatrics 1990a; **86**: 18–26.

Kramer MS, Olivier M, McLean FH, Willis DM, Usher RH. Impact of intrauterine growth retardation and body proportionality on fetal and neonatal outcome. Pediatrics 1990; **86**: 707–13.

Lang JM, Lieberman E, Cohen AP. A comparison of risk factors for preterm labor and term small-for-gestational-age birth. Epidemiology 1996; **7**: 369–76.

Langer O, Damus K, Maiman M, Divon M, Levy J, Bauman W. A link between relative hypoglycemia–hypoinsulinemia during oral glucose tolerance tests and intrauterine growth retardation. American Journal of Obstetrics and Gynecology 1986; **155**: 711–16.

Lechtig A, Delgado H, Lasky R, et al. Maternal nutrition and fetal growth in developing countries. American Journal of Diseases of Children 1975; **129**: 553–6.

Lechtig A, Klein RE. Prenatal nutrition and birth weight: is there a causal association? In: Dobbing J, ed. Maternal nutrition in pregnancy – eating for two? New York: Academic Press, 1981: 131–92.

Li R, Haas J, Habicht J-P. The critical period of maternal nutritional influence during pregnancy on fetal growth. FASEB Journal 1997; **11**: A398(abst).

Lieberman E, Gremy I, Lang JM, Cohen AP. Low birthweight at term and the timing of fetal exposure to maternal smoking. American Journal of Public Health 1994; **84**: 1127–31.

Lumey LH. Decreased birthweights in infants after maternal *in utero* exposure to the Dutch famine of 1944–1945. Pædiatric and Perinatal Epidemiology 1992; **6**: 240–53.

Macarthur C, Knox EG. Smoking in pregnancy: effects of stopping at different stages. British Journal of Obstetrics and Gynæcology 1988; **95**: 551–5.

Misra DP. The effect of the pregnancyinduced hypertension on fetal growth: a review of the literature. Pædiatric and Perinatal Epidemiology 1996; **10**: 244–63.

Mongelli M, Gardosi J. Reduction of false-positive diagnosis of fetal growth restriction by application of customized fetal growth standards. Obstetrics and Gynecology 1996; **88**: 844–8.

Muscati SK, Koski KG, Gray-Donald K. Increased energy intake in pregnant smokers does not prevent human fetal growth retardation. Journal of Nutrition 1996; **126**: 2984–9.

Naeye RL. Maternal blood pressure and fetal growth. American Journal of Obstetrics and Gynecology 1981; **141**: 780–7.

National High Blood Pressure Education Program (NHBPEP). Working Group Report on High Blood Pressure in Pregnancy. 1997; No. 91–3029: (abst).

Olson RK. Developing indicators that predict benefit from prenatal energy supplementation. Ph.D. dissertation. Ithaca (NY): Cornell University, 1994.

Owens JA, Owens PC, Robinson JS. Experimental restriction of fetal growth. In: Anonymous Growth. New York: Cambridge University Press, 1995: 139–75.

Paige DM, Cordano A, Mellits ED, Baertl JM, Davis L. Nutritional supplementation of pregnant adolescents. Journal of Adolescent Health Care 1981; **1**: 261–7.

Pettersson R, Regnström N, Sterky G, Taube A. Birthweight distribution and socioeconomic variables. In: Sterky G, Mellander L, eds. Birthweight distribution – an indicator of social development. Uppsala: SAREC, 1978: 45–53.

Prentice AM, Cole TJ, Foord FJ, Lamb WH, Whitehead RG. Increased birthweight after prenatal dietary supplementation of rural African women. American Journal of Clinical Nutrition 1987; **46**: 912–25.

Quinn VP, Mullen PD, Ershoff DH. Women who stop smoking spontaneously prior to prenatal care and predictors of relapse before delivery. Addictive Behaviors 1991; **16**: 29–40.

Rama Sastry BV. Placental toxicology: tobacco smoke, abused drugs, multiple chemical interactions, and placental function. Reproduction, Fertility, and Development 1991; **3**: 355–72.

Rasmussen KM, Abrams B. Annotation: cigarette smoking, nutrition, and birthweight. American Journal of Public Health 1997; **87**: 543–4.

Rasmussen KM, Mock NB, Habicht J-P. The biological meaning of low birthweight and the use of data on low birthweight for nutritional surveillance. Cornell Nutritional Surveillance Program Working Paper Series No. 43. Ithaca, NY: Cornell University, 1985.

Repke JT, Villar J. Pregnancy-induced hypertension and low birth weight: the role of calcium. American Journal of Clinical Nutrition 1991; **54**: 237S–41S.

Roberts EM. Neighborhood social environments and the distribution of low birthweight in Chicago. American Journal of Public Health 1997; **87**: 597–603.

Robinson JS, Chidzanja S, Kind K, Lok F, Owens P, Owens J. Placental control of fetal growth. Reproduction, Fertility, and Development 1995; **7**: 333–44.

Rosso P, Winick M. Intrauterine growth retardation: a new systematic approach based on the clinical and biochemical characteristics of this condition. Journal of Perinatal Medicine 1974; **2**: 147–51.

Rush D, Alvir JM, Kenny DA, Johnson SS, Horvitz DG. III. Historical study of pregnancy outcomes. American Journal of Clinical Nutrition 1988a; **48**: 412–28.

Rush D, Sloan NL, Leighton J, et al. V. Longitudinal study of pregnant women. American Journal of Clinical Nutrition 1988b; **48**: 439–83.

Rush D, Stein Z, Susser M. A randomized controlled trial of prenatal nutritional supplementation in New York City. Pediatrics 1980; **65**: 683–97.

Saftlas AF, Olson DR, Franks AL, Atrash HK, Pokras R. Epidemiology of preeclampsia and eclampsia in the United States, 1979–1986. American Journal of Obstetrics and Gynecology 1990; **163**: 460–5.

Schneider H. Ontogenic changes in the nutritive function of the placenta. Placenta 1996; **17**: 15–26.

Scholl TO, Miller LK, Salmon JW, Cofsky MC, Shearer J. Prenatal care adequacy and the outcome of adolescent pregnancy: effects on weight gain, preterm delivery, and birth weight. Obstetrics and Gynecology 1987; **69**: 312–16.

Serdula M, Williamson DF, Kendrick JS, Anda RF, Byers T. Trends in alcohol consumption by pregnant women: 1985 through 1988. Journal of the American Medical Association 1991; **265**: 876–9.

Streissguth AP, Grant TM, Barr HM, et al. Cocaine and the use of alcohol and other drugs during pregnancy. American Journal of Obstetrics and Gynecology 1991; **164**: 1239–43.

Viegas OAC, Cole TJ, Wharton BA. Impaired fat deposition in pregnancy: an indicator for nutritional intervention. American Journal of Clinical Nutrition 1987; **45**: 23–8.

Viegas OAC, Scott PH, Cole TJ, Easton P, Needham PG, Wharton BA. Dietary protein energy supplementation of pregnant Asian mothers at Sorrento, Birmingham. II: Selective during third trimester only. British Journal of Medicine 1982a; **285**: 592–5.

Viegas OAC, Scott PH, Cole TJ, Mansfield HN, Wharton P, Wharton BA. Dietary protein energy supplementation of pregnant Asian mothers at Sorrento, Birmingham. I: Unselective during second and third trimesters. British Journal of Medicine 1982b; **285**: 589–92.

Villar J, Belizán JM. The timing factor in the pathophysiology of the intrauterine growth retardation syndrome. Obstetrical and Gynecological Survey 1982a; **37**: 499–506.

Villar J, Belizán J. The relative contribution of prematurity and fetal growth retardation to low birth weight in developing and developed countries. American Journal of Obstetrics and Gynecology 1982b; **143**: 793–8.

Villar J, Belizán J, Spalding J, Klein RE. Postnatal growth of intrauterine growth retarded infants. Early Human Development 1982; **6**: 265–71.

Villar J, Bergsjo P. Scientific basis for the content of routine antenatal care: I. Philosophy, recent studies, and power to eliminate or alleviate adverse maternal outcomes. Acta Obstetricia et Gynecologica Scandinavica 1996; **75**: 1–14.

Villar J, Cogswell M, Kestler E, Castillo P, Menendez P, Repke JT. Effect of fat and fat-free mass deposition during pregnancy on birth weight. American Journal of Obstetrics and Gynecology 1992; **167**: 1344–52.

Villar J, de Onis M, Kestler E, Bolanos F, Cerezo R, Berendes HW. The differential neonatal mortality of the intrauterine growth retardation syndrome. American Journal of Obstetrics and Gynecology 1990; **163**: 151–7.

Villar J, Khoury MJ, Finucane FF, Delgado H. Differences in the epidemiology of prematurity and intrauterine growth retardation. Early Human Development 1986; **14**: 307–20.

Villar J, Rivera J. Nutritional supplementation during two consecutive pregnancies and the interim lactation period: effect on birth weight. Pediatrics 1988; **81**: 51–7.

Villar J, Smeriglio V, Martorell R, Brown CH, Klein RE. Heterogeneous growth and mental development of intrauterine growth-retarded infants during the first 3 years of life. Pediatrics 1984; **74**: 783–91.

Warshaw JB. Intrauterine growth retardation: adaptation or pathology? Pediatrics 1985; **76**: 998–9.

Weathers WT, Crane MM, Sauvain KJ, Blackhurst DW. Cocaine use in women from a defined population: prevention at delivery and effects on growth of infants. Pediatrics 1993; **91**: 350–4.

WHO Expert Committee on Physical Status. Physical status: the use and interpretation of anthropometry. Geneva: World Health Organization, 1995.

Wilcox MA, Johnson IR, Maynard PV, Smith SJ, Chilvers CED. The individualised birthweight ratio: a more logical outcome measure of pregnancy than birthweight alone. British Journal of Obstetrics and Gynæcology 1993; **100**: 342–7.

Winkvist A. Maternal depletion among Pakistani and Guatemalan women. Ph.D. dissertation. Ithaca, NY: Cornell University, 1992.

Zuspan FP. New concepts in the understanding of hypertensive diseases during pregnancy: an overview. Clinics in Perinatology 1991; **18**: 653–9.

7

Impact of prenatal care on intrauterine growth restriction

Linda J. Heffner

Introduction

Intrauterine growth restriction (IUGR), a condition of poor intrauterine fetal growth, affects at least 200 000 pregnancies in the United States annually. It is a major cause of perinatal morbidity and mortality, accounting for over 30 000 fetal and neonatal deaths. Although the etiology of IUGR is complex and poorly understood, it can be recognized, evaluated, and treated, reducing perinatal mortality by over 50% (Hughey, 1984; Kurjak et al., 1980).

Prenatal care can have an important effect in four areas related to IUGR: prevention of unnecessary interventions for otherwise healthy, small infants; prevention of some cases of IUGR by treatment of maternal diseases and high-risk behaviors; diminution of perinatal morbidity and, perhaps, long-term morbidity associated with IUGR; and prevention of fetal death. This chapter describes these areas and details the prenatal care interventions that are most likely to reduce morbidity and mortality associated with IUGR, including accurate diagnosis of IUGR, early delivery, and prevention initiatives such as those related to sickle cell anemia, chronic hypertension, preventable congenital infections, and substance use.

Magnitude of the problem of IUGR

Theoretically, IUGR describes any fetus who fails to reach its full growth potential. Thus, in the strictest definition, the eight-pound term baby delivered of a multipara who previously has had ten-pound babies is likely to have a degree of growth restriction. These infants, however, are rarely at risk for intrauterine or neonatal morbidity or mortality. Instead, the classification of IUGR is usually reserved for those infants whose weight is less than the 10th percentile and who demonstrate other corroborative evidence of suboptimal prenatal growth, such as documented cessation of intrauterine growth, decreased amniotic fluid, or poor prenatal testing. In actuality, the majority of infants whose birth weight is less than the 10th

Table 7.1. Causes of intrauterine growth restriction and their prevalence

---

Genetic (5–15%)
    Chromosomal (aneuploidy) (2–5%)
    Single gene defects (3–10%)
Fetal anomalies (1–2%)
Multiple gestation (2–3%)
Congenital infection (5–10%)
Malnutrition
Drugs/toxins/smoking (15–30%)
Uteroplacental factors (25–30%)

Source: Creasy and Resnik, 1994.

percentile are not truly growth restricted but rather constitutionally small. The true incidence of IUGR is no more than 4 to 8% in developed countries (Creasey and Resnik, 1994). Table 7.1 lists the causes of IUGR and their prevalence.

Of the four million births annually in United States, about 10–12% are low birth weight (< 2500 gm). Of these low birth weight infants, about one-third suffer from IUGR. Perinatal mortality in IUGR is about four to ten times that of appropriately grown fetuses and is comparable to being born prematurely at 28 to 29 weeks of gestation (Callan and Witter, 1990; Galbraith et al., 1979; Hughey, 1984; Wennergren et al., 1988). If the IUGR is undetected during the pregnancy, perinatal mortality is ten to thirty times higher than that of appropriately grown fetuses and is comparable to being born at 27 weeks of gestation (Holzman and Paneth, 1994; Kramer et al., 1990). Fetuses with IUGR are at unusually high risk of stillbirth (Kramer, 1993).

Similarly, both short- and long-term morbidity are increased in IUGR. Fifty to eighty percent of fetuses with IUGR will demonstrate fetal distress in labor, requiring a high proportion of operative deliveries. At least 50% of neonates will experience morbidity in the nursery, including hypoglycemia, polycythemia, pulmonary hemorrhage, and meconium aspiration. The neonates delivered early to prevent stillbirth are at risk for all the morbidity associated with prematurity. Longitudinal follow-up of children born at term with IUGR demonstrates that at least twice as many of them have minimal cerebral dysfunction as do babies without IUGR (Allen, 1984). This rate is even higher if the infants were born preterm. Short- and long-term outcomes of IUGR are discussed further in Chapter 8.

The interventions that can improve health outcomes for growth-restricted infants will help many, but not all such infants. For example, pregnancies in which fetal growth is restricted because of a lethal chromosome aneuploidy will not benefit from prenatal attempts at fetal salvage. Similarly, early delivery of infants with a congenital infection will not improve the long-term outcome. For this reason, an important goal of prenatal care is the recognition of IUGR and identification of an etiology whenever possible. Targeted interventions can then be undertaken.

Interventions most likely to reduce morbidity and mortality from IUGR

Four basic steps reduce the morbidity and mortality of IUGR. These include: (1) detection of the fetus affected by IUGR; (2) correct diagnosis of the etiology of the IUGR; (3) prenatal testing for signs of intrauterine fetal deterioration; and (4) administration of prenatal steroids to those infants at risk of preterm birth. As noted above, detection of IUGR and determination of its etiology permits targeted interventions in those fetuses in which such interventions may improve outcome. Correct diagnosis of the etiology also prevents unnecessary or misdirected interventions. In cases of poor intrauterine perfusion, prenatal testing for fetal well-being permits prolongation of the pregnancy as long as possible, thereby reducing the risks of prematurity. In those infants at risk of premature delivery from IUGR, administration of prenatal corticosteroids may have a disproportionately beneficial effect on reducing the incidence of severe (grades III–IV) intraventricular hemorrhage (IVH), as demonstrated in a prospective observational study where prenatal corticosteroid administration reduced the incidence of severe IVH more in IUGR infants than in well-grown fetuses and in pre-eclamptic compared to normotensive pregnancies (Spinillo et al., 1995). A reduction in serious complications of prematurity in these pregnancies has the potential for dramatically reducing the long-term morbidity seen in the premature infant suffering from IUGR.

Impact of prenatal care on IUGR

Correct diagnosis of IUGR

Ultrasound is the only way to make the diagnosis of IUGR. There are two ways to use ultrasound to screen a population of pregnant women for those fetuses suffering from IUGR. One is to use selective ultrasound assessment based on maternal risk screening to identify factors, such as those in Table 7.2, that increase the probability of IUGR. The other is to routinely assess fetal growth by ultrasound in the third trimester.

Several large studies have compared the proportions of IUGR fetuses detected using the two methods. Routine application of three ultrasounds at 20, 30, and 36

Table 7.2. Maternal risk factors for IUGR

- Hypertension, both chronic and pregnancy-associated
- Multiple gestation
- IUGR in a previous pregnancy
- Antiphospholipid antibody carrier
- Poor maternal weight gain in small women
- Previously unrecognized proteinuria
- Severe maternal anemia
- Drug abuse, including heavy cigarette smoking in older women
- Failure of the maternal fundus to grow or a size/date discrepancy of $\geqslant$ 4 cm
- Diabetes with vascular disease

weeks to a study population of 1600 women improved the detection rate to 57% from the 23% detected in the 13 000 risk-screened women. However, perinatal outcome, including mortality, low Apgar scores, cesarean section rates and mean gestational age at delivery did not differ between the groups (Hughey, 1984). In this population, three of four perinatal deaths that occurred in the routine ultrasound group were in women who were not compliant with their prenatal care. A second, similar study showed a smaller improvement in detection of IUGR with routine ultrasound (74.5%) compared to risk-based screening (54.6%) with no improvement in perinatal mortality (Holmquist et al., 1986). A third study in Scandinavia also increased detection using serial third trimester ultrasounds in the study population without affecting perinatal outcome (Larsen et al, 1992).

Routine ultrasound screening of women at low risk of IUGR is limited by the utility of a single ultrasound to correctly diagnose IUGR in a low-prevalence population. When looking at the function of a screening test, such as ultrasound, in making the diagnosis, one needs to look not only at how many of the affected fetuses are identified by that parameter (sensitivity), but at how well the test excludes fetuses without the problem (specificity). Assuming a prevalence of IUGR of 10%, Benson et al. (1986), from our institution, calculated the sensitivity, specificity, and predictive value of the estimated fetal weight (EFW), amniotic fluid volume, and head circumference/abdominal circumference ratio derived from an ultrasound in diagnosing IUGR in the third trimester (Table 7.3).

Given that the true prevalence of IUGR in the overall obstetrical population is lower than 10%, there is limited utility in a single ultrasound in diagnosing IUGR. Sequential ultrasounds in the low-risk population will increase the detection rate of IUGR, but without improving perinatal outcome. In populations at high risk of IUGR, single ultrasound scans have improved utility in the detection of IUGR. The highest sensitivity and specificity is found in serial scans in high-risk patients. Failure of the fetus to grow over a matter of weeks or the onset of oligohydramnios

Table 7.3. Value of single ultrasound parameters in predicting IUGR (assuming 10% prevalence of IUGR)

	Sensitivity (%)	Specificity (%)	Predictive value positive (%)	Predictive value negative (%)
Low estimated fetal weight	89	88	45	99
Oligohydramnios	24	98	55	92
Elevated head circumference/abdominal circumference	82	94	62	98

Source: Benson et al., 1986.

in the presence of a small fetus strongly support the diagnosis of IUGR. Conversely, linear growth and maintenance of a normal amniotic fluid volume over time suggests that a fetus is constitutionally small and not affected by a pathologic process.

In addition to documenting the presence of a small fetus, prenatal ultrasound is critical in establishing the etiology of the IUGR. The presence of anomalies in an IUGR fetus strongly suggests the presence of an underlying genetic basis for the IUGR and is an indication for a fetal karyotype. Only 2% of structurally normal fetuses with IUGR will have an underlying karyotypic abnormality (Snijders et al., 1993). Cardiovascular anomalies put the fetus at risk for IUGR independent of chromosomal abnormalities.

Use of umbilical Doppler flow velocity waveforms obtained by ultrasound are also useful in determining the etiology of the IUGR as well as in managing the pregnancy. It is the one test that has been shown to reduce perinatal mortality in suspected IUGR (Alfirevic and Nielson, 1995). Increased resistance in the placental circulation will result in diminished, absent, or reversed end-diastolic flow in the umbilical arteries. Absence or reversal of umbilical artery end-diastolic flow is associated with severe compromise of the fetal perfusion; without medical intervention, the natural history of these pregnancies leads frequently to intrauterine death. Similarly, the presence of a normal Doppler umbilical artery waveform in a small fetus is reassuring and associated with less risk of adverse perinatal outcome (Gaziano et al., 1994). Thus prenatal ultrasound evaluation of small fetuses at, or less than, the 10th percentile for weight should include a careful fetal anatomic survey and umbilical cord Doppler velocimetry in order to improve diagnostic accuracy and management.

Targeted interventions

Early delivery will benefit those pregnancies in which a compromised intrauterine environment is present, a situation that occurs in about 75–80% of cases. Early delivery does not help in cases of underlying genetic defects or congenital infections.

Currently, delivery is timed to prevent fetal death. Data on the long-term benefits of early delivery are lacking except as they affect stillbirth. An argument for elective early delivery can be made in that the increasing hypoxia and acidosis resulting from continuing the pregnancy may affect long-term development of the fetal brain (Gaudier et al., 1994). Arguing against early delivery are the increased risks of neonatal death and cerebral palsy associated with prematurity (Bhushan et al., 1993). This dilemma has been underscored by the results of a recent survey in which European obstetricians were asked when they would advise delivery of an IUGR fetus based on gestational age, Doppler flow velocimetry waveforms, and other measures of prepartum fetal well-being (GRIT, 1996). Based on their responses, a zone of collective uncertainty was identified in which obstetricians would be willing to randomize patients to a trial of timed delivery. The pilot phase of this study, known as the European Growth Restriction Intervention Trial (GRIT), is currently underway (GRIT, 1996).

Prevention of IUGR related to maternal risk factors

Because at least two-thirds of cases of IUGR occur in women with risk factors for IUGR (Galbraith et al., 1979), prenatal identification of these women provides the opportunity to treat selective maternal conditions in the hope of actually preventing the IUGR. Table 7.4 summarizes identifiable conditions in which treatment may reduce the risk of IUGR. Women with a history of a previous IUGR infant even in the absence of other risk factors may also benefit from daily low-dose aspirin therapy (Wallenberg and Rotmans, 1987), although as discussed in Chapter 4, recent studies have failed to substantiate this effect (Caritis et al., 1997; CLASP, 1994; ECPPA, 1996; Sibai et al, 1993).

Severe maternal anemia, caused by malaria, is the leading cause of IUGR in the world. Infectious anemia is a rare cause of IUGR in the United States, where inherited hemoglobinopathies, such as sickle cell disease and the thalessemias, are the more prominent causes of anemia. The prevalence of IUGR among patients with sickle cell anemia, the most severe of the sickle cell diseases, is 15% (Koshy et al., 1988). While prophylactic transfusion with normal adult blood is no longer recommended because of unacceptable side effects associated with blood products, including transmission of hepatitis and immune deficiency viruses and isoimmunization, patients with frequent crises and evidence of IUGR may benefit from therapeutic transfusion (Koshy et al., 1988). The impact of other severe

Table 7.4. Potentially treatable conditions associated with IUGR

Maternal conditions
Severe anemia, including hemoglobinopathies
Severe malnutrition
Hyperthyroidism
Cyanotic heart disease
Hypertension
Antiphospholipid antibody syndrome
Medication exposure
    – coumarin
    – dilantin
    – chemotherapy
History of previous IUGR infant
High-risk behaviors
    – cigarette smoking
    – cocaine use
    – heroin use
    – alcohol abuse

Fetal conditions
High-order multiple gestations
Congenital infections

---

maternal anemias on fetal growth is not well described.

Severe malnutrition can be associated with an increased risk of low birth weight; however, studies on the effects of caloric supplementation on birth weight and perinatal mortality have demonstrated only modest increases in maternal weight gain and fetal growth, even in the most undernourished women (Kramer, 1993; see also the discussion in Chapter 6). A weighted mean difference in birth weight of 30 gm in the supplemented group was obtained from the 12 best studies in the field. Stratification for maternal prepregnancy nutritional status failed to demonstrate a larger effect on birth weight among undernourished women. In fact, the effect of balanced energy and protein supplementation on infant birth weight was less in undernourished women compared to adequately nourished women. A dietary intervention study in 1049 twin gestations over 14 years showed a reduction in odds for preterm delivery, but not for IUGR or for perinatal mortality (DuBois et al., 1991).

Maternal hyperthyroidism from Graves' disease is associated with IUGR in about 1% of fetuses, with the poor growth presumably resulting from fetal hypermetabolism (Seely and Burrow, 1994). Maternal administration of antithyroid medications, such as propylthiouracil or methimazole, appears effective in controlling fetal Graves' disease and encouraging fetal growth (Check et al., 1982; Millar et al., 1994).

Maternal cyanotic heart disease is a rare cause of IUGR, but may become more frequent as the increasing number of young women who survive correction of congenital heart disease reach their childbearing years. Their infants are at increased risk of congenital heart disease, an independent cause of IUGR, as well.

Patients with chronic hypertension enter pregnancy with a 25–30% risk of low birth weight from a combination of prematurity and poor growth (Mabie et al., 1986; Sibai and Anderson, 1986). The risk of low birth weight in an individual woman is related to the degree of her hypertension and ranges from a low of 20% with mild hypertension (diastolic blood pressure 90 to 110 mmHg in the first trimester) to 70% when hypertension is severe (blood pressure equal to or greater than 170/110 mmHg in the first trimester) (Sibai et al., 1983; Sibai and Anderson, 1986). The pregnancy is at extremely high risk if the woman develops superimposed pre-eclampsia (Mabie et al., 1986; Sibai et al., 1983; Sibai and Anderson, 1986). Similarly, pregnancy-induced hypertension and pre-eclampsia put patients at increased risk of IUGR and account for more cases on a population basis than do any other medical condition. Women with pre-existing hypertension may benefit from daily low-dose aspirin therapy in reducing the risk of IUGR (Beaufils et al., 1985; Uzan et al., 1991), although a recent large multi-center study failed to demonstrate an effect of the aspirin therapy (Caritis et al., 1997). Similar reductions in risk of pre-eclampsia initially were seen in the initial trials of low-dose aspirin therapy in hypertensive women; the same recent multi-center trial again did not show a benefit in pre-eclampsia prevention (Caritis et al., 1997).

Antiphospholipid antibodies are detectable in the sera of 2% of otherwise healthy pregnant women (Lockwood et al., 1989). These women are at risk of poor pregnancy outcomes, including IUGR. At least 30% of patients with anticardiolipin antibodies will have IUGR. Although controlled studies are lacking, patients with poor pregnancy histories or the antiphospholipid antibody syndrome may benefit from anticoagulation with heparin and low-dose aspirin therapy during pregnancy (Branch et al., 1992; Cowchock et al., 1992).

Preventable congenital infections, such as rubella, cytomegalovirus, and human immunodeficiency virus (HIV), have been associated with increased risk for IUGR (Bulterys et al., 1994; Klein and Remington, 1990). Recent breakdowns in herd immunity have occurred, with increasing numbers of women in their childbearing years demonstrating loss of immunity to rubella after vaccination. This loss of immunity in significant numbers of women puts fetuses at risk for fetal rubella syndrome and emphasizes the need for continuing diligence to the vaccination status of women. Transmission of cytomegalovirus can be reduced by close

Table 7.5. Multi-fetal pregnancy rates using different infertility treatment strategies (%)

Treatment	Twins	Triplets	Higher order
None	1.2	0.015	0.00017
Clomiphene	8–10	< 1	—
Gonadotropins	15	5	0.6
Assisted reproductive techniques (ART)	27.9	5.9	1

Sources: Hardy and Fox, 1995; SART, 1996

attention to hand washing, especially by health care and day care workers. It is not known at this time what effect maternal treatment with zidovudine (AZT) or antiretroviral therapy will have on fetal growth in the HIV-positive woman.

Several medications administered for other serious maternal medical conditions can stunt fetal growth. These include, but are not limited to, coumarin, dilantin, and chemotherapeutic agents (Briggs et al., 1997). These medications should be avoided whenever possible. However, as discussed in Chapter 14, the maternal and fetal risks and benefits must be carefully weighed in each individual instance.

One or more of the fetuses in multiple gestations are generally at significant risk of IUGR. One-third of perinatal losses occurring before 30 weeks in a twin population were due to stillbirth of a twin suffering from IUGR (Fliegner, 1989). The frequency of twins and higher order multiple gestations is increasing in the population as a result of increasing treatment for infertility. Multifetal pregnancy rates are dramatically increased with some forms of infertility treatment (Table 7.5). As the number of fetuses in the uterus increases, so does the risk for IUGR. Attempts to improve pregnancy outcome in high order multiple gestations (triplets and higher) using the technique of selective fetal reduction have not markedly improved the prevalence of IUGR (DuBois et al., 1991) (see Table 7.6). However, selective reduction to twins of higher order multiples has increased overall survival because of the reduced risk of spontaneous preterm delivery (Evans et al., 1995). The risk of IUGR appears proportional to the number of fetuses originally implanted in the uterus.

Maternal smoking affects fetal growth in a dose-dependent manner. In a recent investigation of over one million Swedish women, 5.7% of infants born to mothers who smoked heavily ($\geq$ 10 cigarettes per day) during pregnancy were small-for-gestational-age (SGA), defined as less than the 5th percentile for population norms (Cnattingius, 1997). This was in comparison to 4.6% SGA in women who smoke moderately (up to nine cigarettes per day) and 2.3% SGA in non-smokers. The net increase in risk for SGA is 2.1–fold in moderate smokers and

Table 7.6. Fetal growth in reduced and nonreduced twin gestations

	Nonreduced twins	Twins reduced from triplets	Twins reduced from quadruplets	Twins reduced from > 4
Number of pregnancies	61	113	89	34
Percent with IUGR	19.4	36.3	41.6	50

χ^2 for trend; $P = 0.001$; most pregnancies had only one growth-restricted fetus.
Source: Depp et al., 1996.

2.7–fold in heavy smokers. This effect is further modified by maternal age, independent of parity and family stability. The odds ratio for SGA increased from 1.7 and 2.0 at ages 15–19, to 2.9 and 4.4 at ages 40–44 for moderate and heavy smokers, respectively. Although data are not available on corroborative evidence of IUGR in this study, the strict definition of SGA makes it likely that many of these infants were in a compromised intrauterine environment. The association of cigarette smoking with diminished placental blood flow and the deleterious effect of the carbon monoxide byproducts of cigarette smoking on oxygen-carrying capacity of blood provide two mechanisms by which the intrauterine environment is compromised (Longo, 1977; Rauramo et al., 1983).

Smoking is a prevalent behavior in pregnancy, with population estimates ranging from 20 to 30% of all pregnant women (Cnattingius, 1997). Cnattingius (1989) has attributed 25% of all IUGR to maternal smoking. Unfortunately, all data gathered to date indicate that only about 30% of women stop smoking during pregnancy despite information that smoking cessation will increase birth weight (Cnattingius, 1992; Johnson et al., 1987; Sexton and Hebel, 1984).

Although cocaine use has been reputed to cause multiple adverse perinatal outcomes, including low birth weight, preterm delivery, congenital anomalies, abruptio placentae, sudden infant death syndrome, and perinatal injuries, only its effect on birth weight has been consistently identified (Holzman and Paneth, 1994). The magnitude of cocaine's impact on fetal growth is uncertain; unadjusted analyses have described deficits in mean birth weight of 265–610 gm. Adjusted analyses reduce the deficits into the range of 78–382 gm. In one study, which controlled for maternal age, parity, alcohol and cigarette use, hypertension, and prenatal care, tobacco was found to be a greater fetal growth restrictor than cocaine (McCalla et al., 1991). Prevalence estimates based on meconium sampling place the frequency of use late in pregnancy at 4.6–30.7%. Self-reported cocaine use among women with no prenatal care is as high as 62%.

Heroin use during pregnancy appears to reduce birth weight proportionate to the degree of abuse, with at least 40% of babies below the 10th percentile for gestation (Stone et al., 1971). Methadone therapy appears to promote fetal growth in a similar dose-dependent fashion with the maximum effect present when methadone is started in the first trimester (Kandall et al., 1976). Outpatient methadone programs with the greatest success appear to be those that are directly linked with prenatal care rather than through separate providers (Giles et al., 1989).

Like smoking and cocaine and heroin use, alcohol abuse is associated with IUGR in a dose- and timing-related fashion. Unlike the growth restriction associated with smoking and cocaine and heroin use, however, alcohol-associated IUGR is sustained postnatally for at least a year (Jacobson et al., 1994). Sustained heavy alcohol consumption (more than five drinks per day) throughout pregnancy is associated with a high prevalence of the fetal alcohol syndrome (FAS), which includes fetal growth restriction, craniofacial anomalies, and neurologic disorders including mental retardation (Murray-Lyon, 1985). Moderate alcohol consumption, defined as three or more drinks per week, increased the risk for IUGR 2.3-fold (95% CL = 1.2,4.6) above non-drinking controls (Windham et al., 1995). About 40–60% of problem drinkers intensively counseled about the risk of continued drinking appear to be able to reduce their alcohol consumption by at least 50% (Halmesmaki, 1988; Rosett et al., 1980). Reducing heavy alcohol intake by midpregnancy can reduce the frequency of IUGR, but not of anomalies (Rosett et al., 1983).

Measuring the impact of prenatal care on IUGR in the United States

As detailed above, prenatal care has an impact in four areas related to IUGR: prevention of unnecessary interventions for otherwise healthy, small infants; prevention of some cases of IUGR by treatment of maternal diseases and high-risk behaviors; diminution of perinatal morbidity and, perhaps, long-term morbidity associated with IUGR; and prevention of fetal death.

Calculation of the number of fetal lives that are saved by detecting IUGR ultrasonographically and monitoring the pregnancy closely for signs of fetal deterioration are dependent upon the assumed method used for screening. Assuming that there are a minimum of 200 000 infants afflicted with IUGR annually in the United States, risk factor screening will detect about 37% or 74 000 of them. Aggressive use of "routine" prenatal ultrasound will detect about 67% or 134 000 of the cases. If perinatal mortality is estimated at 24% for undetected IUGR (Hughey, 1984; Kurjak et al., 1980), then 48 000 of these 200 000 infants would be expected to die with no intervention. Detection and intervention will lower perinatal mortality, estimated here for computation purposes to be 6%. Thus, with risk factor screening, 13 320 infant lives could be saved annually by detection and intervention, and with aggressive routine ultrasound of all pregnancies, 24 120 infant lives could be saved.

The potential of prenatal care to prevent perinatal and long-term morbidity is harder to quantify. At the very least, a diagnosis of IUGR should alert pediatricians and neonatologists to look for the metabolic difficulties, such as hypoglycemia, that these newborns may exhibit, thereby preventing them from becoming further compromised in the newborn period. Administration of prenatal corticosteroids to those mothers whose infants are likely to require preterm delivery before 34 weeks may reduce the risk of severe IVH by as much as 50%, thereby reducing the long-term neurologic risk for them. Determination of further reductions in morbidity await the results of the GRIT study in Europe.

Prenatal care offers an important opportunity to provide medical attention and education for underlying conditions and high-risk behaviors that can lead to IUGR. Although individual medical conditions, especially hypertension, may account for 30% of the cases, many still cannot be sufficiently treated to prevent the disorder. However, as described above, intervention can prevent some cases of IUGR.

In contrast, IUGR caused by maternal smoking is preventable. Smoking has been estimated to cause 25% of the cases of IUGR in industrialized countries (Cnattinguis, 1989). Thus, at least 50 000 cases of IUGR are attributable to smoking in the United States annually. Assuming that, under ideal circumstances, we could identify 100% of cases of IUGR caused by smoking, 3000 deaths annually would still occur from smoking alone (assuming the lowest perinatal mortality reported from detected IUGR to be 6%). Because we do not achieve a 100% detection rate, the number of perinatal lives lost annually because of smoking-induced IUGR is probably closer to 12 000. This latter number is equivalent to the number of deaths prevented with a very aggressive (and expensive) program of three routine ultrasounds in each pregnancy and is not a factor in any of the other adverse pregnancy outcomes associated with smoking, such as spontaneous preterm birth and sudden infant death syndrome.

Conclusion

The best of prenatal care can reduce the morbidity and mortality of IUGR, especially in those cases of maternal predisposing disorders, and it can reduce the number of unnecessary interventions for normal, small infants. Given the impact that maternal smoking has on the prevalence of IUGR, improving and expanding prenatal care interventions that target smoking may substantially increase the impact of prenatal care on infant morbidity and mortality.

REFERENCES

Alfirevic Z, Nielson JP. Doppler ultrasonography in high-risk pregnancies: systematic review with meta-analysis. American Journal of Obstetrics and Gynecology 1995; **72**: 1379–87.

Allen, MC. Developmental outcome and follow-up of the small for gestational age infant. Seminars in Perinatology 1984; **8**: 123–56.

Beaufils M, Uzan S, Donsimoni R, Colau JC. Prevention of pre-eclampsia by early antiplatelet therapy. Lancet 1985; **1**: 840–2.

Benson CB, Doubilet PM, Saltzman DH. Intrauterine growth retardation: predictive value of US criteria for antenatal diagnosis. Radiology 1986; **160**: 415–17.

Bhushan V, Paneth N, Kiely JL. Impact of improved survival of very low birthweight infants on recent secular trends in the prevalence of cerebral palsy. Pediatrics 1993; **91**: 1094–100.

Branch WD, Silver RM, Blackwell JL, Reading JC, Scott JR. Outcome of treated pregnancies in women with antiphospholipid syndrome: an update of the Utah experience. Obstetrics and Gynecology 1992; **80**: 614–20.

Briggs GC, Freeman RK, Yaffe SJ. Drugs in pregnancy and lactation, 4th edition. Baltimore: Williams and Wilkins, 1997.

Bulterys M, Chao A, Munyemana S, et al. Maternal human immunodeficiency virus-1 infection and intrauterine growth: a prospective cohort study in Butare, Rwanda. Pediatric Infectious Disease Journal 1994; **13**: 94–100.

Callan NA, Witter FR. Intrauterine growth retardation: characteristics, risk factors and gestational age. International Journal of Gynecology and Obstetrics 1990; **33**: 215–20.

Caritis SN and the MFM Network. Low dose aspirin does not prevent preeclampsia in high risk women. American Journal of Obstetrics and Gynecology 1997, **176**. 35.

Check JH, Rezvani I, Goodner D, Hopper B. Prenatal treatment of thyrotoxicosis to prevent intrauterine growth retardation. Obstetrics and Gynecology 1982; **60**: 122–4.

CLASP. A randomised trial of low-dose aspirin for the prevention and treatment of pre-eclampsia among 9364 pregnant women. Lancet 1994; **3443**: 619–29.

Cnattingius S. Does age potentiate the smoking-related risk of fetal growth retardation? Early Human Development 1989; **20**: 203–11.

Cnattingius S. Smoking during pregnancy: pregnancy risks and socio-demographic characteristics among pregnant smokers. International Journal of Technology Assessment in Health Care 1992; **8**: 91–5.

Cnattingius S. Maternal age modifies the effect of maternal smoking on intrauterine growth retardation but not on late fetal death and placental abruption. American Journal of Epidemiology 1997; **145**: 19–23.

Cowchock FS, Reece EA, Balaban D, Branch DW, Plouffe L. Repeated fetal losses associated with antiphospholipid antibodies: a collaborative randomized trial comparing prednisone with low-dose heparin therapy. American Journal of Obstetrics and Gynecology 1992; **166**: 1318–23.

Creasy RK, Resnik R. Intrauterine growth restriction. In: Creasy RK, Resnick R, eds. Maternal–fetal medicine, 3rd edition. Philadelphia: WB Saunders, 1994: 558–74.

Depp R, Macones GA, Rosenn MF, Yurzo E, Wapner RJ, Weinblatt VJ. Multifetal pregnancy reduction: evaluation of fetal growth in the remaining twins. American Journal of Obstetrics and Gynecology 1996; **174**: 1233–8.

DuBois S, Dougherty C, Duquette M-P, Hanley JA, Moutquin J-M. Twin pregnancy: the impact of the Higgins Nutrition Intervention Program on maternal and neonatal outcomes. American Journal of Clinical Nutrition 1991; **53**: 1397–403.

ECPPA Collaborative Group. ECPPA: randomised trial of low dose aspirin for the prevention of maternal and fetal complications in high risk pregnant women. British Journal of Obstetrics and Gynæcology 1996; **103**: 39–47.

Evans MI, Dommergues M, Johnson MP, Dumez Y. Multifetal pregnancy reduction and selective termination. Current Opinion in Obstetrics and Gynecology 1995; **7**: 126–9.

Fliegner JRH. When do perinatal deaths in multiple pregnancies occur? Australian and New Zealand Journal of Obstetrics and Gynæcology 1989; **29**: 371–4.

Galbraith RS, Karchmar EJ, Piercy WN, Low JA. The clinical prediction of intrauterine growth retardation. American Journal of Obstetrics and Gynecology 1979; **133**: 281–6.

Gaudier FL, Goldenberg RL, Nelson KG, et al. Acid base status and subsequent neurosensory impairment in surviving 500 to 1000 gm infants. American Journal of Obstetrics and Gynecology 1994; **170**: 48–53.

Gaziano EP, Knox H, Ferrara B, Brandt DG, Calvin SE, Knox GE. Is it time to reassess the risk for the growth-retarded fetus with normal Doppler velocimetry of the umbilical artery? American Journal of Obstetrics and Gynecology 1994; **170**: 1734–43.

Giles W, Patterson T, Sanders F, Batey R, Thomas D, Collins J. Outpatient methadone programme for pregnant heroin using women. Australian and New Zealand Journal of Obstetrics and Gynæcology 1989; **29**: 225–9.

GRIT Study Group. When do obstetricians recommend delivery for a high-risk preterm growth-retarded fetus? European Journal Of Obstetrics, Gynecology, and Reproductive Biology 1996; **67**: 121–6.

Halmesmaki E. Alcohol counselling of 85 pregnant problem drinkers: effect on drinking and fetal outcome. British Journal of Obstetrics and Gynæcology 1988; **95**: 243–7.

Hardy RI, Fox J. Infertility Treatment. In: Ryan KJ, Berkowitz RS, Barbieri RL, eds. Kistner's gynecology: principles and practice. 6th edition. St. Louis: Mosby, 1995: 305–29.

Holmquist P, Ingemarsson E, Ingemarsson I. Intra-uterine growth retardation and gestational age. Acta Obstetricia et Gynecologica Scandinavica 1986; **65**: 633–8.

Holzman C, Paneth N. Maternal cocaine use during pregnancy and perinatal outcomes. Epidemiologic Reviews 1994; **16**: 315–34.

Hughey MJ. Routine ultrasound for detection and management of the small-for-gestational-age fetus. Obstetrics and Gynecology 1984; **64**: 101–3.

Jacobson JL, Jacobson SW, Sokol RJ. Effects of prenatal exposure to alcohol, smoking, and illicit drugs on postpartum somatic growth. Alcoholism, Clinical and Experimental Research 1994; **18**: 317–23.

Johnson SF, McCarter RJ, Ferencz C. Changes in alcohol, cigarette, and recreational drug use during pregnancy: implications for intervention. American Journal of Epidemiology 1987; **126**: 695–702.

Kandall SR, Albin S, Lowinson J, Berle B, Eidelman AI, Gartner LM. Differential effects of maternal heroin and methadone use on birthweight. Pediatrics 1976; **58**: 681–5.

Klein JO, Remington JS. Current concepts of infections of the fetus and newborn infant. In Remington JS, Klein JO, eds. Infectious diseases of the fetus and newborn infant. 3rd edition. Philadelphia: W.B. Saunders, 1990: Chapter 1.

Koshy M, Burd L, Wallace D, Moawad A, Baron J. Prophylactic red-cell transfusions in pregnant patients with sickle cell disease. New England Journal of Medicine 1988; **319**: 1447–52.

Kramer MS. Effects of energy and protein intakes on pregnancy outcome: an overview of the research evidence from controlled clinical trials. American Journal of Clinical Nutrition 1993; **58**: 627–35.

Kramer MS, Olivier M, McLean FH, Willis DM, Usher RH. Impact of intrauterine growth retardation and body proportionality on fetal and neonatal outcome. Pediatrics 1990; **85**: 707–13.

Kurjak A, Kirkinen P, Latin V. Biometric and dynamic ultrasound assessment of small-for-dates infants: report of 260 cases. Obstetrics and Gynecology 1980; **56**: 281–4.

Larsen T, Larsen JF, Petersen S, Greisen G. Detection of small-for-gestational-age fetuses by ultrasound screening in a high risk population: a randomized controlled study. British Journal of Obstetrics and Gynæcology 1992; **99**: 469–74.

Lockwood CJ, Romero R, Freiberg RF, Clyne LP, Coster B, Hobbins JC. The prevalence and biologic significance of lupus anticoagulant and anticardiolipin antibodies in a general obstetric population. American Journal of Obstetrics and Gynecology 1989; **161**: 369–73.

Longo LD. The biological effects of carbon monoxide on the pregnant woman, fetus and newborn infant. American Journal of Obstetrics and Gynecology 1977; **129**: 69–103.

Mabie WC, Pernoll ML, Biswas MK. Chronic hypertension in pregnancy. Obstetrics and Gynecology 1986; **67**: 197–205.

McCalla S, Minkoff HL, Feldman J, et al. The biological and social consequences of perinatal cocaine use in an inner-city population: results of an anonymous cross-sectional study. American Journal of Obstetrics and Gynecology 1991; **164**: 625–30.

Millar LK, Wing DA, Leung AS, Koonings PP, Montoro MN, Mestman JH. Low birth weight and preeclampsia in pregnancies complicated by hyperthyroidism. Obstetrics and Gynecology 1994; **84**: 946–9.

Murray-Lyon IM. Alcohol and foetal damage. Alcohol 1985; **20**: 185–8.

Rauramo I, Forss M, Kariniemi V, Lehtovirta P. Antepartum fetal heart rate variability and intervillous placental blood flow in association with smoking. American Journal of Obstetrics and Gynecology 1983; **146**: 967–9.

Rosett HL, Weiner L, Lee A, Zuckerman B, Dooling, Oppenheimer E. Patterns of alcohol consumption and fetal development. Obstetrics and Gynecology 1983; **61**: 539–46.

Rosett HL, Weiner L, Zuckerman B, McKinlay S, Edelin KC. Reduction in alcohol consumption during pregnancy with benefits to the newborn. Alcoholism, Clinical and Experimental Research 1980; **4**: 178–84.

Seely BL, Burrow GN. Thyroid disease in pregnancy. In Creasy RK, Resnick R, eds. Maternal–fetal medicine. Philadelphia: WB Saunders, 1994: 979–1003.

Sexton M, Hebel RH. A clinical trial of change in maternal smoking and its effect on birthweight. Journal of the American Medical Association 1984; **251**: 911–15.

Sibai BM, Abdella TN, Anderson GD. Pregnancy outcome in 211 patients with mild chronic hypertension. Obstetrics and Gynecology 1983; **61**: 571–6.

Sibai BM, Anderson GD. Pregnancy outcome of intensive therapy in severe hypertension in the first trimester. Obstetrics and Gynecology 1986; **67**: 517–22.

Sibai BM, Caritis SN, Thom E, et al. Prevention of pre-eclampsia with low-dose aspirin in healthy, nulliparous pregnant women. New England Journal of Medicine 1993; **329**: 1213–18.

Snijders RJM, Sherrod C, Gosden CM, Nicolaides KH. Fetal growth retardation: associated malformations and chromosomal abnormalities. American Journal of Obstetrics and Gynecology 1993; **168**: 547–55.

Society for Assisted Reproductive Technology (SART). Assisted reproductive technology in the United States and Canada: 1994 results generated from the American Society for Reproductive Medicine/Society for Assisted Reproductive Technology Registry. Fertility and Sterility 1996; **66**: 697–705.

Spinillo A, Capuzzo E, Ometto A, Stronati M, Baltaro F, Iasci A. Value of antenatal corticosteroid therapy in preterm birth. Early Human Development 1995; **42**: 37–47.

Stone ML, Salerno LJ, Green M, Zelson C. Narcotic addiction in pregnancy. American Journal of Obstetrics and Gynecology 1971; **109**: 716–23.

Uzan S, Beaufils M, Breart G, Bazin B, Capitant C, Paris J. Prevention of fetal growth retardation with low-dose aspirin: findings of the EPREDA trial. Lancet 1991; **337**: 1427–31.

Wallenberg HCS, Rotmans N. Prevention of recurrent idiopathic fetal growth retardation by low-dose aspirin and dipyridamole. American Journal of Obstetrics and Gynecology 1987; **157**: 1230–5.

Wennergren M, Wennergren G, Vilbergsson G. Obstetric characteristics and neonatal performance in a four-year small for gestational age population. Obstetrics and Gynecology 1988; **72**: 615–20.

Windham GC, Fenster L, Hopkins B, Swan SH. The association of moderate maternal and paternal alcohol consumption with birthweight and gestational age. Epidemiology 1995; **6**: 591–7.

8

Short- and long-term outcomes of intrauterine growth restriction

Kathleen G. Nelson

Introduction

There is considerable controversy in interpreting data relating intrauterine growth restriction (IUGR) both to short-term health effects occurring during infancy and childhood and to longer-term consequences throughout the lifespan. This chapter reviews areas of debate and presents current information on these effects. The discussion begins with the link between IUGR and infant mortality and morbidity. Next, the evidence of effects of IUGR on growth through infancy and childhood is discussed, followed by a review of the evidence describing the impact of IUGR on neurological development. We then turn to the controversial subject of longer-term effects of IUGR in adulthood, reviewing Barker's programming theory and the studies supporting it, as well as the critiques of this theory.

IUGR and infant mortality and morbidity

IUGR is one of the known leading causes of death in infants. As the degree of growth restriction increases, so too does the risk of death. Infants weighing 2000–2499 gm at birth are approximately four times as likely to die in the neonatal period than are infants weighing 2500–2999 gm, who in turn are twice as likely to die than are infants weighing 3000–3499 gm. This relative risk of death in each 500 gm birth weight interval has been found to hold true across different populations (Tebers et al., 1988).

The association between IUGR and increased infant mortality extends into the post-neonatal period and holds for such causes of death as sudden infant death syndrome and infection. The risk of post-neonatal deaths in infants weighing 2000–2499 gm is twice that of infants weighing 2500–2999 gm, which is also twice the post-neonatal death risk of infants weighing 3000–3499 gm.

Studies of infant mortality in IUGR infants are frequently complicated by vast differences in socioeconomic status among study participants, particularly in community-based studies and studies in developing countries. Families with

IUGR infants are often at a disadvantage with regard to income and education as compared with families of appropriately grown infants, and the infants may also have more infections or receive less than satisfactory medical care. Even in the few studies where socioeconomic and other confounders could be controlled for, an increased mortality of about 30% remains.

Among growth-restricted infants, the type of growth restriction appears to be significantly associated with infant mortality and morbidity. Proportionally small, or symmetrically growth restricted infants (those who are small in both length and weight) have a higher neonatal mortality than those who are asymmetrically growth-restricted (thin relative to height) (Cuttini et al., 1991). Symmetrical growth restriction is associated with a higher incidence of chromosomal abnormalities and with a poorer prognosis both for growth and neurodevelopmental outcome (Brar and Rutherford, 1988).

Current research

Several relatively recent large-scale studies have examined the relationship between IUGR and infant morbidity and mortality. For example, in a study of nearly 9000 infants born at Montreal's Royal Victoria Hospital between 1980 and 1986, Kramer and colleagues (1990) assessed the specificity of prognosis by degree of growth restriction. They defined intrauterine growth on the basis of fetal growth ratio, which is the ratio of the observed birth weight to the mean birth weight for gestational age for this hospital population. Levels of growth restriction were based on a definition of mild IUGR as a fetal growth ratio of 0.80 to < 0.85, moderate growth restriction as a fetal growth ratio of 0.75 to < 0.80, and severe growth restriction as a fetal growth ratio of < 0.75. Poor outcomes were stillbirth, abnormal fetal heart rate monitoring, hypoglycemia, hypocalcemia, polycythemia, passage of meconium, a one-minute Apgar of 1, and a five-minute Apgar of less than 7.

The authors of this study concluded that the association of IUGR and poor outcome appears to be "dose related" because the risk of morbidity and mortality increased with increasing severity of IUGR. This risk was particularly high in infants with severe growth restriction. The study did not uncover strong evidence that outcome within a given degree of growth restriction varied as a function of the cause of growth restriction. However, the study may not have been able to detect this relationship because infants with congenital malformations, known chromosomal abnormalities, or other major malformations were excluded. The study did not find a major role for symmetrical versus asymmetric growth restriction in determining poor outcome.

In another study, Piper and colleagues (1996) looked at all preterm pregnancies delivered during a 15–year period (1970–1985) in San Antonio, Texas. They found significantly higher rates of fetal and neonatal deaths in the infants classified as small-for-gestational-age (SGA). Stratification revealed higher rates of neonatal deaths for SGA groups compared with an appropriate-for-gestational-age (AGA) group even within gestational age category. The authors of this study found that fetal heart rate abnormalities occurred more commonly in SGA pregnancies, and SGA infants had a higher rate of hyaline membrane disease than did AGA infants of a similar gestational age. However, SGA infants had a lower rate of hyaline membrane disease than did AGA infants of a similar birth weight. After examining this population, which included over 1000 preterm, growth-restricted infants, the authors found that growth-restricted infants had a uniformly higher risk of death in the fetal, neonatal, and overall perinatal periods, which outweighed their risk of mortality associated with their prematurity at all preterm gestational ages.

In another study, Cuttini and colleagues (1991) in Milan, Italy, examined neonatal mortality and morbidity in 2600 SGA infants. Approximately 40% of these infants and 64% of the preterm infants were described as proportionately small. The authors found that the risk of death for the first month of life was increased from two- to five-fold for proportionately small as compared with disproportionately small infants.

Studies evaluating infant immunocompetence also demonstrate an association with IUGR: the greater the fetal growth restriction, the more impaired the immunocompetence (Piper et al., 1996). Part of this immunodeficiency is due to the fact that growth-restricted infants have fewer mature thymocytes and do not have a clear demarcation between the cortex and the medulla of the thymus. They also have decreased placental transfer of immunoglobulins and impaired lymphocyte response to mitogenetic stimulation. It appears that there is significant improvement in immune response as IUGR infants age.

Growth in infancy and childhood

Growth in infancy is affected by growth status at birth. This was shown in a study by Nelson and colleagues (1977) of a cohort of 949 singleton births, 294 of whom were categorized as SGA. Among these infants, significant differences were demonstrated in weight, height, and head circumference between those who were SGA and those who were not. Although the rate of growth of SGA children for length and head circumference surpassed those of the non-SGA, significant differences still remained at one year of age. Very little is known about the effects of IUGR on skeletal or sexual maturation. The limited evidence suggests no differences in timing of peak height velocity or sexual maturation with respect to non-IUGR subjects. In addition, radiographic bone age appears similar in IUGR and non-IUGR subjects.

Although IUGR subjects generally remain shorter during childhood and adolescence than those born at term without IUGR (Gluckman, 1993), many growth-restricted infants experience catch-up growth over time. A study by Karlberg and Albertsson-Wikland (1995) followed a Swedish cohort of healthy full-term singletons from birth to final height at 18 years old. Looking at SGA defined either by height or weight, these investigators found that the majority of infants plotted on growth curves were within the range of normal height during the first six to twelve months of life. By age one year, only 13% of those categorized as SGA by length were below two standard deviations of the reference populations' means in height. By 18 years of age, this percentage had decreased to 7.9%. Of the total short population at age 18, 22% had been short at birth, and 14% had been SGA as defined by birth weight. Infants who were SGA by length had a seven-fold higher risk of short final stature compared to the non-SGA group.

The relationship of long-term growth potential in symmetrically growth-restricted versus asymmetrically growth-restricted infants has commanded significant attention over the past several years. Presumably, symmetrically growth-restricted infants are affected early in pregnancy, while growth restriction in asymmetric infants occurs later in gestation, usually during the third trimester. For this reason, symmetrically growth-restricted infants have a poorer growth prognosis than asymmetrically growth-restricted infants (Brar and Rutherford, 1988). However, some symmetrically growth-restricted children are born to parents who are small. Their growth restriction is consistent with their genetic potential for growth, and these children probably have a better prognosis than similarly sized children with greater genetic growth potential. Catch-up growth is more likely to occur with infants who were asymmetrically growth restricted than those symmetrically growth restricted (Brar and Rutherford, 1988).

Neurodevelopmental outcome

There remains a great deal of controversy about whether or not IUGR infants differ significantly from infants born AGA with regard to their neurodevelopmental outcomes. It is very difficult to compare the population involved in one study to the population of those in another because of differences in the definitions of IUGR. As was discussed in Chapter 6, although IUGR is frequently defined using the 10th percentile birth weight for gestational age, other standards for this cut-off are also used. Race- and sex-specific qualifiers needed for cross-study comparison also are not frequently described. In addition, because preterm SGA infants may have different neurodevelopmental outcomes than term SGA infants, gestational age ranges can have an important effect on study outcomes and must be specified if comparisons are to be valid.

Many of the factors associated with IUGR may have a direct effect on neurologic or neurosensory development, making it difficult to separate the specific effect of growth restriction. For example, many infants with chromosomal abnormalities are born small-for-gestational-age. These infants also have neurodevelopmental handicaps, but it would seem inappropriate to consider the IUGR as the cause of the neurodevelopmental handicap. This is also true of other risk factors, such as congenital infection, maternal drug use, and smoking, which cause growth restriction and may also cause neurodevelopmental problems, in addition to their effects on growth.

It is also unclear whether poor neurodevelopmental outcomes associated with SGA are related to the growth restriction or to hypoxia. Poor placental function is a cause of a significant portion of the IUGR. SGA infants are more likely to have perinatal complications, including asphyxia, and may have passed meconium in utero. They are at greater risk for hypoglycemia and hypothermia as neonates, both of which can affect long-term neurologic outcome. Data from the National Collaborative Perinatal Project showed that in the absence of hypoxia-related factors, IUGR children were not at higher risk for neurologic morbidity compared to non-IUGR children. However, in the presence of perinatal hypoxia-related factors, IUGR children were found to be more neurologically abnormal; children with symmetric IUGR have a greater association with this slightly higher risk of neurologic dysfunction than do those with asymmetric IUGR (Berg, 1989). A study by Uvebrant and Hagberg (1992) found that for IUGR infants born at term, an increase in cerebral palsy is associated with an increased risk of asphyxia at term. In our own institution, we looked at almost 300 term SGA infants matched for socioeconomic status, race, and sex and found that those with growth restriction scored four to five points below their non-SGA peers on intelligence tests, a statistically significant difference (Goldenberg et al., 1996).

In examining other adverse neurodevelopmental outcomes, such as cerebral palsy, it is clear that the incidence is dependent on gestational age. Babies born at term who are subsequently diagnosed with cerebral palsy tend to be smaller than those who do not have cerebral palsy, even though most small babies are not born with cerebral palsy and most children with cerebral palsy are of normal birth weight. In general, being IUGR appears to double or triple the risk of cerebral palsy for full-term babies. For preterm infants, those who are SGA appear to have less cerebral palsy than those who are AGA at similar gestational ages. Most SGA preterm infants are born to women with maternal pre-eclampsia, and many studies suggest a protective effect of pre-eclampsia on preterm SGA with regard to subsequent disability (Uvebrant and Hagberg, 1992).

Although Uvebrant and Hagberg (1992) determined that cerebral palsy was more common in late preterm (i.e., gestational age of 34–36 weeks) and term SGA infants than in AGA children of similar gestational ages, all other investigators do not share these conclusions. In studying infants weighing less than 1500 gm who were born at less than the 10th percentile, Robertson and colleagues (1990) found that preterm SGA infants were not at greater risk to be disabled with cerebral palsy than were AGA birth weight or gestational-age-matched control children, but all were substantially at greater risk than a term AGA comparison group. Hack and colleagues (1996) observed an 8% rate of cerebral palsy in AGA infants with birth weights less than 1500 gm but only a 3% rate in the SGA group. Sung (1993) showed that SGA infants weighing less than 1500 gm had less cerebral palsy than preterm AGA infants of the same weight. Thus, in cohorts defined by birth weights, SGA infants have less cerebral palsy, though in cohorts defined by gestational age, SGA infants have higher rates of cerebral palsy.

A study by Hutton and colleagues (1997) of preterm infants of less than 32 weeks gestation born in the early 1980s, and followed until age nine, found that effects on motor and cognitive development differed depending on whether the child was preterm or SGA. Cognitive ability as measured by IQ and reading comprehension was negatively associated with the degree of fetal growth restriction. Motor ability was positively associated with gestational age and negatively associated with the degree of fetal growth restriction. Reading speed and reading accuracy were not associated with either gestational age of growth restriction but were socially determined.

Other, more subtle forms of neurologic dysfunction, including attention deficit disorder and "soft signs" of neurologic disease, are more likely to occur in SGA populations. Hadders-Algra and Touwen (1990) showed that, at age six, 24% of full-term SGA infants had signs of minor neurologic dysfunction compared to 15% of full-term AGA infants. The most severe SGA infants had more than double the rate of "soft neurologic" signs (41%) as compared to the term AGA infants (16%). In a study of Israeli Army recruits, those born small-for-gestational-age had about 50% more minor neurologic abnormalities as compared to AGA peers, even after adjusting for socioeconomic status, birth order, and intrapartum events (Paz et al., 1995).

In summary, being born with intrauterine growth restriction is associated with an increase in neurologic dysfunction. Major motor and cognitive disabilities are rare, but are probably statistically significantly increased when large populations are evaluated. Boys are more affected than girls, and children born in lower socioeconomic circumstances are more affected than other children. Early onset intrauterine growth restriction that affects head growth appears to have more of an impact on neurologic function than does later intrauterine growth restriction. Intrauterine growth restriction accompanied by asphyxia is more commonly associated with neurodevelopmental abnormalities. There does not seem to be a major relationship between IUGR status and hearing or vision defects.

Long-term consequences of IUGR

Much of the work on long-term outcomes of intrauterine growth restriction comes from the studies of D.J.P. Barker and colleagues in the United Kingdom (Barker, 1994, 1995; Barker et al., 1993c). This work has related intrauterine growth restriction to increased subsequent incidence of coronary heart disease, hypertension, and diabetes mellitus. Barker and colleagues believe that undernutrition in utero permanently changes the body's structure and function and "programs" the appearance of disease in later life. They observed that in England and Wales, high infant death rates in the early years of the century were correlated with the small size of the babies. Several decades later, in similar geographic areas, high death rates from coronary artery disease occurred. Barker and his colleagues hypothesized that alteration in fetal growth secondary to periods of undernutrition may permanently reduce the number of cells in particular organs depending on when this undernutrition occurs. This may result in long-lasting changes in the size of the organs and in the distribution of cell types, hormonal feedback, metabolic activity, and organ structure. Animal experiments also seem to support this hypothesis. For example feeding rats low protein intakes during pregnancy results in persistently raised blood pressure in their offspring (Langley and Jackson, 1994).

To examine the programming hypothesis in humans, Barker and his colleagues investigated three populations in Britain – those in Hertfordshire, Preston, and Sheffield (Barker, 1994, 1995; Barker et al., 1993a; Law et al., 1992). Birth weights were available on almost 16 000 Hertfordshire residents born between 1911 and 1930. Death rates from coronary heart disease were significantly greater in those individuals with birth weights less than 2500 gm. By examining residents who still live in these three communities, they determined that infants who were small have, as adults, increased blood pressure, raised serum cholesterol and plasma fibrinogen, and impaired glucose tolerance. They determined an inverse relationship between blood pressure and birth weight in 17 separate studies of men, women, and children and found that differences in blood pressure associated with birth weight that appeared small in childhood were magnified throughout life. These investigators also demonstrated that in a group of men and women in Preston, where placental weights were known, adult systolic pressure at ages 46–54 years tended to rise at any birth weight as placental weight increased, so that the highest pressures were in people who, in fetal life, had allocated more resources to placental development (Barker et al., 1990). According to Barker, placental en-largement is a general marker for fetal malnutrition. Studies in Sheffield showed that disorders of cholesterol metabolism and blood coagulation in adults were linked to disproportionate size at birth, that is, a short body in relation to the size of head (Barker et al., 1993c).

Supportive of the Barker hypothesis is the speculation by Mackenzie and Brenner (1995) that adult hypertension may be due to a decreased number of nephrons occurring in the kidneys of low birth weight individuals. Low birth weight from intrauterine growth restriction has been shown to be associated with deficiencies of nephron number of up to 20%, even in pregnancies that go to term. Brenner also argues that the "thrifty genotype hypothesis" may explain hyperten-sion. In times of famine, reductions in capacity of nephrons as well as pancreatic islet cells could represent an integrated metabolic adjustment favoring ready availability of energy sources to meet metabolic needs and the achievement of electrolyte conservation at minimal renal energy expenditure. Conversely, in times of plenty, appropriate programming would endow the kidney with greater re-serves of nephrons to meet greater excretory demands. In the pancreas, a greater capacity to secrete insulin thereby shifts metabolism toward synthesis growth and energy storage. Although some observers believe that increased adult blood pressure in former low birth weight children may be a result of vascular smooth muscle cell growth resulting in increased peripheral vascular resistance (Lever and Harrap, 1992), the deficit in nephron number provides a compelling alternative explanation. The extent to which normal distribution of nephron numbers follows the normal distribution of blood pressure in the general population awaits studies of autopsies of adults to compare nephron numbers to blood pressures.

IUGR and diabetes/Syndrome X

Barker and colleagues (1993a) also determined that the prevalence of non-insulin-dependent diabetes and impaired glucose tolerance differs markedly between men who were small at birth and men who were large. Those with birth weights of less than 2500 gm had an odds ratio of 6.6 for impaired glucose tolerance compared to those with birth weights of more than 4300 gm. This relationship held even when current body mass index was taken into account, with those individuals of lowest birth weight and highest body mass index having substantially increased glucose intolerance compared to those of high birth weight and high adult body mass index. The lowest two-hour plasma glucose concentrations were seen among men who were large at birth and remained thin. The highest concentrations were among men who were small at birth and became fat as adults.

These investigators (1993a) have hypothesized that there is a reduced number of pancreatic beta cells and a reduced capacity to make insulin in people who are small at birth and who subsequently become obese. They believe that there is evidence that small babies become insulin resistant. Barker demonstrated that Syndrome X, a condition characterized by diabetes, hypertension, and increased triglyceride concentrations, occurs at a relative risk 10 times higher among people who were less than 2955 gm at birth than those who were more than 4300 gm. Syndrome X is an insulin resistance syndrome, and it appears to be associated not only with low birth weight, but more specifically with a low ponderal index at birth. Barker also demonstrated that below average weight and a decreased abdominal circumference at birth, associated with decreased growth of the liver, is subsequently associated with raised concentrations of cholesterol and raised death rates from coronary heart disease. However, the converse of this situation, that is, babies of large birth weight with large abdominal circumferences, has also been linked to later coronary heart disease.

Studies by groups other than Barker's seem to support the programming hypothesis. Curhan and colleagues (1996) looked at a cohort of almost 23 000 U.S. male health professionals. He demonstrated that low birth weight was associated with an increased risk of hypertension and diabetes and that high birth weight was associated with an increased risk of obesity. Although this study was conducted using a questionnaire and included only self-reported measurements of weight, height, and blood pressure, the study is significant because almost 1200 of the respondents had low birth weight and they represented a wide geographic distribution within the United States. Though the study was not able to look at gestational age, but only birth weight, it found that the adult body mass index had no effect on the association of low birth weight and risk of hypertension and diabetes. This finding suggests that in low birth weight infants, the association between hypertension and non-insulin-dependent diabetes mellitus is independent of obesity. Similarly, a study by Valdez and colleagues (1994) of almost 600 Mexican American and non-Hispanic white men and women participants in the San Antonio Heart Study supports the programming hypothesis and extends it to a broader population. These authors found that in normotensive non-diabetic adults, birth weight was inversely associated with fasting insulin and truncal fat. They also determined that blood pressure decreased as birth weight increased. The findings were independent of sex, ethnicity, and current levels of socioeconomic status or obesity and indicated that low birth weight could be a major independent risk factor for adult chronic conditions associated with insulin resistance.

IUGR and other diagnoses

Other provocative relationships between growth restriction and subsequent outcomes concern the relation between low birth weight and schizophrenia. Rifkin and colleagues (1994) demonstrated that in 167 patients with schizophrenia or affective psychoses, a birth weight of less than 2500 gm was significantly more common than in other patients. This was particularly marked after controlling for sociodemographic confounders. In monozygotic twins, the schizophrenic patients were significantly more likely to be lighter than their twins.

Other studies have looked at second-generation consequences of SGA birth. For example, Klebanoff and colleagues (1989) studied 1154 Swedish women born between 1955 and 1965 who gave birth to children between 1972 and 1983. Women who were themselves small-for-gestational-age at birth were at an increased risk of giving birth to an SGA infant (odds ratio 2.21, 95% confidence interval = 1.4, 3.48). Women who had been categorized as SGA had an even greater incidence in risk of giving birth to a preterm infant than were women who were preterm at birth. These latter women were not at increased risk of either preterm or SGA births. They concluded that the long-term effects of intrauterine growth restriction may extend into the next generation. That is, women that were SGA themselves may be at increased risk of giving birth to growth-restricted as well as preterm infants.

Challenges to the programming theory

Since the publication of Dr. Barker's hypothesis, a number of investigators have challenged its validity. For example, investigators have noted that twins do not appear to demonstrate effects similar to those hypothesized by Barker, despite their frequent small size at birth. Vagaro and Leon (1994) examined the linkage between IUGR infants and later adverse outcomes by analyzing data from the Swedish Twin Registry. Although these studies did not include specific birth weight data, the authors posited that twins should be expected to have substantially higher coronary heart disease mortality if the programming hypothesis were true. However, the data demonstrated that twins' mortality from coronary heart disease was not greater than coronary heart disease mortality in the general population.

A second challenge has come in examinations of links between fetal undernutrition and disease rates across different countries. Fetal undernutrition and coronary heart disease do not have the same distribution worldwide. In China, although infants are of low birth weight as compared to Western infants, coronary heart disease is rare. Barker believes that this is because infants in China are proportionately growth restricted and this pattern of fetal growth is not associated with coronary heart disease, but with raised blood pressure. Furthermore, country-specific, age-adjusted mortality rates from coronary heart disease do not appear to reflect patterns in birth weight and fetal growth. The highest recorded rates of coronary heart disease mortality occur in Scotland, Northern Ireland, Finland,

England, Wales, New Zealand, Norway, and Denmark, countries that have had among the world's highest birth weight distributions for many decades (Thom, 1989). Studies by Elford and colleagues (1990) in the British Regional Heart Study have looked at the effect of migration within the U.K. on coronary heart disease. The risk of high blood pressure or coronary heart disease reflects the place migrated *to* rather than the place migrated *from*, despite the fact that men born in Scotland who subsequently migrated to the south of England were shorter on average than men born in the south of England. Thus, the early life factors that shaped height seemed less important than the factors associated with the place to which the men migrated.

A third challenge is based on examinations of disease rates over time. Coronary heart disease rates in England and Wales have declined in every age group from the youngest to those over 75 years of age, after increasing steadily from the postwar period to the early 1970s. If gradually improving infant and fetal health were responsible for the decline in coronary heart disease, then it could be expected that the younger cohorts would have greater declines than the older ones. However, the decline in coronary heart disease is period-related and not mediated by increasing reductions in coronary heart disease rates among successive birth cohorts.

Perhaps the most significant critique of Barker's work comes from Joseph and Kramer (1996), who have reviewed the substantive and methodological issues relevant to this area of research. Because of the preponderance of studies that demonstrate that socioeconomic factors are important determinants of coronary heart disease, Joseph and Kramer assert that adjustment for socioeconomic factors, such as income, nutrition, smoking, physical activity, and stress, is mandatory. Unfortunately, socioeconomic status is not easily and precisely measured in longitudinal studies and they express concern over the techniques of adjustment for socioeconomic factors in Barker's work. In most of these studies, the sole measure of socioeconomic status is social class, when it is used at all. In contrast, a link between birth weight and socioeconomic status has been consistently demonstrated in numerous studies across decades and countries. Joseph and Kramer also have focused on potential selection bias due to losses to follow up and have looked at the inconsistencies in the hypotheses tested and in the analytic procedures used. For example, they note that the cohort studies in Hertfordshire represented only about 36% of all eligible births during the period under study. Of the 15 000 subjects, only 5700 were available for analysis. They point out that initial reports on 5654 subjects and subsequent reports on 5718 subjects showed strikingly different death rates from specific causes between those traced early and those traced subsequently. This finding raises the possibility that the sample of the cohort studied was not representative of the original cohort with regard to absolute rates of cause-specific mortality.

Other investigators have also demonstrated that the ecologic correlation between infant mortality rates and coronary heart disease is not restricted to past infant mortality rates. Rather, infant mortality rates drawn from the same period as the birth records of those who died from coronary heart disease correlate well, thus implicating socioeconomic factors. A study in 43 counties in England and Wales by Ben-Schlomo and Smith (1991), looked at infant mortality rates between 1895 and 1908 and cause-specific mortality between 1969 and 1973. They demonstrated that although infant mortality rates were associated with recent mortality from specific causes, these associations were abolished or attenuated by adjustment for current socioeconomic factors.

Conclusion

The data presented here indicate that intrauterine growth restriction is responsible for considerable short-term morbidity to the fetus. These infants can be shown to have increased risk for mortality and morbidity in the neonatal period. In addition, most studies also reveal that intrauterine growth restriction may affect neurodevelopmental function and, for a significant number of children, subsequent growth. Studies looking at intrauterine growth restriction as a cause of adult disease are more problematic. The difficulty of ascertaining outcomes for large populations over several decades is a significant one. Animal data and many of the population-based studies that have been performed seem to indicate that there is an association between low birth weight and Syndrome X. Because of the large number of studies particularly from one institution, reporting to demonstrate the causal relationship, and because of the potential policy implications of such a conclusion, it is important that studies be undertaken in other populations where follow up can be assured.

REFERENCES

Barker DJP. Outcome of low birth weight. Hormone Research 1994; **42**: 223–30.

Barker DJP. Fetal origins of coronary heart disease. British Journal of Medicine 1995; **311**: 171–4.

Barker DJP, Bull AR, Osmond C, et al. Fetal and placental size and risk of hypertension in adult life. British Journal of Medicine 1990; **301**: 259–62.

Barker DJP, Hales CN, Full CH, et al. Type 2 diabetes mellitus, hypertension and hyperlipidema relative to reduced fetal growth. Diabetologia 1993a; **36**: 62–7.

Barker DJP, Martyn CN, Osmond C, et al. Growth in utero and serum cholesterol concentration in adult life. British Journal of Medicine 1993b; **307**: 1524–7.

Barker DJP, Osmond C, Simmonds SJ, et al. The relation of small head circumference and thinness at birth to death from cardiovascular disease in adult life. British Journal of Medicine 1993c; **306**: 422–6.

Ben-Schlomo Y, Smith GD. Deprivation in infancy or in adult life: which is more important for mortality risk? Lancet 1991; **337**: 530–4.

Berg AT. Indices of fetal growth-retardation, perinatal hypoxia-related factors and childhood neurological morbidity. Early Human Development 1989; **19**: 271–83.

Brar HS, Rutherford SE. Classification of intrauterine growth retardation. Seminars in Perinatology 1988; **12**: 2–10.

Curhan GC, Willett WC, Rimm EB, et al. Birth weight and adult hypertension, diabetes mellitus, and obesity in US men. Circulation 1996; **94**: 3246–50.

Cuttini M, Cortinovis I, Bossi A, de Vonderweid U. Proportionality of small for gestational age babies as a predictor of neonatal mortality and morbidity. Pædiatric and Perinatal Epidemiology 1991; **5**: 56–63.

Elford J, Phillips AN, Thomson AG et al. Migration and geographic variations in blood pressure in Britain. British Journal of Medicine 1990; **300**: 291–5.

Gluckman PD. Intrauterine growth retardation: future directions. Acta Pædiatrica. Supplement 1993; **388**: 96–9.

Goldenberg RL, DuBard MB, Cliver SP, et al. Pregnancy outcome and intelligence at age five years. American Journal of Obstetrics and Gynecology 1996; **175**: 1511–15.

Hack M, Weissman B, Borawski-Clark E. Catch-up growth during childhood among very low-birth-weight children. Archives of Pediatrics and Adolescent Medicine 1996; **150**: 1122–9.

Hadders-Algra M, Touwen B. Body measurements, neurological and behavioral development in six-year-old children born preterm and/or small-for-gestational-age. Early Human Development 1990; **22**: 1–13.

Hutton JL, Pharoah POD, Cooke RWI, et al. Differential effects of preterm birth and small gestational age on cognitive and motor development. Archives of Disease in Childhood 1997; **76**(2SI): F75–F81.

Joseph KS, Kramer MS. Review of the evidence on fetal and early childhood antecedents of adult chronic disease. Epidemiologic Reviews 1996; **18**: 158–74.

Karlberg J, Albertsson-Wikland K. Growth in full-term small-for-gestational-age infants: from birth to final height. Pediatric Research 1995; **38**: 733–9.

Klebanoff MA, Meirik O, Berendes HW. Second-generation consequences of small-for-dates birth. Pediatrics 1989; **84**: 343–7.

Kramer MS, Oliver M, McLean FH, et al. Impact of intrauterine growth retardation and body proportionately in fetal and neonatal outcome. Pediatrics 1990; **86**: 707–13.

Langley SC, Jackson AA. Increased systolic blood pressures in adult rats induced by fetal exposure to maternal low protein diets. Clinical Science 1994; **86**: 217–22.

Law CM, Barker DJP, Osmond C, et.al. Early growth and abdominal fatness in adult life. Journal of Epidemiology and Community Health 1992; **46**: 184–6.

Lever AF, Harrap SB. Essential hypertension: a disorder of growth with origins in childhood? Journal of Hypertension 1992; **10**: 101–20.

Mackenzie HS, Brenner BM. Fewer nephrons at birth: a missing link in the etiology of essential hypertension? American Journal of Kidney Diseases 1995; **26**: 91–8.

Nelson KG, Goldenberg RL, Hoffman HJ, Cliver SP. Growth and development during the first year in a cohort of low income term-born American children. Acta Obstetricia et Gynecologica Scandinavica 1997; **165**(Suppl.): 87–92.

Paz I, Gale R, Laor A, et al. The cognitive outcome of full-term small for gestational age infants at late adolescence. Obstetrics and Gynecology 1995; **85**: 452–6.

Piper JM, Xenakis EM-J, McFarland M, et al. Do growth-retarded premature infants have different rates of perinatal morbidity and mortality than appropriately grown premature infants? Obstetrics and Gynecology 1996; **87**: 169–74.

Rifkin L, Lewis S, Jones P, et al. Low birth weight and schizophrenia. British Journal of Psychiatry 1994; **165**: 357–62.

Robertson X, Etches P, Kyle J. Eight year school performance and growth of preterm, small for gestational age infants: a comparison study with subjects matched for birth weight or for gestational age. The Journal of Pediatrics 1990; **116**: 19–26.

Sung IK, Vohr B, Oh W. Growth and neurodevelopmental outcome of very low birth weight infants with intrauterine growth retardation: comparison with control subjects matched by birth weight and gestational age. The Journal of Pediatrics 1993; **123**: 618–24.

Tebers AJ, Walther FJ, Pena IC. Mortality, morbidity and outcome of the small for gestational age infant. Seminars in Perinatology 1988; **12**: 84–94.

Thom TJ. International mortality from heart disease: rates and trends. International Journal of Epidemiology 1989; **18** (3 Suppl. 1): 520–8.

Uvebrant P, Hagberg G. Intrauterine growth in children with cerebral palsy. Acta Pædiatrica 1992; **81**: 407–12.

Vagero D, Leon D. Ischaemic heart disease and low birth weight: a test of the fetal-origins hypothesis from the Swedish Twin Registry. Lancet 1994; **343**: 260–3.

Valdez R, Athens MA, Thompson GH, et al. Birth weight and adult health outcomes in a biethnic population in the USA. Diabetologia 1994; **37**: 624–31.

Part IV

Preventing and Treating Birth Defects

9

Prevalence and etiology of birth defects

Joan M. Stoler

Introduction

The impact of birth defects on the affected individual, his or her family, and society in general is immense, encompassing mortality, morbidity, lost productivity, and medical care costs. In countries with low infant mortality, over 20% of infant deaths are due to birth defects (Shepard et al., 1989) and 18–30% of pediatric hospitalizations are due to congenital defects (Soltan and Craven, 1981; Weatherall, 1991). Risks of postnatal mortality, of prolonged hospitalization for children up to one year of age, and of neurologic abnormalities of children up to seven years of age are all increased in the presence of congenital abnormalities. Clearly, if there was a way to prevent the occurrence of birth defects, the benefits would be enormous.

This chapter first presents various ways in which birth defects are commonly defined and describes current knowledge of their frequency, as derived from various data sources including birth defect surveillance programs. The chapter then discusses our understanding of the etiology of birth defects from several perspectives and presents a case for addressing their prevention on primary, secondary, and tertiary levels.

Defining birth defects

There are numerous inconsistencies in defining birth defects, particularly in distinguishing between major and minor malformations. This lack of consistency has led to difficulties in tabulating congenital defects. The frequency of birth defects can vary greatly in different studies if, for example, one study includes all malformations, major and minor, while another excludes minor malformations.

There also is confusion among the different terms used to describe birth defects, which include "malformation," "anomaly," "deformation," and "disruption." A birth defect has been defined as "an abnormal structural variant originating during prenatal life." A malformation is "a morphologic defect of a part of the body resulting from abnormal prenatal development" (Smith, 1977). For all practical purposes, malformation and anomaly are equivalent and will be considered synonymous (Holmes, 1976). While a malformation is considered a primary defect originating from poor formation of tissue, a deformation is defined as a secondary defect caused by "unusual forces on normal tissue," and a disruption is a secondary defect caused by breakdown of normal tissue (Graham, 1988). For example, a congenital heart defect such as Tetralogy of Fallot would be considered a malformation. Contractures of the limbs from prolonged oligohydramnios would be considered a deformation, and a limb body wall defect secondary to an amniotic band sequence would be classified as a disruption. All malformations, deformations, and disruptions are considered birth defects.

Malformations are classified according to whether they are major or minor. There has been little disagreement about the definition of a major malformation, with most investigators in the field agreeing that major defects are those responsible for increased morbidity, handicap, and/or mortality (Chung and Myrinathopoulos, 1987). However, disagreement has arisen on the definition of minor malformations. Smith (1971) defined minimal malformations as "morphologic anomalies of neither medical nor cosmetic significance." A year earlier, Hook and Petry (1970) defined them as "anatomic variants occurring in low frequency in the normal population." In a 1985 editorial, Opitz added to the discussion by suggesting that malformations be divided into severe or mild and that mild malformations be distinguished from minor anomalies. He defined mild malformations as abnormal but relatively common defects and minor anomalies as not distinguishable from normal variants (Opitz, 1985).

We have found the following distinctions to be the most useful: a major malformation has either surgical, medical, or cosmetic significance, while a minor malformation does not (Holmes, 1976). In addition, a minor malformation is distinguished from a "normal variant" by the fact that the feature in question occurs in 4% or less of infants of the same race (Holmes, 1976). Examples of minor malformations would be epicanthal folds and fifth finger clinodactyly (incurving of the finger).

Determining the frequency of birth defects

The true incidence of birth defects is not known because many embryos with malformations are lost. The prevalence of a birth defect is therefore the measure used to reflect the frequency of its occurrence.

Many studies have been conducted to determine the prevalence of birth defects. However, the methodology of these studies varies widely, leading to different estimates of frequency. When analyzing the results of such studies, attention should be paid to the following questions:

- How were the data obtained and from what sources?
- What population was targeted, and over what time period?
- What is being used as the base population (as the denominator in the frequency calculations)?
- How are the defects categorized? Are minor malformations included in the tabulations?

Registry of surveillance programs

Most studies rely on data obtained from birth defect registries or surveillance programs. These programs collect data actively or passively, or they may use both methods. In active programs, registry personnel retrieve the data themselves. Passive programs depend upon transmission of data to them by physicians and other hospital staff. There can be incomplete ascertainment of cases in passive surveillance programs because all cases may not be reported. There can also be bias in ascertaining cases if only the most severe defects are reported. However, an advantage of passive registries is that they can cover wide populations, detect regional clustering of birth defects, and are less expensive than active surveillance programs. With active surveillance, incomplete ascertainment may be less of a concern than with passive programs. However, such programs are by necessity smaller in scope due to the greater expense and time commitment required to acquire the data (Cordero, 1992).

In the United States, there are many different birth defect surveillance programs, both population-based and hospital-based. Information from these programs has been used to study the occurrence, trends, and in some cases, the etiology of birth defects (Khoury, 1995). For example, the federal Centers for Disease Control and Prevention (CDC) has a national program, the Birth Defects Monitoring Program (BDMP), that is a passive registry and obtains data from newborn discharge summaries reported from participating hospitals. In addition, 20 states each have their own statewide birth defects surveillance programs (Khoury, 1995). One example is the California Birth Defects Monitoring Program (Hexter et al., 1990), an active surveillance system in which the staff visit each hospital to register children with birth defects detected in the first year of life. There are also smaller programs, such as those at the city level (e.g., the Metropolitan Atlanta Congenital Defects Program run by the Centers for Disease Control and Prevention) and those at the hospital level (e.g., the Malformation Surveillance Program at the Brigham and Women's Hospital in Boston, Massachusetts).

The CDC has an International Clearinghouse for Birth Defects Monitoring

Systems, which is comprised of 25 birth defects surveillance systems (Cordero, 1992; Khoury, 1995). In Europe there are regional registries from various countries that are part of the European Registration of Congenital Anomalies (EURO-CAT) system. These systems facilitate worldwide comparisons and pooling of data from studies of rare defects from registries in 13 European countries (Francannet et al., 1993).

Data from passive and active surveillance programs are sometimes comparable. For example, data on the frequency of spina bifida at birth from 1983 to 1990 obtained from the CDC BDMP was compared to data from 16 more active state programs and found to indicate a similar prevalence (Lary and Edmonds, 1996). The state programs reported 4.6 cases per 10 000 births compared to 4.4 cases per 10 000 from the BDMP data. Of course, it is possible that both methods under-ascertained the cases. The data from these registries can be considered as minimum frequencies of the defect in question.

When comparing birth defect frequency data, it is important to note the base population that is used as the denominator in calculations. For population-based programs, the denominator is the number of births to residents of the defined area. In a hospital-based program, the denominator is the total number of births at a particular hospital. Hospital-based programs have the disadvantage of having a smaller denominator. However, their ascertainment of cases may be more complete than those of larger population-based programs (Cordero, 1992).

If a hospital-based program is at a tertiary referral center, then adjustment must also be made for referrals made to the center. The malformation surveillance program at the Brigham and Women's Hospital, for example, adjusts for this potential bias by determining whether the woman intended to deliver at that hospital or was referred. Cases of infants with birth defects whose mothers fall into the referral category (referred to as "transfers") are excluded from the tabulations (Nelson and Holmes, 1989).

Data sources for registries and surveillance

Sources of data for birth defect registries and surveillance programs include discharge diagnoses, medical records, postmortem reports, delivery log books, information from cytogenetic laboratories, records from genetic counseling clinics, parental interviews, and birth, death, and stillborn certificates. While some programs limit their data collection to certificates or discharge diagnoses, many others use more than one resource.

Using birth certificates or discharge diagnoses as a sole source of data is problematic, as illustrated by an Atlanta study of the sensitivity and positive predictive value of birth certificates for the detection of congenital defects. The investigators compared 771 birth certificates that reported birth defects to 2427 liveborn infants ascertained in a birth defects registry. Only 14% of the cases from the registry had the defects listed on their birth certificates, resulting only in a sensitivity of 28% and a positive predictive value of 77% (Watkins et al., 1996). Similarly, discharge diagnoses are also often inaccurate either in terms of the wrong diagnosis or in excluding multiple diagnoses (Hexter et al., 1990). Hexter and colleagues (1990) showed that the discharge diagnosis omitted one-third to one-half of cases with a diagnosis and had a high percentage of false positive diagnoses. Hexter and Harris (1991) also showed that hospitals with many births report lower birth defect rates than do hospitals with fewer deliveries. This was attributed to the fact that the larger hospitals' source of information was usually the obstetrician rather than the pediatrician.

In order to compare the frequencies across different programs, it is important to see how each study categorizes the various defects. Many programs have strict definitions of the different types of defects and some have used modifications of the ICD-9 Diagnoses Code in order to provide consistency in the categorization of defects (Barbujani et al., 1989; Nelson and Holmes, 1989).

Target population and time period of detection

Deriving an accurate estimate of the prevalence of birth defects is also dependent on the target population chosen and the time period selected for analysis. Birth defects diagnosed in the newborn period will underestimate the prevalence of defects because a number of defects are not commonly diagnosed until later in infancy. These include defects of the internal organs, such as the heart and kidneys, or central nervous system (Graham, 1992). Extending the time period of detection up to one year of age will double the percentage of total congenital malformations diagnosed (Graham, 1992).

Many studies do not include data on spontaneous abortions, stillbirths, and terminations. Between 10 to 20% of stillborn fetuses and 19% of spontaneously aborted fetuses have been found to have birth defects (Khoury, 1995). Infants who die in the newborn period also have a higher rate of malformations than do other newborns (Chung and Myrinathopoulos, 1987). With the improvement of pre-natal diagnosis of birth defects, elective termination of an affected fetus is possible. Accordingly, the number of liveborn infants with birth defects could decrease over time.

Geographic/ethnic distribution of birth defects

Data from surveillance programs have shown that the total malformation rate is similar across diverse populations, and is in the range of 1–4% (Table 9.1). These rates take into account the potential differences in methodology among the

Table 9.1. Frequency of birth defects in different populations

Country	Time period	Birth defect frequency (%)	Type of study
Belgium	1975–1984	2	Hospital-based
Canada	1970–1981	4	Population-based
China	1988–1991	1.02	Hospital-based
England	1960–1964	2.39	Population-based
Finland	1963–1970	1.22	Population-based
Iran	1972–1975	1.84	Hospital-based
Israel	1959–1960	1.32	Population-based
Japan	1948–1990	1.07	Hospital-based
United States	1978–1988	3.6	Atlanta area

Sources: Halevi, 1967; Imaizumi et al., 1991; Lowry et al., 1986; Mili et al., 1991; Naderi, 1979; Saxen and Klemetti, 1973; Smithells, 1968; Van Regemorter et al., 1984; Wu et al., 1995.

different studies. However, in some discrete populations, the rate of total birth defects may differ, such as the rate of 6% found in Quebec compared to 4% in the rest of Canada (Murnan, 1973).

While the total rate of malformations and the rate of chromosomal abnormalities are the same in differing populations, there may be clustering of specific malformations in different populations and/or geographic areas (Smithells, 1968). Neural tube defects (NTDs) are good examples of this phenomenon. In Great Britain, the frequency of NTDs differs between the north and south (Carter, 1976; Hall, 1988). In the United States, the overall rates range from 0.4/1000 to 1.2/1000 (CDC, 1992a; Yen et al., 1992). NTDs in the U.S. also appear to vary by ethnicity. Hispanics have the highest birth prevalence of spina bifida followed by non-Hispanic whites. The lowest rates are found among African Americans and Asians (CDC, 1992a).

Other examples of defects that vary by race are postaxial polydactyly type B and cleft lip with or without cleft palate. Postaxial polydactyly occurs in about 1.2% of African Americans in comparison to 0.09% in American Caucasians (Woolf and Myrinathopoulos, 1973). The frequency of cleft lip and/or palate in the Native American population is 3.6/1000 (Gorlin et al., 1990) while that in France is much lower (0.67/1000) (Long et al., 1992). Similarly, a Canadian study showed that Native Americans of British Columbia had lower rates of hypospadias and foot abnormalities and higher rates of congenital heart disease, cleft lip and/or palate, and cleft palate alone than did non-Native residents (Lowry et al., 1986). Correa-Villasenor and colleagues (1991) showed that the frequency of certain congenital

Table 9.2. Frequency of a sampling of specific defects

Birth defects	Frequency
Neural tube defects:	
U.S., 1970	1.3/1000
U.S., 1989	0.6/1000
Hungary, 1960	2.95/1000
Congenital heart defects:	
Overall	1/100
Ventricular septal defect	2.5–5/1000
Tetralogy of Fallot	0.7/1000
Transposition of the great vessels	0.4/1000
Ebstein's anomaly	0.12/1000
Facial clefts:	
Cleft lip +/− cleft palate	1/500 – 1/1000
Cleft palate alone	1/2500
Other:	
Clubfoot	1.82/1000

Sources: Bower and Ramsay, 1994; CDC, 1992a; Czeizel, 1973; Harper, 1988; Leck, 1976; Yen et al., 1992.

heart defects differs between Caucasians and African Americans and by socioeconomic status. Table 9.2 illustrates the varying frequency of selected birth defects.

Associations with birth defects

Epidemiologic research has demonstrated specific associations with some birth defects. In some cases, these are clues to the etiologies of the defect.

Birth weight

Low birth weight infants have a higher frequency of birth defects than do higher birth weight babies. Mili and colleagues (1991) found an inverse relationship between birth defects and birth weight, ranging from a 16.2% frequency of birth defects among infants weighing less than 1500 gm and 13.2% in infants weighing 1500–1990 gm to 2.8% in those 4000 gm or more. The birth defects in the low birth weight infants added to their morbidity and mortality and were unrelated to infant gender or maternal age. This association included most birth defects with the exception of prematurity-related defects (e.g., patent ductus arteriosus, patent foramen ovale, hydrocephalus associated with hemorrhage, and undescended testicles), which are complications of the prematurity, and certain other defects (e.g., hypoplastic left heart, endocardial cushion defect, coarctation of the aorta, esophageal atresia, and bladder exstrophy), which were not seen in increased frequency among low birth weight infants as compared to non-low birth weight infants.

Twinning

A higher frequency of malformations is seen in monozygotic twins. This may be a part of the monozygotic twinning process itself (Schinzel et al., 1979). These defects include early embryonic malformations and malformation complexes such as sirenomelia (a malformation associated with severe genitourinary and gastrointestinal defects in which there is a single malformed midline lower extremity), holoprosencephaly (a severe brain malformation in which the brain fails to cleave into the cerebral and lateral hemispheres), and anencephaly. Defects that are thought to be secondary to vascular disruptions are also increased in monozygotic twins. Examples of this type of defect include limb amputations, aplasia cutis (a localized area in which the skin and underlying subcutaneous tissue are missing), and intestinal atresias.

Gender

In general, males have a higher overall frequency of birth defects, although this may vary by defect. For example, bilateral cleft lip and palate are more common in males, while anencephaly is more common in females (Carter, 1976).

Consanguinity

There is a higher rate of birth defects in the offspring of consanguineous couples. In general, there is about a doubling of the baseline rate of birth defects in the offspring of first cousins (Harper, 1988). An Iranian study showed a rate of 1.66% of congenital abnormalities in newborns of non-consanguineous couples versus 4.02% in the newborns of consanguineous couples (Naderi, 1979). These figures included major and multiple malformations as well as prematurity and perinatal mortality rates.

Number of birth defects

Over 12% of children with birth defects have two types of malformations (Myrianthopoulos and Chung, 1974). Furthermore, stillborn fetuses have a higher frequency of multiple malformations (Shepard et al., 1989).

Etiology of birth defects

The etiologies of birth defects are almost as varied as the malformations themselves. In many cases, the exact etiology is not known. This makes it difficult to develop preventive strategies, because the etiology and/or pathophysiology of the defects in question must be known if rational efforts at prevention are to be devised.

Birth defects can have multiple etiologies (Holmes, 1974). For example, a ventricular septal defect can be found in children with chromosomal abnormalities, such as trisomy 21 and 22q11 deletion and in children who have had teratogenic exposures, such as in maternal diabetes, maternal PKU or maternal alcohol abuse. It also can be part of a single gene malformation syndrome.

Nelson and Holmes (1989) tabulated the etiologies of 1549 infants with malformations born at the Brigham and Women's Hospital over a 10-year period from 1972 to 1975 and from 1979 to 1985. Of these cases, genetic etiologies were identified for 27.7%: 10.1% had chromosomal abnormalities, 3.1% had single mutant gene disorders, and 14.5% had familial disorders (but without a recognized inheritance pattern). Of other etiologies identified, 23% were multifactorial inheritance, 3.2% were teratogenic, 2.5% were uterine factors, and 0.4% were twinning. Of note, was the fact that 43% of the birth defects were of unknown etiology.

Chromosomal abnormalities

Chromosomal abnormalities are a major cause of malformations both in newborns and in stillborn fetuses. They are found in 20.6% of preimplantation embryos, 50% of spontaneous abortions, and 2.5–8% of children with birth defects (Gardner and Sutherland, 1996). These abnormalities include abnormalities of chromosome number and/or structure.

Abnormalities of chromosome number

These abnormalities (the aneuploidies) include the trisomies and monosomies. Practically all monosomies result in embryonic demise. The one exception is 45,X (Turner syndrome), which, however, has an extremely high perinatal mortality. Birth defects seen in association with 45,X include cardiac defects (e.g., bicuspid aortic valve, coarctation of aorta), renal defects (e.g., horseshoe kidneys), and gonadal dysgenesis.

Trisomies are common, with the trisomies 21, 18, 13 and the sex chromosome trisomies XXY and XXX being the most common in liveborn infants. The livebirth prevalence figures for these trisomies are 1 in 800, 1 in 8000, 1 in 25 000, respectively, and 1 in 1000 for the sex chromosome aneuploidies (Thompson et al., 1991). The true incidence is lower at birth than at conception because of substantial fetal losses. Many other trisomies, such as trisomy 16, may be detected prenatally, but rarely result in liveborn infants.

The birth defects associated with the aneuploidies depend upon the chromosome involved. Trisomy 21 (Down's syndrome) may be associated with congenital heart disease, gastrointestinal defects such as duodenal atresia, tracheoesophageal fistula, and skeletal abnormalities. Infants with trisomy 13 usually have multiple birth defects, including cleft lip and palate, polydactyly, holoprosencephaly, eye abnormalities, and omphalocele, among many other possible defects. By contrast, the sex chromosome aneuploidies (47,XXX and 47,XXY) are not typically associated with birth defects.

Trisomies are usually sporadic, and the only known association is with advanced maternal age. Families in which there are multiple individuals who have offspring with trisomies have been noted (Empu et al., 1985). Whether this is due to chance or whether there are individuals who are genetically predisposed to nondisjunction in their germ cells is not known at the present time.

Abnormalities of chromosome structure

These abnormalities include translocations, inversions, deletions, and duplications. Although individuals with balanced translocations and inversions may be asymptomatic, their offspring are at increased risk of inheriting an imbalance in the karyotype (the chromosomal constitution of the cell nucleus), with deletion and/or duplication of chromosomal material. Such an imbalance usually results in some type of birth defect and developmental delay.

Deletions can be either microscopic (visible on a standard karyotype) or submicroscopic (requiring specialized DNA probes for diagnosis). They may result in contiguous gene syndromes in which there is a pattern of defects associated with the absence of multiple genes. For example, a child with a deletion of part of the short arm of chromosome 5 (called the 5p- or Cri du Chat syndrome) can have various skeletal and internal malformations. The majority of these cases – 85% – occur de novo while 15% are the consequence of a balanced parental translocation involving chromosome 5 (Gardner and Sutherland, 1989). An example of a submicroscopic deletion is the 22q11 deletion, which has varied manifestations including DiGeorge syndrome (infantile hypocalcemia, thymic aplasia, interrupted aortic arch), velocardiofacial syndrome, and conotruncal heart defects. This deletion can occur de novo or can be inherited from a parent who may be mildly affected, or from an unaffected parent who carries a balanced translocation (Motskin et al., 1993).

Similarly, duplications can arise de novo or from malsegregation of a balanced translocation and can be microscopic or submicroscopic. For example, duplication of a particular portion of the long arm of chromosome 11, can be seen in association with Beckwith–Wiedemann syndrome (macrosomia, hypoglycemia, omphalocele).

Single gene disorders

Another category of birth defect involves mutation of a single gene, in contrast to the chromosomal abnormalities, which involve many genes. These can be autosomal dominant (when the condition is due to one abnormal copy of a gene), autosomal recessive (when the condition is due to two abnormal copies of a gene), or X-linked disorders (when the responsible gene is located on the X chromosome).

A malformation syndrome due to an autosomal dominant gene can be familial, meaning that the mutant gene is already present in the family, and the affected child inherited it from a parent. A child also can have the disorder as the result of a new mutation. From then on the disorder can be inherited if the disorder does not affect the individual's reproductive fitness.

An example of an autosomal dominant malformation syndrome is Holt–Oram syndrome. This is a disorder due to a defect in the gene TBX-5 (Li et al., 1997), which results in malformations of the hands and the heart. Apert syndrome, the craniosynostosis syndrome with major hand malformations, is another example of an autosomal dominant condition. Although it can be familial, most of the cases are due to new mutations.

New mutations in Apert syndrome as well as 12 other autosomal dominant conditions have been associated with older paternal age (Olshan et al., 1994). Recently, one study analyzed the association of birth defects with parental age and estimated that 5% of cardiac defects, such as ventricular septal defect, may be due to advanced paternal age (> 35 years of age), perhaps secondary to new dominant mutations (McIntosh et al., 1995). This same group of investigators also showed a pattern of increasing adjusted relative risk estimates for neural tube defects, congenital cataracts, limb reduction defects, and Down's syndrome with increasing paternal age. They hypothesized that a certain proportion of malformations of unknown etiology is actually due to new dominant mutations of paternal origin.

Recurrence risks (the risk for another individual in the family to be affected) for autosomal dominant conditions depend on whether the condition is familial (50% recurrence risk for the offspring of an affected parent) or sporadic (where the recurrence risk is low).

Malformation syndromes can also be inherited as autosomal recessive conditions in which both parents are heterozygous for the gene. The recurrence risk in this situation is 25% for each pregnancy; the new mutation rate is not as much a factor as with autosomal dominant disorders. An example of such a recessive condition is Bardet–Biedl syndrome in which there may be polydactyly, hypogonadism, vaginal atresia, obesity, and retinitis pigmentosa.

Other malformation syndromes may be due to X-linked genes and, therefore, have an increased frequency in males. Females may have some manifestations of the disorder, but are generally much less severely affected than males. An example of this is X-linked hydrocephalus, in which males may have massive hydrocephalus and the carrier females are asymptomatic.

Multifactorial inheritance

In multifactorial inheritance, genetic factors interact with environmental exposures or agents to cause birth defects. There may be several genes involved (a "polygenic" disorder), or there may be direct interaction of different genes with the environment, for example, a change in an individual's susceptibility to a teratogenic agent. Neural tube defects, cleft lip, and/or palate and pyloric stenosis are thought to be inherited in this manner. Recurrence risks for first and second-degree relatives of an affected individual are higher than the general background population risk, but lower than those of the single gene disorders.

Similar conditions that have differing etiologies may be mixed within this group. Such genetic heterogeneity, especially if there are different inheritance patterns, can confuse understanding of the mode of inheritance. For example, if malformations that can occur as the result of a new autosomal dominant mutation or homozygosity of a recessive gene are similar, they may be lumped together and the recurrence risks of the combined disorders would be lower than what would be quoted for the single gene disorder.

Multifactorial inheritance patterns may involve alternative forms of a gene or genes with differing activity levels in those forms (alleles). By virtue of the differing activity level, these alleles may render an individual more or less susceptible to the action of an environmental agent. This situation has been seen with a particular allele of the gene for transforming growth factor alpha. When a woman with this particular allele smokes cigarettes, the risk of her having a child with an oral cleft is increased over the general population risk (Hwang et al., 1995). It may also turn out that this is the case with neural tube defects and that individuals who have a particular form of an enzyme involved in folate metabolism may be at increased risk for having a child with a neural tube defect. However, to date this has not been shown to be the case, and the mechanism behind folate metabolism and the development of birth defects has yet to be determined.

Teratogens

Teratogens include medications, substances of abuse, maternal conditions, maternal infections, medical procedures, maternal nutrition, and environmental

Table 9.3. Examples of teratogens

Type of agent	Specific agent	Birth defect
Antiepileptic medications	Valproic acid	Spina bifida
	Carbamazepine	Spina bifida
Antihypertensive medications	Angiotensin-converting enzyme (ACE) inhibitors	Renal dysplasia
Antithyroid agents	Propylthiouracil	Goiter
Anticoagulants	Warfarin	Nasal hypoplasia
Psychotropic agents	Lithium	Congenital heart defects
Maternal infections	Rubella	Cataracts
Chronic maternal disorders	Insulin-dependent diabetes	Congenital heart defects
	Maternal PKU	Congenital heart defects
	Maternal lupus	Congenital heart block
Substance abuse	Alcohol	Fetal alcohol syndrome
	Toluene	Toluene embryopathy
	Cocaine	Vascular disruptions
Medical procedures	Chorionic villus sampling	Transverse limb defects
	Radiation therapy	Microcephaly

Sources: Brent et al., 1993; Chernoff, 1980; Firth et al., 1991; Hersh, 1989; Holmes, 1992; Volpe, 1992

exposures. Most cause malformations, although some can cause disruption defects. For example, chorionic villus sampling and cocaine may both cause limb defects secondary to vascular disruptions (Firth et al., 1991; Volpe, 1992). The mechanism of action is known for only a small fraction of teratogens, and most available data involve maternal exposures. There are very few data on the effects of paternal exposures, and research has focused on this area only recently (Olshan and Mattison, 1994).

It is commonly assumed that the list of teratogens is endless. However, at this time, the list of documented teratogens includes only about 50 agents or procedures (Holmes, 1992). Table 9.3, which lists a sampling of these teratogens and specific birth defects with which they have been associated, demonstrates that there is a wide variety of different teratogenic agents (Brent et al., 1993; Chernoff, 1980; Firth et al., 1991; Hersh, 1989; Holmes, 1992; Volpe, 1992). For some of these agents, the listed birth defect is not the only one associated with the teratogen.

Other potential teratogens include defects in maternal nutrition, such as folate deficiency, which is related to the development of such birth defects as neural tube defects and conotruncal heart defects. Interestingly, an association also has been noted between maternal obesity and neural tube defects (odds ratio of 1.9) (Watkins et al., 1996).

Maternal substance abuse can cause significant fetal defects. Prenatal alcohol exposure is one of the most common causes of mental retardation, cognitive deficits, and birth defects (CDC, 1995a). Cocaine has effects on size, may cause disruption defects secondary to vascular constriction, and may have additive effects with alcohol (Napiorkowski et al., 1996).

Uterine structural anomalies can cause deformation defects, such as clubfeet. Crowding in the uterus, such as may occur with multiple pregnancy, can also cause such defects.

In determining whether a substance is teratogenic, investigators must tease out the effect of the agent in question versus any background risk. To assist in this process, teratologists have established the following guidelines (Brent et al., 1993; Holmes, 1992):

- Does the exposure produce a specific defect or pattern of defects? An increase in a specific defect or group of defects is more likely to be the result of a teratogen than an increase in the overall number of diverse birth defects.
- Is there a dose-response relationship between the exposure and the effects?
- Is there a biologically sound proposed mechanism for the agent? For example, Nora and colleagues (1978) reported an association between oral contraceptives and various birth defects, including congenital heart defects. However, these agents require interaction with specific receptors for their action and such receptors are not found in the heart, making the association unlikely (Brent, 1994). In fact, subsequent studies have reported that there is no association between oral contraceptives and congenital heart defects (Bracken, 1990).
- Is there an animal model? While animal studies can be useful, one must view the results of these studies with caution. The doses used in animal studies are often vastly greater than the human dosage and the routes of administration are not comparable to the oral route. There are also differences in susceptibility to teratogens among species. For example, thalidomide, a potent human teratogen, is not teratogenic in rodents. Investigators must also ask whether there are genetic differences in susceptibility. One strain of inbred mice is quite susceptible to the effects of alcohol, for example, while others are not (Chernoff, 1980).

Studies on some known teratogenic agents do not fulfill all of these criteria. Nonetheless they are useful guidelines to judge such agents. One must analyze studies on teratogenicity carefully, and ask the following questions:

- Were possible confounders accounted for?
- Was there bias of ascertainment in the recruitment of cases?
- Was the sample size adequate to see potential effects?

Unknown causes

The largest etiologic category of birth defects continues to be those of unknown cause. With time, the discovery of new genes, new gene–environment interactions, and genetic susceptibilities should decrease the number of defects due to unknown causes. Some investigators have speculated that environmental and occupational exposures account for some of the birth defects of unknown etiology (Lynberg and Khoury, 1993; Sever, 1994). The possible association of environmental estrogens and male genital abnormalities, such as hypospadias, is used as a possible example (Jensen et al., 1995). In this particular instance, a case-control study of infants is being conducted by the CDC Atlanta Birth Defects Surveillance program to try to identify causative agents. The study consists of maternal interviews detailing diet, substance abuse, and possible environmental exposures, including pesticides and aflatoxins. Blood and urine are collected from both the mothers and infants to test for cocaine and its metabolites, maternal folate levels, and other micronutrients (such as zinc) and to save DNA for future gene studies (Lynberg and Khoury, 1993).

Trends in birth defect prevention efforts

Primary prevention

Over the last 20 years, there has been some progress in preventing the occurrence of birth defects (Czeizel, 1995b). In the 1980s, progress included: (1) an increased avoidance of exposure to teratogenic agents; (2) genetic counseling for the increased number of recognizable single gene defects; and (3) a greater emphasis on adequate control of maternal disorders, such as insulin-dependent diabetes mellitus and maternal phenylketonuria, before and during pregnancy, based on increased recognition of the effects of these disorders on the fetus.

In the 1990s, investigators clarified the association between folate and certain birth defects affecting the neural tube, heart, and possibly the urinary tract (Botto et al., 1996; Czeizel, 1995a; Mulinare, 1993). This offered an important opportunity for primary prevention. Folate was found to decrease the occurrence of isolated neural tube defects and of nonsyndromic NTDs associated with other birth defects by 50%. It also was associated with a decreased recurrence of neural tube defects in subsequent pregnancies (Khoury et al., 1996). This research led to the recommendation that all women of child-bearing age consume 0.4 mg of folate per day during the preconception period (CDC, 1992b).

Secondary prevention

In the last 20 years, secondary prevention of birth defects by prenatal diagnosis has improved dramatically. This has involved the development of maternal serum alpha-fetoprotein (MSAFP) screening during pregnancy to detect open fetal defects of the spine and abdomen, improved ultrasound resolution, and amniocentesis.

Maternal serum screening

The major use of the MSAFP screening is in the detection of neural tube defects and ventral abdominal wall defects (including gastroschisis and omphaloceles). Depending on the cut-off selected by the laboratory, about 85% of cases of open spina bifida and 95% of cases of anencephaly are detected. Similarly, about 98% of cases of gastroschisis and 70–80% of cases of omphaloceles will be detected (Knight, 1991).

The recognition that lower serum MSAFP levels in about 30% of pregnancies were correlated with Down's syndrome fetuses resulted in the development of the additional analytes for screening for Down's syndrome, which are human chorionic gonadotropin (hCG) and unconjugated estriol (uE3). A combination of these three analytes detects approximately 60% of Down's syndrome fetuses in women less than 35 years old and a higher percentage in women over 35 years of age (Benn et al., 1996). It was found that this triple screen can also detect approximately 60% of pregnancies with trisomy 18 fetuses (Staples et al., 1991).

Ultrasound

Improved ultrasound resolution and recognition of certain physical features on ultrasound has improved the detection rate of many birth defects. For example, the combination of a short femur, nuchal fold (a widened area on the posterior aspect of the fetal neck), and a bright papillary muscle (an area in the fetal heart) has improved the detection rate of fetuses with Down's syndrome in women who would otherwise not have been considered high risk (Benacerraf et al., 1994).

The findings of birth defects on ultrasound may result in an amniocentesis being offered, with subsequent improved detection of other chromosome abnormalities, such as trisomy 13 and 18 and 45,X.

Transvaginal ultrasonography has improved the detection of specific features in the first trimester, such as a nuchal translucency, which is highly correlated with chromosomal abnormalities if detected at 14 weeks or less of gestation (Reynders et al., 1997).

Many other birth defects can be detected by prenatal ultrasound. This detection may result in further testing, termination of the pregnancy, or arrangement for delivery at a center that has experience in treating the condition, such as centers that can perform surgical treatment for diaphragmatic hernia. The use of ultra-sound to detect birth defects is discussed further in Chapters 10 and 11.

Amniocentesis

Amniocentesis has resulted in the identification of chromosomal etiologies of many birth defects. Of course, the benefit of the amniocentesis must be weighed against the risk of the procedure (1/200 for miscarriage). It is offered routinely only to women at high risk, such as advanced maternal age, abnormal maternal serum screening, abnormalities detected by ultrasound, family history of a chromosomal abnormality (such as a translocation) or a neural tube defect.

With the advent of more genes being identified as the etiologies for many conditions, prenatal diagnosis is available in some cases using DNA obtained from the amniocentesis. Direct DNA analysis is possible if the responsible gene and its various mutations are known (either the one responsible for the disorder in the specific family or those mutations that occur most commonly in the disorder). However, in many situations, the gene location but not the actual gene responsible is known, or the mutations are unique to each family and not known in the family at risk. Indirect testing by linkage analysis (that is, trying to identify which chromosome carries the abnormal gene in the family, using chromosomal markers in the vicinity of the gene) is possible in some cases. The use of markers and other diagnostic technologies involving molecular genetics are described further in Chapter 10.

However, only a certain number of genes implicated in the pathogenesis of congenital malformations are known. In a review by Wilkie and colleagues (1994), 139 gene loci and 65 specifically identified genes were cited as being known causes of congenital malformations. With the identification of more genes, the possibility of prenatal diagnosis for more conditions will increase substantially with time.

Despite these recent advances, there are still significant limitations to prenatal diagnosis for birth defects. One study in England showed that only 51% of NTDs were detected by ultrasound, with 64% of those detected at less than 24 weeks and 36% later in the pregnancy (Chambers et al., 1995). Some of this was due to late presentation for prenatal care, declines in the numbers of women being screened, and false negative results of the testing. A group in Italy also analyzed the sensitivity of ultrasound as a prenatal diagnostic tool and found that, overall, only 18% of the defects diagnosed in utero were detected before 24 weeks (Baroncigni et al., 1995).

Tertiary prevention

Therapies for children with birth defects have improved dramatically over the past decade. Some serious conditions, such as congenital diaphragmatic hernia, can now be repaired surgically. Others, including metabolic conditions such as phenylketonuria, galactosemia, congenital adrenal hyperplasia, congenital hypothyroidism, maple syrup urine disease, and homocystinuria, can be detected through neonatal screening and medically treated. All newborns are screened for these conditions and, if positive, treated immediately. Such efforts have dramatically improved the outcome for these affected individuals.

Changes over time

Has there been any decrease in birth defects over time as a result of prevention efforts? The example of neural tube defects provides a good way to answer this question. A 7.5% per year decline in NTDs has been detected by state surveillance programs and a 3.5% per year decline has been detected by the CDC Birth Defects Monitoring Program (Lynberg et al., 1993). This decline reflects successes in primary and secondary prevention, as well as a decrease in the baseline prevalence of NTDs that preceded these efforts. The impact of prevention strategies differs by region. Studies in Arkansas show that only 9% of NTDs diagnosed prenatally were terminated in that state, versus 42% in Atlanta and Hawaii (Cragan et al., 1995).

Other conditions that appear to have been affected by prenatal diagnosis are the chromosomal abnormalities such as Down's syndrome and other trisomies. Olsen and colleagues (1996) showed that prenatal screening maintained the birth prevalence of Down's syndrome in New York state at 10.4/10 000 from 1983 to 1992. They calculated that in the absence of prenatal screening, the increased birth rate among women over 30 years of age and the decreased birth rate among younger women would have resulted in an increase in the birth prevalence of Down's syndrome to 15.3/10 000.

An important set of conditions that are potentially amenable to prevention are defects caused by maternal alcohol and cocaine abuse. To date, efforts directed to preventing fetal alcohol syndrome such as warning labels on alcoholic beverages do not appear to have decreased the prevalence of this condition (Hankin et al., 1996). These efforts appear to have their main effect on light drinkers; the number of heavy drinkers and the amount consumed at conception has not changed substantially (CDC, 1994, 1995b).

Conclusion

Although many advances have been made in the detection of birth defects and in determining their etiology, much work remains. The causes of many birth defects remain unknown, and without more knowledge of etiology, efforts at primary prevention remain rudimentary.

Over time, researchers are gradually discovering more about the vast block of birth defects of unknown cause. The concepts of genetic susceptibility, gene–environment interactions, environmental exposures, new dominant mutations of paternal origin, and the discovery of microdeletion syndromes have advanced progress in this area. Techniques for detecting many birth defects, such as ultrasound, are now available. Although these techniques have limitations, they have expanded options for secondary prevention and treatment of birth defects.

Future efforts should investigate factors associated with various birth defects in order to better illuminate their pathophysiology and etiology. The example of folate supplementation and its potential to decrease the frequency of serious birth defects serves as an inspiration for further research. We also should strive to improve early access for prenatal care for all women, so that the opportunity for secondary and tertiary prevention will not be missed.

REFERENCES

Barbujani G, Russo A, Farabegoli A, Calzolar E. Influences on the inheritance of congenital anomalies from temporal and spatial patterns of occurrence. Genetic Epidemiology 1989; **6**: 537–52.

Baronciani D, Scaglia C, Corchia C Torcetta F, Mastroiacovo P. Ultrasonography in pregnancy and fetal abnormalities: screening or diagnostic test? IPIMC 1986–1990 register data. Indagine Policentrica Italiana sulle Malformazioni Congenite. Prenatal Diagnosis 1995, **15**(12). 1101–8.

Benacerraf BR, Nadel A, Bromley B. Identification of second-trimester fetuses with autosomal trisomy by use of a sonographic scoring index. Radiology 1994; **193**(1): 135–40.

Benn PA, Horne D, Craffey A, Collins R, Ramsdell L, Greenstein R. Maternal serum screening for birth defects: results of a Connecticut regional program. Connecticut Medicine 1996; **60**(6): 323–7.

Botto KD, Khoury MJ, Mulinare J, Erickson JD. Periconceptual multivitamin use and the occurrence of conotruncal heart defects: results from a population-based case-control study. Pediatrics 1996; **98**(5): 911–17.

Bower C, Ramsay JM. Congenital heart disease: a 10 year cohort. Journal of Pædiatrics and Child Health 1994; **30**(5): 414–18.

Bracken MB. Oral contraception and congenital malformations in offspring: a review and meta-analysis of the prospective studies. Obstetrics and Gynecology 1990; **76**(3 Pt 2): 552–7.

Brent RL. Cardiovascular birth defects and prenatal exposure to female sex hormones: importance of utilizing proper epidemiological methods and teratologic principles. Teratology 1994; **49**(3): 159–61.

Brent RL, Beckman DA, Lundel CP. Clinical teratology. Current Opinion in Pediatrics 1993; **5**(2): 201–11.

Carter CO. Genetics of common single malformations. British Medical Bulletin 1976; **32**(1): 21–6.

Centers for Disease Control and Prevention (CDC). Update: Trends in fetal alcohol syndrome – United States, 1979–1993. Morbidity and Mortality Weekly Report 1995a; **44**: 249–51.

Centers for Disease Control and Prevention (CDC). Sociodemographic and behavioral characteristics associated with alcohol consumption during pregnancy – United States, 1988. Morbidity and Mortality Weekly Report 1995b; **44**: 261–4.

Centers for Disease Control and Prevention (CDC). Spina bifida incidence at birth – United States, 1983–1990. Morbidity and Mortality Weekly Report 1992a; **41**(27): 497–500.

Centers for Disease Control and Prevention (CDC). Recommendations for the use of folic acid to reduce the number of cases of spina bifida and other neural tube defects. Morbidity and Mortality Weekly Report 1992b; **41**(RR-14): 1–7.

Centers for Disease Control and Prevention (CDC). Frequent alcohol consumption among women of childbearing age – Behavioral Risk Factor Surveillance System, 1991. Journal of the American Medical Association 1994; **271**: 1820–1.

Chambers SE, Geirsson RT, Stewart RJ, Wannapirak C, Muir BB. Audit of a screening service for fetal abnormalities using early ultrasound scanning and maternal serum alpha-feto protein estimation combined with selective detailed screening. Ultrasound in Obstetrics and Gynecology 1995; **5**(3): 168–73.

Chernoff GI. The fetal alcohol syndrome in mice: maternal variables. Teratology 1980; **23**: 72–5.

Chung CS, Myrinathopoulos NC. Congenital anomalies: mortality and morbidity, burden and classification. American Journal of Medical Genetics 1987; **27**: 505–23.

Cordero JF. Registries of birth defects and genetic disease. Pediatric Clinics of North America 1992; **39**(1): 65–77.

Correa-Villasenor A, McCarter R, Downing J, Ferencz C. White–black differences in cardiovascular malformations in infancy and socioeconomic factors. The Baltimore–Washington Infant Study Group. American Journal of Epidemiology 1991; **134**(4): 393–402.

Cragan JD, Roberts HE, Edmonds LD, et al. Surveillance for anencephaly and spina bifida and the impact of prenatal diagnosis – United States, 1985–1994. MMWR. Morbidity and Mortality Weekly Report CDC Surveillance Summaries 1995; **44**(4): 1–13.

Czeizel A. Incidence and recurrence risk of common congenital malformations in Budapest in the sixties. Acta Universitatis Carolinae Medica Monographia 1973; **LVI–LVII**, 49–51.

Czeizel AE. Nutritional supplementation and prevention of congenital abnormalities. Current Opinion in Obstetrics and Gynecology 1995; **7**(2): 88–94.

Czeizel AE. Congenital abnormalities are preventable. Epidemiology 1995b; **6**(3): 205–7.

Empu D, McDonald D, Zackai E. Down syndrome: rate in second degree relatives. American Journal of Human Genetics 1985; **37**: A132.

Firth HV, Boyd PA, Chamberlain P MacKenzie IZ, Lindenbaum RH, Huson SM. Severe limb abnormalities after chorion villus sampling at 56–66 days gestation. Lancet 1991; **337**: 762–3.

Francannet CF, Lancaster PA, Pradat P, Cocchi G, Stoll C. The epidemiology of three serious cardiac defects. A joint study between five centres. European Journal of Epidemiology 1993; **9**(6): 607–16.

Gardner RJM, Sutherland GR. Other aneuploidies: full and partial. In: Chromosome abnormalities and genetic counseling. New York: Oxford University Press, 1989: 144 59.

Gardner RJM, Sutherland GR. Pregnancy loss and infertility. In: Chromosome abnormalities and genetic counseling. New York: Oxford University Press, 1996: 311–21.

Gorlin RJ, Cohen M, Levin LS. Orofacial clefting syndromes: general aspects. In: Syndromes of the head and neck. New York: Oxford University Press, 1990: 693–700.

Graham J. Congenital anomalies. In: Levine MD, Carey WB, Crocker AC (eds). Developmental-behavioral pediatrics. Philadelphia: W.B. Saunders Co., 1992: 229–43.

Graham JM, Jr. Introduction. In: Smith's recognizable patterns of human deformation. Philadelphia: W.B. Saunders Co., 1988: 1–3.

Halevi HS. Congenital malformations in Israel. British Journal of Preventive and Social Medicine 1967; **21**: 66–77.

Hall JG. Clinical, genetic and epidemiological factors in neural tube defects. American Journal of Human Genetics 1988; **43**: 827–37.

Hankin JR, Firestone IJ, Sloan JJ, Ager JW, Sokol RJ, Martier SS. Heeding the alcoholic beverage warning label during pregnancy: multiparae versus nulliparae. Journal of Studies on Alcohol 1996; **57**: 171–7.

Harper PS. Speical problems in genetic counselling. In: Practical genetic counselling. London: Wright Publishers, 1988: 112–21.

Hersh J. Toluene embryopathy: two new cases. Journal of Medical Genetics 1989; **26**: 333 7.

Hexter AC, Harris JA. Bias in congenital malformations: information from the birth certificate. Teratology 1991; **44**(2): 177–80.

Hexter AC, Harris JA, Roeper P, Croen LA, Krueger P, Gant D. Evaluation of the hospital discharge diagnoses index and the birth certificates as sources of information on birth defects. Public Health Reports 1990; **105**(3): 296 307.

Holmes LB. Inborn errors of morphogenesis: a review of localized hereditary malformations. New England Journal of Medicine 1974; **291**: 763–73.

Holmes LB. Current concepts in genetics: congenital malformations. New England Journal of Medicine 1976; **295**: 204–7.

Holmes LB. Fetal environmental toxins. Pediatrics in Review 1992; **13**(10): 364–70.

Hook EB, Petry JJ. Single hit etiology of human minor malformations unassociated with major congenital malformations. Nature 1970; **227**: 847–8.

Hwang S, Beaty TH, Panny SR, et al. Association study of transforming growth factor alpha (TGFα) Taq1 polymorphism and oral clefts: indication of gene–environment interaction in a population-based sample of infants with birth defects. American Journal of Epidemiology 1995; **141**: 629–36.

Imaizumi Y, Yamamura H, Nishikawa M, Matsuoka M, Moriyama I. The prevalence at birth of congenital malformations at a maternity hospital in Osaka City 1948–1990. Japanese Journal of Human Genetics 1991; **36**: 275–87.

Jensen TK, Toppari J, Keiding N, Skakkebock NE. Do environmental estrogens contribute to the decline in male reproductive health? Clinical Chemistry 1995; **41**(12 Pt2): 1896–901.

Khoury MJ. Commentary: Contributions of epidemiology to the study of birth defects in humans. Teratology 1995; **52**: 186–9.

Khoury MJ, Shaw GM, Moore CA, Lammer EJ, Mulinare J. Does periconceptual vitamin use reduce the risk of NTD associated with other birth defects? Data from two population-based case-control studies. American Journal of Medical Genetics 1996; **61**: 30–6.

Knight GJ. Maternal serum α-fetoprotein screening. In: Hommes FA ed. Techniques in diagnostic human biochemical genetics: a laboratory manual. New York: Wiley-Liss, Inc., 1991: 491–5.

Lary JM, Edmonds LD. Prevalence of spina bifida at birth – United States, 1983–1990: a comparison of two surveillance systems. Morbidity and Mortality Weekly Report CDC Surveillance Systems 1996; **45**(2): 15–26.

Leck I. Descriptive epidemiology of common malformations. British Medical Bulletin 1976; **32**(1): 45–52.

Li QY, Newbury-Ecobo RA, Terrett JA, et al. Holt-Oram syndrome caused by mutations in TBX5, a member of the Brachyury (T) gene family. Nature Genetics 1997; **15**: 21–9.

Long S, Robert E, Lauman B, Pradert E, Robert JM. Epidemiology of cleft palate and cleft lip in the Rhone Alps/Aubergne/Jura region. Apropos of 903 cases reported 1978–1987. Pediatrie 1992; **47**(2): 133–40.

Lowry RB, Thuren NY, Silven M. Congenital anomalies in American Indians of British Columbia. Genetic Epidemiology 1986; **3**: 455–67.

Lynberg MC, Khoury MJ. Interaction between epidemiology and laboratory sciences in the study of birth defects: design of birth defects risk factor surveillance in Metropolitan Atlanta. Journal of Toxicology and Environmental Health 1993; **40**(2–3): 435–44.

McIntosh GC, Olshan AF, Baird PA. Paternal age and the risk of birth defects in offspring. Epidemiology 1995; **6**(3): 282–8.

Mili F, Edmonds LD, Khoury MJ, McClearn AB. Prevalence of birth defects among low-birth-weight infants. A population study. American Journal of Diseases of Children 1991; **145**: 1313–18.

Motskin B, Marion R, Goldberg R, Sphrintzen R, Saenger P. Variable phenotypes in velocardiofacial syndrome with chromosomal deletion. The Journal of Pediatrics 1993; **123**: 406–10.

Mulinare J. Epidemiological association of multivitamin supplementation and occurrence of NTDs. Annals of the New York Academy of Science 1993; **678**: 130–6.

Murnan L. Congenital defects in Quebec. Lancet 1973; **7813**: 1191.

Myrianthopoulos NC, Chung CS. Congenital malformations in singletons: epidemiologic survey. In: Bergsma D, ed. Birth defects original article series, symposia specialist for the National Foundation March of Dimes Miami: National Foundation March of Dimes, 1974; **10**: 1.

Naderi S. Congenital abnormalities in newborns of consanguineous and nonconsanguineous parents. Obstetrics and Gynecology 1979; **53**(2): 195–9.

Napiorkowski B, Lester BM, Freier MC, et al. Effects of in utero substance exposure on infant neurobehavior. Pediatrics 1996; **98**: 71–5.

Nelson K, Holmes LB. Malformations due to presumed spontaneous mutations in newborn infants. New England Journal of Medicine 1989; **320**: 19–23.

Nora JJ, Nora AH, Blu J, et al. Exogenous progestrogen and estrogen implicated in birth defects. Journal of the American Medical Association 1978; **240**(9): 837–43.

Olsen CL, Cross OK, Gensburg LJ, Hughes JP. The effects of prenatal diagnosis, population aging and changing fertility rates on the live birth prevalence of Down syndrome in New York State, 1983–1992. Prenatal Diagnosis 1996; **16**(11): 991–1002.

Olshan AF, Mattison DR, eds. Male-mediated developmental toxicity. New York: Plenum Press, 1994.

Olshan AF, Schnitzer PG, Baird PA. Paternal age and the risk of congenital heart defects. Teratology 1994; **50**(1): 80–4.

Opitz JM. Invited editorial comment: study of minor anomalies in childhood malignancy. European Journal of Pediatrics 1985; **144**: 252–4.

Reynders CS, Pauker SP, Benacerraf BR. First trimester isolated fetal nuchal lucency: significance and outcome. Journal of Ultrasound in Medicine 1997; **16**(2): 101–5.

Roberts HE, Moore CA, Cragan JD, Fernhoff PM, Khoury MJ. Impact of prenatal diagnosis on the birth prevalence of neural tube defects, Atlanta, 1990–1991. Pediatrics 1995; **96**(5Pt1): 880–3.

Saxen L, Klemetti A. The Finnish register of congenital malformations. Acta Universitatis Carolinæ Medica 1973; **LVI–LVII**: 23–30.

Schinzel AAGL, Smith DW, Miller Jr. Monozygotic twinning and structural defects. The Journal of Pediatrics 1979; **95**(6): 921–30

Sever LE. Congenital malformations related to occupational reproductive hazards. Occupational Medicine 1994; **9**(3): 471–94.

Shepard TH, Fantel AG, Fitzsimmons. Congenital defect rates among spontaneous abortuses: twenty years of monitoring. Teratology 1989; **39**: 325–31.

Smith DW. Minor malformations: their relevance and significance. In: Hook EB, Janerich DT, Porter IH (eds). Monitoring birth defects and environments. New York: Academic Press, 1971: 169–75.

Smith DW. An approach to clinical dysmorphology. The Journal of Pediatrics 1977; **91**(4): 690–2.

Smithells RW. Incidence of congenital abnormalities in Liverpool, 1960–64. British Journal of Preventive and Social Medicine 1968; **22**: 36–7.

Soltan HC, Craven JL. The extent of genetic disease in human populations. Canadian Medical Association Journal 1981; **124**: 427–9.

Staples AJ, Robertson EF, Ranieri EN, Ryall RG, Haan EA. A maternal serum screen for trisomy 18: an extension of maternal serum screening for Down syndrome. American Journal of Human Genetics 1991; **49**: 1025–33.

Thompson MW, McInnes RR, Willard HF. Clinical cytogenetics: general principles and autosomal abnormalities. In: Genetics in medicine. Philadelphia: W.B. Saunders, 1991: 224–6.

Van Regemorter N, Dodion J, Druart C, et al. Congenital malformations in 10 000 consecutive births in a university hospital: need for genetic counseling and prenatal diagnosis. The Journal of Pediatrics 1984; **104**: 386–90.

Volpe JJ. Effect of cocaine use on the fetus. New England Journal of Medicine 1992; **327**: 399–407.

Watkins ML, Edmonds L, McClearn A, Mullins L, Mulinare J, Khoury MK. The surveillance of birth defects: the usefulness of the revised U.S. standard birth certificate. American Journal of Public Health 1996; **86**: 731–4.

Watkins ML, Scanlon KS, Mulinare J, Khoury MJ. Is maternal obesity a risk factor for anencephaly and spina bifida? Epidemiology 1996; **7**(5): 507–12.

Weatherall DJ. The frequency and clinical spectrum of genetic diseases. In: The new genetics and clinical practice. New York: Oxford University Press, 1991: 32–8.

Wilkie AOM, Amberger AS, McKusick VA. A gene map of congenital malformations. Journal of Medical Genetics 1994; **31**: 507–17.

Woolf CM, Myrinathopoulos MC. Polydactyly in American negroes and whites. American Journal of Human Genetics 1973; **25**(4): 397–404.

Wu T, Zeug M, Yu C, et al. Analyses of the prevalence for NTD and cleft lip and palate in China from 1988–1991. Hua Hsi I Ko Ta Hsueh Hsueh Pao (Journal of West China University of Medical Sciences) 1995; **26**(2): 215–18.

Yen IH, Khoury MJ, Erickson JD, James LM, Waters GD, Berry RJ. The changing epidemiology of neural tube defects. United States, 1968–1989. American Journal of Diseases of Children 1992; **146**(7): 857–61.

10

Developing fetal diagnostic technologies

Richard B. Parad

Introduction

Congenital anomalies, defined as malformations, deformations, and inherited disorders, account for 22% of infant deaths in the first year of life, and are currently the number one cause of infant mortality (Peters et al., 1997). This percentage has steadily increased as the relative importance of such public health problems as infectious diseases and malnutrition has diminished and as survival of preterm infants has increased.

Understanding the basic science of human development may provide some practical solutions for preventing congenital anomalies. For example, supplementing maternal folate intake prior to and during pregnancy may lower the risk of fetal neural tube defects, and avoiding exposure to identified toxic agents may prevent other malformations in the developing embryo. Many developmental abnormalities cannot be prevented, however, in particular those that disrupt the integrity of the blueprint provided to the embryo by its genetic material. Abnormalities with genetic etiologies may either be passed down by parents or may develop, de novo, during early stages of development.

Once an anomaly is destined to occur, the potential value of its identification in the fetus is to provide information that may be acted upon by the clinician and the parents. With means for early diagnosis, one might consider three options: First, for a lethal irreparable or potentially devastating anomaly, early termination might be a reasonable option to discuss with parents, within an appropriate social and religious context. Second, for potentially correctable problems, in utero therapies, such as gene therapy (Ballard et al., 1995; Coutelle et al. 1995; Fletcher and Richter, 1996; Holzinger et al., 1995; Sekhon and Larson, 1995; Tanswell and O'Brodovich, 1997) or surgical intervention (Flake, 1996; Longaker et al., 1991; Mychaliska et al., 1996), may be or might become available. Finally, for an anomaly that is potentially treatable or correctable after birth, such as diaphragmatic hernia, transposition of the great arteries, or cystic fibrosis (CF) with bowel obstruction, the clinician can prepare parents and encourage delivery plans that will improve outcome (Nichols and Bianchi, 1996). Although attenuation of the parental shock experienced at the birth of a child with unsuspected anomalies may be of significant value, this has not been well studied.

Whatever technologic advances occur, it remains vital that the information generated be used and presented appropriately. One major challenge resulting from rapidly advancing diagnostic technologies is the ability of the clinician to keep up with the principles underlying the use of these tools and the interpretation of reported output. This is particularly true in the realm of molecular genetics, where knowledge of what genes have been identified, and what mutations should be screened for in what disease, become outdated so fast that few clinicians, except for geneticists, are capable of keeping up with the pace of newly generated information.

This chapter describes these rapidly developing diagnostic technologies, which include the use of ultrasound and a number of techniques that employ the principles of molecular genetics. The chapter concludes with two examples that illustrate how these technologies can be combined to provide an accurate prenatal diagnosis to guide the parents of a fetus with an anomaly.

Technologies

The generation of information on which counseling and intervention are based relies upon the accuracy of the technologies used in fetal diagnosis. Technologies that have improved most dramatically in recent years include ultrasound imaging, magnetic resonance imaging (MRI), cytogenetic techniques, and DNA analysis. These techniques have broadened capabilities for prenatal testing, newborn screening, and population screening of genetically based disorders.

Imaging

The quality and resolution of ultrasound imaging for prenatal diagnosis has significantly improved since it was first introduced. Real time imaging developed in the early 1980s, when advances in transducer technology allowed for an array of resonating crystals that could provide a continuous image. Reduction in transducer size now allows for high-resolution imaging, which adds greater detail to fetal images (Nelson et al., 1993). Ultrasound units are now equipped with Doppler capability, which allows quantitative assessment of vascular flow and thereby provides important information about the blood supply to fetal organs and from the placenta (Nyberg et al., 1990). Three-dimensional reconstruction is the next era of ultrasound imaging and will further improve detection of anomalies. However, this technique is currently limited in its ability to capture a clear image of a fetus in motion. The development of ultrasound as a diagnostic technique is also described in Chapter 11.

Ultrasound screening is valuable in the identification of congenital anomalies, correction of gestational dating errors, early diagnosis of multiple gestation, and in the detection of fetal growth disorders. Used in these ways, ultrasound can provide the basis for improved prenatal care. In experienced hands, the structural fetal survey conducted during ultrasound screening provides an accurate assessment of fetal anatomy and growth. Deviation from the norm either in size or structure often signals that an abnormality is present.

Fast magnetic resonance imaging (MRI) now allows high-resolution images of the fetus (Levine et al., 1996). Although not yet routine, in some cases fetal MRI can improve the detection of some congenital anomalies, especially those involving the central nervous system.

In well-trained hands, fetal screening using these imaging technologies can detect malformations of the brain, lungs, heart, bowel, kidneys and skeleton, suggest the presence of aneuploidy, and signal that the fetus should be further assessed by cytogenetic or DNA analysis.

Technologies that employ the principles of molecular genetics
Background on cellular and molecular biology

When abnormal imaging, family history, or risk profile suggests the possibility of a syndrome or disorder known to be associated with a specific chromosomal or DNA etiology, a specific diagnostic investigation for chromosome, gene, or gene product abnormalities may be indicated. In recent years, a number of new diagnostic technologies have been developed that are based on the principles of molecular genetics. These will be described following a brief background discussion of cell and molecular biology.

With the exception of mature red blood cells, each of the approximately 100 trillion cells in the human body contains a copy of the entire human genome. This information is encoded in 3 billion base pairs of deoxyribonucleic acid (DNA), with egg and sperm cells containing half this amount. Inside each cell nucleus is about 1.8 metres of DNA packaged into 23 pairs of chromosomes. One chromosome in each pair comes from each parent. Each of the 46 human chromosomes contains DNA coding for hundreds or thousands of individual genes (50 000–100 000 total in each nucleus). Each of these genes is a segment of double-stranded DNA that holds the recipe for making a specific molecule, usually a protein. These recipes are spelled out in varying sequences of the four chemical bases that make up DNA: adenine (A), thymine (T), guanine (G), and cytosine (C). These bases form interlocking pairs that can fit together in only one way: G pairing with C and A pairing with T. Proteins are composed of amino acids, which are coded for by series of three DNA base pair clusters (triplets) by way of ribonucleic acid (RNA) intermediates.

Genomic DNA is the form of DNA from which chromosomes are constructed. It contains small regions that code for genes, interspersed with long sequences of unknown function that are probably involved with structure and regulation. Within the regions that contain genes, there are two types of DNA sequences: exons and introns. Exons code for the final protein sequence. One intronic segment usually follows each exon, creating a series of exons with intervening introns. An editing process termed "splicing" occurs when the intronic segments in gene-containing copies of transcribed genomic DNA are removed, and the exonic segments are linked together. This final editing leads to a sequence that is transcribed into a messenger RNA, which can then be translated into the final protein.

When cells replicate, the genomic DNA must be copied. The two strands of the genomic DNA, the sense and the antisense strands, are complementary, with a G and C or an A and T always paired. Enzymes known as DNA polymerases function to copy each of these strands by extending the complementary matching sequence for each unwound strand by one base pair at a time.

Diagnostic identification of normal and abnormal DNA sequences has become feasible with the ability to amplify the number of copies of the sequence in question. For example, the polymerase chain reaction (PCR) takes advantage of the function of Taq polymerase, a thermally stable DNA polymerase. This enzyme allows the extension of a short synthesized strand of nucleotides known as an oligonucleotide or a primer. Primer sequences are complementary to segments of DNA that flank the region one wishes to increase in copy number (amplify). Once the synthesized oligonucleotide strand has been mixed with genomic DNA and binds to its complementary sequence in that genomic DNA, the polymerase can extend that short strand by adding on bases. Repeated cycles of heating (denaturation) allow separation, followed by duplication of the DNA strands. Multiple cycles of duplication lead to an exponential increase in the number of desired sequence copies. The length of the amplified segment is defined by the oligonucleotides that frame the sequence of interest. Within a brief period of time, millions of copies can be made of the specific desired DNA sequence. Once a large enough quantity of this specific DNA is available, various means of detection can be employed to search that sequence for specific abnormalities.

Techniques for detecting genetic abnormalities

Amplified DNA provides substrate for several different approaches through which anticipated sequence alterations may be detected:

Use of markers

Efforts by the National Human Genome Research Institute at the National Institutes of Health (NIH) are resulting in the mapping and characterization of an increasing proportion of genes and the complete DNA sequence encoded on human chromosomes. The use of "markers" has been an important research tool since the early stages of gene mapping. Markers result from even minute DNA sequence differences between individuals and are valuable when discrepant between those who are and are not affected by a disease. They can be detected at specific locations in the genome by variants in gel electrophoresis band patterns from either small regions of variable length repeated nucleotide sequences or from digested DNA (DNA broken down into several fragments of different size). A marker functions as a pointer to a region on the molecular map. If a gene location is imagined to be equivalent to a house number on a street, the marker is analogous to the name of the city where that house is located. Markers are useful for tracking the presence of abnormal genes in disease-affected individuals when the gene itself has not been identified. A specific marker pattern passed down in the same inheritance pattern as a disease can be assumed to be in the neighborhood of the abnormal gene that is associated with the disease. Markers are being less widely used as diagnostic tools now as researchers identify more genes and specific sequence alterations responsible for diseases.

Before the cloning of the factor VIII gene, hemophilia A was an early example of a disease followed with markers for carrier detection and diagnosis. In this disease, affected males inherit an abnormal X chromosome from the carrier mothers. Tests of digested DNA hybridized with a labeled probe show a pattern difference. The sequence difference does not have to be within the actual gene; it may be in a region adjacent to the abnormal gene. If disease marker information is available from other affected family members, a marker can be useful in the prenatal diagnosis of disorders for which a gene has not been identified. A major drawback of marker-based diagnosis is its dependence on informative genetic data from other family members. This approach is sometimes only useful for the assessment of individual families rather than as a diagnostic tool to detect disease in the population.

Cytogenetics-based tests

The anatomic parts of the chromosome include the centromere (separating two arms), a long arm, and a short arm (or Q and P arm). Further addresses within these arms are specified by a complex numbering system that refers to bands visualized along the arms. Genes are now being mapped to specific bands on each chromosome. In a karyotype, the 23 pairs of chromosomes are lined up to confirm that their visible structures match a normal pattern. Pattern analysis of karyotypes is the foundation of cytogenetics, as it allows investigators to determine whether each chromosome has a missing or extra portion relative to a standard or to the chromosome's partner. As new cytogenic technologies are being developed, much more fine anatomy can now be discerned.

One new technique is fluorescence in situ hybridization (FISH), which uses fluorescent signals from tagged oligonucleotide probes to locate specific DNA sequences. DNA strands are separated, which allows for the binding of the fluorescently labeled probe. Probes are designed to bind only when there is an exact match to the DNA sequence. An image of the probe/chromosome complex can then be visualized and captured by photograph. For example, on a karyotype of a patient with DiGeorge sequence, the chromosomes can be stained with two different fluorescent probes that are specific to small regions of chromosome 22. One labeled probe is targeted to a region that should be present both in normal individuals and DiGeorge syndrome patients, and the other probe is targeted for the 22q11 region known to be deleted in some DiGeorge patients. Fluorescence microscopy would reveal that one chromosome 22 carries both signals but the other is missing one signal. This suggests that on the abnormal one-signal chromosomes, the 22q11 probe was unable to bind and thus the sequence must be deleted. This level of resolution was not previously available using standard karyotype banding techniques.

Another use of fluorescent probes is "chromosome painting," a process in which the probes are bound to sequences on each of the 22 sets of autosomal chromosomes and each of the sex chromosomes. Computer-assisted spectral analysis of the output from special fluorescent microscopes allows visualization of chromosome images (Speicher et al., 1996). Each chromosome is identified by a unique color. "Painting" the chromosomes not only allows an easier and more specific mechanism for identifying chromosome pairs, but more importantly may readily allow recognition of the translocation of one portion of one chromosome to another. For instance, a small piece of yellow chromosome 3 translocated onto red chromosome 7 could be readily detected; this abnormality might not have been visible on previous forms of karyotypes. This new technology is increasingly available and will allow for more rapid identification of chromosomal rearrangements that may lead to fetal abnormalities.

Mutation analysis

Mutation analysis, another type of diagnostic approach based on molecular genetic techniques, uses the knowledge of known normal DNA sequences to assess potentially abnormal subjects.

Southern blotting, an early mutation analysis tool, has been used to identify variations in DNA sequence (Sambrook et al., 1989). This technique can be performed without knowledge of the gene or its sequence. DNA can be broken into fragments using a family of proteins known as restriction enzymes. There are hundreds of these enzymes available. Each enzyme recognizes a specific short

DNA sequence (approximately six nucleotides). The enzyme binds to DNA with a matching sequence and cuts the DNA strand. The enzyme will not cut the DNA if a mutation has altered the sequence at even one base pair. When resulting DNA fragments generated from a patient with a disease who is known to carry an abnormal gene are separated in an electric field, the fragments from the abnormal DNA yield a different pattern than does normal DNA undergoing the same process. After traveling through an electrophoresis gel, the DNA fragments, or bands, are transferred to a nitrocellulose filter. Oligonucleotide probes, usually labeled with radioactive phosphorus, are then applied to the nitrocellulose filter. The probe binds to its complementary sequence in the DNA. After washing off free, unbound probe, the filter is applied to x-ray film, and a signal is generated onto the film by bound probe. The digestion or nondigestion of the probed DNA sequence provides DNA fragments of different size. Fragment patterns from individuals with and without the disease are compared, and patterns deviating from normal can be used for diagnosis.

More recent mutation analysis techniques include allele-specific oligonucleotide (ASO) detection, a technique that requires PCR amplification (Saiki et al., 1988). In ASO, primers flanking regions surrounding a known mutation in a specific gene are added to a patient's genomic DNA. After PCR-amplified genomic DNA is bound to a nitrocellulose filter, probes with either radioactive or fluorescent label are bound to the filter. Two probes are added to the filter, one with a sequence that matches the known normal sequence, and one that matches the known abnormal sequence. Binding only occurs when there is an exact match of probe to amplified DNA. Because each patient carries two copies of a given gene, three possible combinations exist: two normal copies, two abnormal copies, or one normal and one abnormal copy. Based on the pattern of probe binding, one can distinguish a homozygous normal patient from a heterozygote or a homozygous abnormal patient. This technique is commonly used by commercial laboratories for gene mutation screening. Other currently available mutation analysis techniques are listed in Table 10.1.

If available, a patient's DNA sequence can be used to detect the presence of a mutation. Rather than the classic dideoxy sequencing process (Sambrook et al., 1989), newer technologies for DNA sequencing have developed in which fluorescent probes label each of the four base pairs and fluorescent dye peaks are scanned on the sequencing gel. Computer analysis of these colored peaks provides a most likely sequence. DNA sequencing is becoming increasingly practical to perform on short amplified DNA fragments. An amplified 500 base pair PCR product can be rapidly sequenced to search for a specific mutation. Although this process is still labor intensive, improving technology is bringing down the cost, size, and complexity of automated sequencers that can be used for clinical diagnosis.

Table 10.1. Examples of mutation analysis techniques

Single Stranded Conformation Polymorphism (SSCP)
Density Gradient Gel Electrophoresis (DGGE)
Chemical cleavage
Sequencing-cloned DNA or PCR products
Polyacrylamide gel electrophoresis
Restriction Fragment Length Polymorphism (RFLP)
Allele Specific Oligonucleotide (ASO)
Amplification Refractory Mutation System (ARMS)
High density oligonucleotide arrays (DNA chips)
Multiplex Allele Specific Diagnostic Assay (MASDA)
Cleavage Fragment Length Polymorphism (CFLP)

Source: Eng and Vijg, 1997.

As the understanding of the role that genetic mutations play in disease has grown, both the utility and the limitations of mutation analysis have become clear. For example, the *BRCA1* gene has been associated with some forms of breast cancer. It was identified by an approach known as positional cloning (Ezzell, 1994). Unfortunately, as is now being found with many diseases, multiple mutations in each gene are found to be associated with the same disease (Harrison, 1997). With close to 200 mutations identified in the *BRCA1* gene, simple mutation analysis becomes impossible (Collins, 1996). While it is relatively straightforward to use basic mutation analysis techniques to identify a few to several dozen mutations, it is not possible, on a population-wide basis, to screen for all known mutations when hundreds of mutations must be assessed.

Furthermore, more than one gene may be involved in the generation of a single disease. For example, in some colon cancers, approximately seven genes may be involved. When all are mutated, malignant disease results (Jessup et al., 1997). A patient born with a few of those mutations may have quiescent disease until somatic cell mutations, perhaps environmentally induced, develop later in life. Once beyond a critical mass of mutations, the cancer is unleashed. Our prior notion that an abnormality of a single gene product leads to a single disease, and that a single gene mutation is responsible for that abnormal protein, must be adjusted.

The need for broader approaches to mutation analysis has led to the newest wave in DNA sequencing technology, the "chip." Through rapid sequencing of either an entire gene, or a portion of a gene, chip technology may be able to provide some solutions to this diagnostic problem. The chip is a square of glass the size of a dime on which a grid of oligonucleotides has been synthesized. Each small square of the grid contains a different oligonucleotide and each oligonucleotide may differ by one base pair from the adjacent sequences. DNA added to this glass chip will bind to complementary oligonucleotide sequences. Binding leads to the generation of fluorescent signals. The fluorescence pattern is detected by a sensor and is analyzed by computer in the context of the surrounding signal pattern. The computer analysis can either determine the exact sequence of a gene, or identify the presence of specific sequences (normal or abnormal) present in the DNA sample. Chip output could provide a comparison of a known normal DNA sequence to an individual's sequence.

Chips have been developed for HIV testing, CF mutation analysis, and *BRCA1* mutation analysis. Current chip technology can allow for the rapid evaluation of approximately 250 000 base pairs at a time, which would potentially allow for screening sequences of portions of hundreds of different genes. Such an approach could be used to screen fetal or newborn DNA samples for disorders amenable to early therapies. Chips could also be used to screen for common diseases that have an inherited component that will develop either during childhood or later in life, such as hypertension, atherosclerotic heart disease, or diabetes. It could become possible to estimate life-time risk for developing these common disorders from the output of such chips. Very small amounts of DNA would be required, though the cost of this hypothetical assessment would be quite high because the chips are costly and not widely available. In addition, all of the DNA sequences that will be needed to calculate these risks have not yet been identified (Douglas, 1997). This technology holds much promise. However, until genetic privacy is better protected legally, the positive value of the information obtainable will be overshadowed by concerns.

Combining technologies for prenatal diagnosis

Two examples demonstrating the current state of prenatal diagnostic technologies are presented below. They illustrate how high-resolution ultrasound can provide a warning signal that can be further evaluated with molecular techniques. In pursuing this course, one of the first and most important considerations is obtaining the actual DNA sample. The clinician must determine who is best tested, the parents as carriers, or the affected fetus. Acquisition of fetal genomic DNA and chromosomes is necessary for molecular and cytogenetic diagnosis. Traditionally, these samples have been supplied by amniocentesis. More recently, PUBS (Percutaneous Umbilical Blood Sampling) and Choroid Villus Sampling (CVS) also have been used. Less invasive sampling of fetal DNA derived from maternal blood is under study (Bianchi, 1995), as amniocentesis, PUBS, and CVS are all associated with complications.

Several fetal cell types exist in the maternal circulation at a ratio of approximately 1 per 10 000 maternal cells. These are identifiable by about 5 weeks' gestation. While studies have used the Y chromosome as a marker of male cells in the maternal circulation, other cells that can serve as markers for fetal cells are needed in order to assess female fetuses. Although it is technically challenging to isolate these cells, separation can be accomplished with fluorescent automated cell sorters. Isolated cells can have FISH performed on them for rapid diagnosis of a specific disorder. For example, a National Institute of Child Health and Human Development trial nearing completion has been assessing the use of fetal cells in maternal circulation for identification of trisomy 21 (Bianchi, 1995). If this approach becomes a practical reality, a 10 cm^3 maternal blood sample drawn when the fetus is at 5 to 10 weeks gestational age would be adequate to provide enough DNA to PCR amplify, apply to a chip, and screen for mutations in the most common disorders that one might want to evaluate in a fetus. The chip would be inserted in a reader the size of a desktop computer that would provide an answer within a matter of moments. Such an approach may not be far from reality.

Cystic fibrosis

Cystic fibrosis (CF), a disease affecting lungs, pancreas, and gastrointestinal and genitourinary tracts, is the most common lethal autosomal recessive disorder in Caucasians, occurring in 1 in 2500 live births. Approximately 3 to 4% of Caucasians are carriers. Over 800 mutations have been reported in this disease (CF Genetic Analysis Consortium, 1997). The most common is named Delta F508 because of the absence of a phenylalanine at position 508 in the CFTR protein. Recently, an NIH consensus statement was issued that recommended prenatal screening for CF carrier status of couples of childbearing age (NIH, 1997). Population screening will be extremely difficult, however, because the distribution of these mutations differs based on ethnicity and geographical location.

The diagnosis of CF can be suspected in the fetus in the setting of several ultrasound findings. Echogenic bowel appears brighter than adjacent structures, and may appear to be as bright as bone. Echogenic bowel is associated with a five-fold increased risk of aneuploidy and a 20- to 200-fold increase in CF risk (Slotnick and Abuhamad, 1996). Amniocentesis for karyotype and CF gene mutation analysis is usually indicated. In the CF fetus, abnormal meconium blocks the distal ileum, leading to dilation of bowel loops. One-third of fetuses with dilated bowel have CF. For a fetus identified on ultrasound as having echogenic bowel, the diagnosis can be further refined by testing the parents' DNA for CF carrier status. Buccal cells are non-invasively collected by cheekbrush scraping (Richards et al., 1993). The DNA from these buccal cells is extracted, and regions in the CFTR gene are assessed by one of the PCR amplification and mutation detection techniques listed in Table 10.1. If one or both parents are found to be a carrier of a CFTR gene mutation, similar mutation analysis on the fetal DNA may reveal the presence of two abnormal CFTR alleles, and thus confirm the diagnosis.

Down's syndrome

Although Down's syndrome is a disorder that occurs with increasing frequency as maternal age increases, 80% of cases are born to mothers who are less than 35 years of age. It has been proposed that biochemical screens such as the "Triple screen" and/or ultrasound screening be used early to detect this disorder in the fetus (Phillips et al., 1992).

Sonography may suggest Down's syndrome by a number of abnormal fetal findings, including a nuchal fold, flattened facial profile, short femur lengths, pyelectasis, and others (Nyberg, 1990). A standard karyotype, which would show three copies of chromosome 21, takes days to complete because of the time required for a sufficient number of cells to grow for the test. A much faster approach is to process cells from an amniocentesis for a FISH, which requires only 24–48 hours for completion.

Conclusion

With the continuing success of the NIH's Human Genome Project, the list of genetic disorders that might lend themselves to screening by the described techniques, either at the parental, fetal, or newborn levels, are increasing daily. Once the hurdles of chip technology and other rapid sequencing capabilities have been passed, it may become fast and perhaps relatively inexpensive to perform an automated DNA screening panel. Very little DNA would be required to provide an individual with either a definitive diagnosis, or an estimated risk for developing these disorders. From the medical viewpoint, if such tests are accurate, one could minimize the morbidity of the diseases that will develop by initiating early prevention strategies. If parents knew their carrier status, early prenatal diagnostic techniques could be instituted. The fetus also could have its own early screening panel from a maternal blood sample. This genetic report card would have positive and negative aspects. Privacy, insurability of those tested, and other issues related to the social, legal, and ethical aspects of genetic testing will need to be addressed in a comprehensive and sensitive manner as part of the development of these important technologies.

REFERENCES

Ballard PL, Zepeda ML, Schwartz M, Lopez N, Wilson JM. Adenovirus-mediated gene transfer to human fetal lung ex vivo. American Journal of Physiology 1995; **268**: L839–L845.

Bianchi DW. Prenatal diagnosis by analysis of fetal cells in maternal blood. Journal of Pediatrics 1995; **127**: 847–56.

CF Genetic Analysis Consortium. Personal Communication [abstract]; 1997.

Collins FS. BRCA1 – lots of mutations, lots of dilemmas. New England Journal of Medicine 1996; **334**: 186–8.

Coutelle C, Douar AM, Colledge WH, Froster U. The challenge of fetal gene therapy. Nature Medicine 1995; **1**: 864–6.

Douglas MG. The human genome project: gateway to managed health. IVD Technology 1997; **46**: 50–6.

Eng C, Vijg J. Genetic testing: the problems and the promise. Nature Biotechnology 1997; **15**: 422–6.

Ezzell C. Breast cancer genes: cloning BRCA1, mapping BRCA2. The Journal of NIH Research 1994; **6**: 33–6.

Flake AW. Fetal surgery for congenital diaphragmatic hernia. Seminars in Pediatric Surgery 1996; **5**: 266–74.

Fletcher JC, Richter G. Human fetal gene therapy: moral and ethical questions. Human Gene Therapy 1996; **7**: 1605–14.

Harrison MR. Genetics of breast cancer. Mayo Clinic Proceedings 1997; **72**: 54–65.

Holzinger A, Trapnell BC, Weaver TE, Whitsett JA, Iwamoto HS. Intraamniotic administration of an adenoviral vector for gene transfer to fetal sheep and mouse tissues. Pediatric Research 1995; **38**: 844–50.

Jessup JM, Menck HR, Fremgen A, Winchester DP. Diagnosing colorectal carcinoma: clinical and molecular approaches. CA: A Cancer Journal for Clinicians 1997; **47**: 70–92.

Levine D, Hatabu H, Gaa J, Atkinson MW, Edelman RR. Fetal anatomy revealed with fast MR sequences. American Journal of Roentgenology 1996; **167**: 905–8.

Longaker MT, Golbus MS, Filly RA, Rosen MA, Chang SW, Harrison MR. Maternal outcome after open fetal surgery. A review of the first 17 human cases. Journal of the American Medical Association 1991; **265**: 737–41.

Mychaliska GB, Bullard KM, Harrison MR. In utero management of congenital diaphragmatic hernia. Clinics in Perinatology 1996; **23**: 823–41.

National Institutes of Health (NIH). [Consensus statement 106 on-line: http://odp.od.nih.gov/consensus/statements] Genetic testing for cystic fibrosis. 1997; **15**(4) 1–37.

Nelson NL, Filly RA, Goldstein RB, Callen PW. The AIUM/ACR antepartum obstetrical sonographic guidelines: expectations for detection of anomalies. Journal of Ultrasound in Medicine 1993; **12**: 189–96.

Nichols VG, Bianchi DW. Prenatal pediatrics: traditional speciality definitions no longer apply. Pediatrics 1996; **97**: 729–32.

Nyberg DA, Mahoney BS, Pretotius DH. Diagnostic ultrasound of fetal anomalies. St Louis: Mosby, 1990.

Peters KD, Martin JA, Ventura SJ, Maurer JD. Monthly Vital Statistics Report. 1997; **10**: 1–38 [abstract].

Phillips OP, Elias S, Shulman LP, Andersen RN, Morgan CD, Simpson JL. Maternal serum screening for fetal Down syndrome in women less than 35 years of age using alpha-fetoprotein, hCG, and unconjugated estriol: a prospective 2-year study. Obstetrics and Gynecology 1992; **80**: 353–8.

Richards B, Skoletsky J, Shuber AP, et al. Multiplex PCR amplification from the CFTR gene using DNA prepared from buccal brushes/swabs. Human Molecular Genetics 1993; **2**: 159–63.

Saiki RK, Chang C-A, Levenson CH, et al. Diagnosis of sickle cell anemia and β-thalassemia with enzymatically amplified DNA and nonradioactive allele-specific oligonucleotide probes. New England Journal of Medicine 1988; **319**: 537–41.

Sambrook J, Fritsch EF, Maniatis T. Molecular cloning: a laboratory manual. Cold Spring Harbor (NY): Cold Spring Harbor Press, 1989.

Sekhon HS, Larson JE. In utero gene transfer into the pulmonary epithelium. Nature Medicine 1995; **1**: 1201–3.

Slotnick RN, Abuhamad AZ. Prognostic implications of fetal echogenic bowel. Lancet 1996; **347**: 85–7.

Speicher MR, Ballard SG, Ward DC. Karyotyping human chromosomes by combinatorial multi-fluor FISH. Nature Genetics 1996; **12**: 368–75.

Tanswell AK, O'Brodovich HM. The present and future role of gene therapy in the newborn. Current Opinion in Pediatrics 1997; **9**: 141–5.

11

Options following the diagnosis of a fetal anomaly

Mark I. Evans, Yuval Yaron, Ralph L. Kramer and Mark P. Johnson

Introduction

Technology has afforded us the opportunity to diagnose an ever increasing number and proportion of anomalies. The decision to terminate or continue such pregnancies has become increasingly complex, as the dramatic increases in our ability to detect birth defects has challenged our capability to counsel about and to treat or ameliorate these problems. This chapter reviews the issues involved in the decision-making process surrounding discovery of a fetal anomaly and describes some of the recent advances in fetal therapies to correct and treat these conditions, including endoscopic procedures, fetal surgery, medical fetal therapies, and gene therapies.

The development of modern prenatal diagnostic procedures

Modern prenatal diagnosis began in the early 1970s with the use of amniocentesis for the diagnosis of cytogenetic and biochemical disorders (Nadler, 1968). Essentially, these procedures were done blindly, and were generally not performed until about 17 weeks of gestation to minimize the risks of damage to the fetus. Ultrasound also began to identify anomalies in the early 1970s, but it was not until the early 1980s that the quality of ultrasound imagery was sufficient for it to become a significant component of invasive procedures, thus enhancing their safety (Evans and Johnson, 1992).

A limited number of centers began to offer prenatal diagnostic services in the early to mid 1970s. However, the number of physicians who had the technical competence to perform the invasive procedures, and the number of laboratories that could handle the specimens, were small. Consequently, testing had to be restricted to patients thought to be at highest risk and to those whose prenatal management would be changed by the data obtained. Thus, it was commonplace to insist as a condition of testing that patients agree to terminate if an abnormality were detected (Larsen and MacMillin, 1989). Requests for prenatal diagnosis by patients who were unwilling to consider such an option were often denied as a "pointless waste" of valuable resources.

As the field of prenatal diagnosis evolved and services became more widely accessible, the fundamental principles of modern genetic counseling began to be applied. These included the notion that testing was for information purposes only and the associated implication that a woman's decision about what to do with the information on the status of her pregnancy should be independent of her choice to undergo testing. By the late 1970s and early 1980s, a consensus had emerged in the United States that linking the offer of prenatal diagnosis with a willingness to consider termination was unacceptable, and in fact, below the standard of care (Wertz and Fletcher, 1989).

A second, related principle also came to be widely shared among practitioners. This was the concept of parental autonomy in reproductive decision-making. In other words, parental decisions should be based on non-directive counseling. Patients should be educated about the fetus' condition and issues related to it, such as differential diagnosis, the limitations of diagnostic technology, the consequent levels of uncertainty, prognosis, anticipated disabilities, emotional and financial burdens, and management options (termination vs. continuation). Parents should be supported in whatever decisions they made (Wertz and Fletcher, 1988).

Throughout the 1980s and 1990s, the quality of ultrasound detail increased radically, to the point where there are now many findings on ultrasound that can alter the risks of chromosomal abnormalities (Johnson et al., 1993; Nicolaides et al., 1993). Some authorities, such as Devore and Benacerraf, have suggested that the majority of chromosomal abnormalities can, in fact, be "detected" by ultrasound findings, obviating the need for invasive procedures (Devore and Alfi, 1995). Because there are now many more specialists in maternal fetal medicine than there are obstetricians who are also qualified in genetics, the general thrust of prenatal diagnosis in most centers around the United States has shifted away from a genetics base to an ultrasound perinatal base. Consequently, there is a lower level of understanding of syndromes related to ultrasound findings and a less rigorous application of non-directive counseling.

Over the years there has been a slow decrease in referrals to tertiary genetic centers for prenatal evaluation and testing. This may, in part, be due to improved sonographic technology, which lowers the level of skill needed to interpret the scan and has led to the presence of more ultrasound machines in private physician's offices. Over the last decade, increased use of ultrasonography in this setting and their consequent financial implications (i.e., their cost and income generation potential) have been generally observed. As the multicenter "RADIUS" study has shown, however, this "improved" service by the clinician has had its drawbacks, as a large proportion of major abnormalities have not been recognized, or have been misdiagnosed (Ewigman et al., 1993). In addition, without appropriate genetic counseling, additional genetic issues are failing to be identified, resulting in inappropriate risk assessment, inappropriate recommendations for further testing, or incorrect prenatal testing.

Finding an abnormality

A significant fetal anomaly is detected in about 2% of all pregnancies and in 5% of pregnancies seen at centers specializing in high-risk pregnancies. These can be divided into anomalies that are chromosomal and those that are structural. In some of these instances, it is possible to give the pregnant woman and her family precise information on the outcome. For example, in certain aneuploidies such as trisomies 13, 18, and triploidy, there is extremely little variation in their usually lethal course. Thus, while the information relayed is unpleasant, the caregivers can have great confidence in the reliability of their counseling. For other conditions, however, there is great variability in expected outcomes and consequently, considerable reluctance to describe specific outcomes.

Decisions after the detection of an anomaly

After choosing to undergo prenatal testing, a minority of women will be faced with the news that there is, or appears to be, something wrong with the fetus they are carrying. Whether there is an abnormality in the chromosomal constituents of the nucleus (the karyotype), the biochemical, or molecular genetic constituents of fetal tissues, or the fetal structure, the patient must decide among very difficult options, all of which she will perceive as inadequate. In limited, carefully selected cases and at only a few centers, she may be offered fetal therapy as an option. In most cases, however, her options will be to continue the pregnancy ("allowing nature to take its course") or to terminate the pregnancy, if legally permissible.

In January 1973, the United States Supreme Court ruled in two related decisions, *Roe* v *Wade* (410 US 113, 1973) and *Doe* v *Bolton* (410 US 179, 1973), that there was an inherent right of privacy, under which auspices a decision about continuation or termination of pregnancy in the first trimester was to be strictly a matter between patient and physician. In the late second trimester, when the mortality rate of abortion procedures approached that of normal childbirth, the state had a right to impose additional "regulations reasonably related to the preservation and protection of maternal health" (*Roe* v *Wade* 410 US 113, 1973). It was only in the third trimester of pregnancy when fetal viability was a possibility, that the state could assert its compelling interests in protecting the fetus. Thus, the right to choose to terminate pregnancy was to be protected in all states. Safe, legal abortion became accessible to most women in the United States.

Today, in most jurisdictions in the United States, women can choose to terminate a pregnancy up to 24 weeks gestation. There are deep divisions in the United States over the abortion issue, and many patients, particularly those of limited financial means, can have significant roadblocks put in the way of accessing such care.

Questions about how women reach their decisions about undergoing prenatal diagnosis per se, how they perceive their reproductive risks, and in the event of discovering a fetal anomaly, how they make choices about continuing or terminating the pregnancy or, in selected cases, pursuing experimental fetal therapy, are extremely complex and consequently difficult to study effectively. Although much has been written and published, the literature does not present a clear picture of the factors influencing reproductive decision-making. Studies tend to be fraught with methodologic problems, are of variable quality, frequently are phenomenologic rather than quantitative, and often address or emphasize esoteric and widely divergent concerns.

The decision to terminate for fetal abnormality

The decision to terminate an otherwise wanted pregnancy because of fetal anomalies is difficult for most parents (Furlong and Black, 1984; Jorgenson et al., 1985) and has various psychological effects on the couple (Kenyon et al., 1988; Leon, 1992) and their family (Black and Furlong, 1987). Issues that are thought to affect decision-making relate to the timing of the diagnosis (first versus second trimester), the nature of the anomaly (type and severity of the anomaly and the level of certainty about the diagnosis and prognosis), and the religious and moral convictions of the parents (Table 11.1).

Timing of diagnosis

It is widely held that the decision to abort an abnormal fetus may be less difficult in the first trimester after chorionic villus sampling (CVS), rather than in the second trimester after amniocentesis or ultrasound. Several authors have reported data supporting this hypothesis (Blumberg and Golbus, 1975; Verp et al., 1988). Suggested explanations relate to the increasingly physically evident nature of the midtrimester developing fetus; fetal movement and ultrasound bonding may be significant. In addition, societal pressure from family and friends may influence the process of decision-making. By contrast, a first trimester diagnosis allows privacy in reproductive decisions because the pregnancy is not yet physically evident, and the announcement of the pregnancy to family and friends may be

Table 11.1. Summary of data on termination decision outcomes after fetal diagnosis of aneuploidy

Reference	Autosomal aneuploidy (%)	Sex chromosomal aneuploidy (%)	"Balanced" de novo translocation (%)
Verp et al. (1988)	87.5	41.2	0
Verp compilation of 24 amniocentesis series	96.0	67.0	31.0
Verp compilation of 13 CVS series	99.0	88.0	Unreported
Southeastern Regional Genetics	82.0	41.0	Unreported
Drugan et al. (1990)	91.0	55.0	20.0

delayed until prenatal evaluation is completed. Moreover, first trimester termination of pregnancy is known to be safer and is thought to be less damaging emotionally than second trimester termination.

Whether or not these factors translate into any effect on the outcome of decision-making is controversial. In an analysis of termination decisions after the diagnosis of fetal chromosomal anomalies, one group reported a tendency to terminate more readily in cases diagnosed in the first trimester by CVS than in cases diagnosed later by standard midtrimester amniocentesis (Duikman and Goldberg, 1992). In contrast, the experience from our own clinic with patients carrying fetuses diagnosed with either fetal aneuploidy (Drugan et al., 1990) or structural anomalies in the absence of aneuploidy (Pryde et al., 1992) is that gestational age within the legal limits for termination does not affect maternal abortion decision outcomes. This is not to say that the very real concerns about safety and the emotional effects of late versus early termination of pregnancy are not issues with our patients. In fact, anecdotally, our team has observed that women experiencing late second trimester abortions are powerfully affected both by fear of the procedure itself and the dread of choosing the death of their increasingly apparent fetus.

Abortion decisions for chromosomal abnormality

Several investigators have shown that, for fetal aneuploidy, the specific karyotype and its prognosis are the major determinants of the parental decision to abort (Table 11.2) (Drugan et al., 1990; Verp et al., 1988; Vincent et al., 1991). All studies demonstrated a high rate of termination of pregnancy for "severe" autosomal aneuploidy (e.g., trisomies 13, 18, and 21; hydropic monosomy X; and unbalanced translocations). For chromosomal abnormalities known to be of less severity with

Table 11.2. Fetal prognosis and the decision to terminate after ultrasound detected abnormalities in nonaneuploid pregnancies

Prognosis	n	Terminated	Continued
Mild	29	0 (0%)	29 (100%)
Uncertain	69	8 (11.6%)	61 (88.4%)
Severe	61	40 (65.6%)	21 (34.2%)
Total	159	48 (30.2%)	111 (69.8%)

Mild: Ultrasound findings suggestive of anatomic abnormalities, the consequences of which were counseled to be neither disabling nor life-threatening (e.g., isolated unilateral ureteropelvic junction obstruction, or a unilateral choroid plexus cyst).
Uncertain: Ultrasound demonstration of abnormalities having natural histories known to be variable, and outcomes difficult to predict (e.g., bilateral hydronephrosis without oligohydramnios, or caudal neural tube defects), or findings suggestive, but not definitively diagnostic, of a worrisome abnormality (e.g. unexplained nonvisualization of the stomach, isolated nuchal membrane, echogenic bowel).
Severe: Ultrasound findings predicting with a large degree of certainty the outcome of a lethal or markedly disabling abnormality for which either no adequate therapy is available or extensive surgery, often of uncertain benefit or high morbidity, will be required (e.g., anencephaly, encephalocele, hypoplastic left heart, nonimmune hydrops fetalis).
ANOVA; $P < 0.0001$.
Source: Pryde et al., 1992.

regard to typical phenotypic outcomes (e.g., sex chromosome aneuploidy, with the exception of Turner mosaics), termination rates were lower. For karyotypes in which outcomes typically, but not certainly, are "normal" (e.g., de novo "balanced translocations," and "marker chromosomes" each having "fetal anomaly risk" empirically estimated (Warburton, 1984) in the 10% range), the sparse data available for this relatively rare group indicated that termination rates are still lower.

The group of women with pregnancies affected by chromosomal anomalies that are associated with a relatively small risk of significant fetal malformation represents a special dilemma and deserve additional comment. The question of "what is too high a risk to take" is a very personal one. One report suggested that such decisions may be based primarily on parental perceptions of the social, family, and emotional consequences of the potential negative outcome, with less consideration of the true risk of that outcome occurring (Lyon, 1988). In our own series, six of eight pregnancies in which chromosomal anomalies were diagnosed with a low but uncertain risk were continued, and two were terminated. In one case a de novo, apparently "balanced" 13:22 translocation was diagnosed by early CVS.

Although the parents were very concerned and strongly considered terminating the pregnancy, they postponed the decision until mid-second trimester, when holoprosencephaly was diagnosed on ultrasound, thus facilitating their difficult decision. In a second case, an inherited (maternal) paracentric inversion of chromosome X was diagnosed in a male fetus. The parents were counseled that, although inherited, whatever effects the inversion might have might be attenuated in the mother as a function of preferential inactivation of the abnormal X chromosome (Beeson and Golbus, 1985) and that its effects on the male fetus therefore could not be assumed to be similarly benign. After prolonged discussions, these parents declined the option of waiting for a detailed ultrasound in the second trimester and decided to terminate the pregnancy immediately. Overall, it has been the experience in our program, and others (Holmes-Seidel et al., 1987), that in cases for which the chromosome results are difficult to interpret or have a considerable degree of prognostic uncertainty, a detailed ultrasound offering additional information seems to help the parents decide whether to terminate or continue the pregnancy.

Termination decisions for fetal anatomic abnormalities

There are fewer data on the issue of maternal termination decisions following an ultrasound discovery of structural abnormalities in the karyotypically normal fetus. With the increasing sophistication of high resolution ultrasound (Chervenak et al., 1992) and the application of color flow Doppler (Sepulveda et al., 1994), the ability to diagnose a wide variety of even subtle anomalies is revolutionizing the era of prenatal anatomic diagnosis. Several authors have commented on the psychological impact of ultrasound imaging on mothers, both with normal findings (Cox et al., 1987; Fletcher and Evans, 1983) and after the detection of structural abnormalities (Jorgenson et al., 1985; Mathews, 1990). However, until recently, there have been no studies specifically evaluating decisions made by women faced with abnormalities.

We have previously published an analysis of our experience in managing women in whom a prenatal diagnosis of nonaneuploid fetal structural malformation had been established (Pryde et al., 1992). In this study, demographic features, including age, gravidity, and parity, were found to have no significant correlation with the decision to terminate or to continue. Socioeconomic status, religious affiliation, and education were not addressed in the study and will be the subject of future inquiry. As it is analogous to the findings in studies about abortion decisions after a prenatal diagnosis of fetal chromosomal aberrations, the prognostic severity of the ultrasound diagnosis was the most significant determinant of the decision to terminate a euploid pregnancy abnormality. Unlike the findings in the chromosomal anomaly studies, however, there was a relatively low rate of termination for structural defects. Taking all ultrasound-diagnosed anomalies as a group, the rate of decision to terminate was only 30%. When stratifying the subjects into groups of "mild," "uncertain," and "severe," according to prognostic severity of the diagnosis, the rates of termination were 0%, 12%, and 66% respectively (Table 11.2).

The generally low rate of termination in this study population was an unanticipated finding, particularly in light of the much higher rates seen in aneuploid fetuses, as shown previously (Drugan et al., 1990; Verp et al., 1988). At the time of writing, the reasons for this can only be speculated about and require further study. Certainly, in wanted pregnancies, there is a powerful reluctance on the part of the mother and father to accept that their fetus is abnormal and, more so, to make the difficult decision to terminate. In our study group, mothers faced with prognostic ambiguity were more likely to continue pregnancy and "hope for the best," despite knowledge in many cases of potential catastrophic outcomes. Still, this does not seem to be a complete explanation, particularly for some of the potentially more severe disorders. Additional factors appear to be operating. We speculate that the increasing availability of potential neonatal and prenatal therapies has modified decision-making after the diagnosis of a variety of fetal disorders. In cases for which neonatal therapy of clear demonstrated benefit could be offered (e.g., omphalocele and gastroschisis), there was virtually a universal choice to continue. In cases for which fetal or neonatal therapy of an investigational nature (e.g., in utero vesicoamniotic shunting for obstructive uropathy) or uncertain outcome (e.g., early neonatal repair of spina bifida), there was a high rate of continuation of pregnancy (61%) despite counseling concerning the spectra of potential outcomes ranging from good to very poor, or even lethal. Both of these situations contrast sharply with the circumstance of clearly defined severe fetal anomalies for which no therapy could be offered and in which very high rates of termination (94%) were predictably observed.

In our service, the major variation in likelihood to terminate between "severe" and "mild to moderate" abnormalities has not changed during the 1990s. More than 80% of patients whose fetuses have severe abnormalities have chosen to terminate regardless of when in gestation the diagnosis was made. The average termination rate for fetuses whose "mild to moderate" disorders were discovered through CVS was 37%, versus 20% for those whose disorders were discovered through amniocentesis. This difference approached but did not reach significance. There has been a slight trend in the "mild to moderate" group toward a lower rate of pregnancy termination over the past several years, although the trend is not statistically significant.

Despite the vastly increased use of ultrasound study in the intervening decade since our first data set, patients' decisions about continuing or terminating a pregnancy with an abnormality have not changed. We speculate that as patients have become more used to seeing ultrasound figures early in gestation, the emotional impact of the bonding from such may not be as great as it was in the early 1980s (Cox et al., 1987; Fletcher and Evans, 1983) and may play a somewhat smaller role in patients' decision-making about problems as they are diagnosed.

In a pluralistic society, patients confronted with emotionally charged issues, such as the diagnosis of a fetus with a significant anomaly, can be expected to have differing initial reactions and thoughts about continuation or termination. Our data suggest that, on balance, patients whose fetuses have severe anomalies are more likely to choose termination. Such data should not be surprising. In fact, such data are reassuring of the quality and non-directiveness of the genetic counseling process that allows couples to reach their own decisions.

Fetal therapy

The ability to detect increasing numbers of fetal abnormalities early in gestation has led to a unique opportunity, that of attempting to fix selected birth defects. While it is true that for many disorders, such as chromosome abnormalities, current technology does not permit correction of the multisystem imbalances that are seen, for selected problems there is experience and some hope that the birth defects can be corrected.

Endoscopic fetal surgery

Attempts to shunt excessive fluid on the brain and bladder achieved significant media coverage in the early 1980s, particularly for the work on fetal hydro-cephalus. Unfortunately, particularly for hydrocephalus, an insufficiently rigorous approach, in retrospect, toward patient selection led to many bad outcomes. These were caused predominantly by patients who had fetal hydrocephalus as well as many other anomalies. When these fetuses were subjected to invasive therapy, the hydrocephalus might have been relieved, but the other problems were not resolved. Instead of the hoped-for outcome of babies who would have been impaired becoming normal, several babies who would have otherwise died, became severely handicapped survivors. Thus, treatment for fetal hydrocephalus fell into disfavor. However, recent appreciation of the poor outcomes of progressive hydrocephalus occurring without any other anomalies, suggests that such fetuses should again be considered for shunting.

Fetal lower urinary tract obstruction (LUTO) affects one in 5000–8000 males. Untreated, the obstruction may lead to hydronephrosis, renal dysplasia, and perinatal death (Evans et al., 1991). Prenatally diagnosed cases of posterior urethral valves have a 30–50% mortality. Death is attributable to pulmonary hypoplasia and/or renal dysplasia.

The sonographic diagnosis of fetal lower urinary tract obstruction is suggested by the presence of a dilated and thickened bladder, hydroureters, hydronephrosis, and oligohydramnios. These findings, in the presence of a male fetus, are highly suggestive of posterior urethral valves. However, other etiologies, such as urethral stricture or atresia, urethral agenesis, ureteral reflux, persistent cloaca, and megalourethra, can present with a very similar sonographic image. Thus, precise diagnosis can only be made after birth (Freedman et al., 1996).

The management of patients with sonographic findings of lower urinary tract obstruction is complex. A careful ultrasound examination is performed to rule out associated major congenital anomalies. Sonographic evidence of renal cystic dysplasia and the volume of amniotic fluid are also noted, as they have prognostic value by determining the concentrations of sodium, calcium, β_2 microglobulin, and total protein in fetal urine as well as its osmolality (Johnson et al., 1994, 1997). Serial vesicocenteses are performed to assess the functional status of the fetal kidneys. A single vesicocentesis may not adequately reflect the renal reserve, because two consecutive samples may be on different sides of the normal cut-off level.

Since 1982, ultrasound-guided vesico amniotic shunts have been suggested for the treatment of fetuses with LUTO. The diversion of fetal urine into the amniotic cavity serves a dual purpose: it prevents the renal damage that may result from the urinary obstruction, and it allows normal pulmonary development. The rationale for this therapy is based on animal studies in which ligation of the ureters or of the urethra and urachus of fetal lambs in mid-gestation produced renal dysplasia and pulmonary hypoplasia. Decompression of the obstruction resulted in resolution of the urinary obstruction and improved pulmonary status at birth. Experience with percutaneous vesico-amniotic shunting in humans, collected by the International Fetal Surgery Registry, shows a 5% procedure-related loss, and a 48% survival rate (40 of 83 treated fetuses). Of the treated fetuses, 74% with posterior urethral valves survived, in contrast to a 55% fetal survival rate reported in untreated fetuses. Survivors with total urethral obstruction, as with urethral atresia or agenesis, are extremely rare.

Treatment of fetuses with LUTO with urinary diversion procedures has significant limitations. First, they are palliative measures that defer the final treatment of the obstruction until the birth of the child. Second, vesico-amniotic shunts may become obstructed or displaced in up to 25% of cases, requiring additional interventions to replace the shunt, with their attendant complications. Fetal vesicostomy or ureterostomy by way of open fetal surgery have been proposed to overcome the problems associated with the percutaneous shunts, but they have not gained support.

We have introduced the concept of performing percutaneous fetal cystoscopy to evaluate fetuses affected with LUTO (Quintero et al., 1995a,b). This procedure uses the same techniques and skills as fetal vesicocentesis. A thin endoscope is passed through the lumen of the needle or trocar to observe the fetal bladder at the time of the vesicocentesis. The elements in the bladder trigone can be identified, and the diagnosis of urethral obstruction can be confirmed or ruled out. The endoscope is then removed, and the bladder is drained. Fetal cystoscopy may also be used therapeutically. Indeed, we have performed ablation of posterior urethral valves in a fetus at 24 weeks of gestation. To accomplish this, we inserted an operating endoscope toward the posterior urethra and advanced an electrode through the operating channel of the endoscope. The valves were electrocauterized under direct endoscopic visualization, and urethral patency was confirmed by instilling physiologic solution into the amniotic cavity transurethrally. We have subsequently used YAG laser energy to ablate the valves, with documentation of urethral patency. The techniques are still in the early learning phase. With increased experience, it will be possible to compare these new techniques against more established shunt procedures.

We hypothesize that percutaneous fetal cystoscopy may allow a more precise prenatal diagnosis and prognosis in fetuses with lower urinary tract obstruction. Since this procedure can be performed at the time of diagnostic vesicocentesis, it should not pose additional risks to the standard assessment of fetal renal function. In addition, those fetuses truly identified as having posterior valves may fare better if the obstruction can be eliminated in utero, avoiding the complications of vesico-amniotic shunts or the morbidity of open fetal surgery. These ideas are currently the subject of intense investigation at our Center for Fetal Diagnosis and Therapy.

Other endoscopic approaches

Similarly, endoscopic fetal surgery is being developed in our center and others for the treatment of umbilical cord ligation in acardiac twins, for laser ablation in twin-to-twin transfusion, for early fetal blood sampling, and as an adjunct to in utero fetal muscle biopsy.

The next several years will be exciting, particularly as new modifications to these techniques make the procedures safer, more reliable, quicker, and therefore more commonplace. It is likely that many applications of open fetal surgery will in fact be modified to be done endoscopically as experience continues.

Open fetal surgery

Open fetal surgery, which involves performing a maternal laparotomy, opening up the uterus, taking out the fetus, operating on the fetus, and then putting everything back, was developed by Dr. Michael Harrison's group at the University of California, San Francisco. Several dozen attempts at the correction of diaphragmatic hernia have been performed by this method.

The original approach of a full fetal laparotomy has been replaced with a much more limited procedure of placing a tracheal clip to trap the pulmonary secretions within the lungs. The lungs then expand, pushing the bowel out of the chest. Further developments in our understanding of the pathophysiology and treatment of diaphragmatic hernia reveals that the milder cases (those that do not have liver in the chest wall), do well enough with postnatal treatment. The "liver up" cases who do not do well naturally or with classic surgery are the ones for whom the clip approach is used. More data are necessary to evaluate the appropriate use of these procedures.

Delivery of fetuses with clips must be accomplished and the clip removed before the fetus can breathe. The EXIT procedure was developed in which the mother is anesthetized and a cesarean incision is made. The incision is then made through the primary one in the uterus, and the fetus is partially removed. The clips are removed and the fetus intubated while oxygen flow is still obtained from the placenta. The use of the EXIT procedure has expanded, and it is now also used to help in the management of neonates with craniofacial tumors, and some other anomalies.

Open surgery is also used in the management of lung malformations (congenital, cystadenomatoid malformations) and saccrococcygeal teratomas. The general thrust is to try to do as many procedures as possible endoscopically so that the degree of medical invasiveness, incision size, etc., can be reduced.

Medical fetal therapies

The treatment of fetal cardiac arrhythmias has been the most common fetal intervention performed to date. Fetuses with cardiac arrhythmias can go into heart failure, which can lead to significant hydrops and fetal death. It has been shown that when there is no structural anomaly, the ability to cardiovert abnormal rhythms is excellent, and a majority of these fetuses will respond clinically with favorable outcomes. Biochemical abnormalities, such as congenital adrenal hyperplasia, have also been treated prenatally with amelioration of the female genital masculinization that is otherwise seen. Thus, a birth defect can be prevented. Other endocrine conditions, such as fetal goiters, can be treated with intra-amniotic injections of thyroxine, and recently, Smith–Lemlin–Optiz syndrome has been treated with cholesterol.

Gene therapy

Medical and surgical treatments are aimed at patients' signs and symptoms. If one is able to give a child or even an embryo the ability to make its own missing product, for example, hemoglobin A in sickle cell anemia or hexosaminidase A in Tay Sachs Disease, it will be possible to cure that disease completely. If the gene for such a product were injected early enough into the embryo, it might be incorporated into that person's own gametes, and might prevent the disease for the future. Work toward such a goal has already been accomplished in animals, and selected cases will be attempted in humans in the not too distant future.

We have successfully used hematopoietic stem cell therapy to treat a fetus with X-linked severe combined immunodeficiency disease (SCIDS, or "bubble baby" disease) by injecting paternal bone marrow that was T-cell depleted to avoid graft versus host disease. The injection of stem cells must be done early in pregnancy to be incorporated before about 15–16 weeks, at which time the fetus will become immunocompetent. In our patient, who is now three years of age and has developed apparently complete engraftment and immunocompetence, the cells became incorporated into the genome of the fetus. All of his T-cells are his father's, and his B-cells are his own. This approach can be the prototype for fetal treatment of several inborn errors of metabolism, but emphasizes the need for early diagnosis to facilitate the opportunities for therapy.

Conclusion

Technology has afforded us the opportunity to diagnose an ever-increasing number and proportion of anomalies. The decision to terminate or continue such pregnancies has become increasingly complex and requires understanding, compassion, and non-directiveness. In some instances, the further component of fetal therapy can be included, with all its hopefulness, which must be tempered with realistic expectations.

REFERENCES

Beeson D, Golbus MS. Decision making: whether or not to have prenatal diagnosis and abortion for x-linked conditions. American Journal of Medical Genetics 1985; **20**: 107–14.

Black RB, Furlong R. Prenatal diagnosis: the experience in families who have children. American Journal of Medical Genetics 1987; **19**: 729–39.

Blumberg BD, Golbus MS. Psychological sequelae of elective abortion. Western Journal of Medicine 1975; **123**: 188–93.

Chervenak FA, Isaacson GA, Streltzoff J. Second trimester ultrasound. In: Evans MI, ed. Reproductive risks and prenatal diagnosis. Norwalk (CT): Appleton & Lange, 1992: 151–74.

Cox DN, Wittman BK, Hess M, Ross AG, Lind J, Lindahl S. The psychological impact of diagnostic ultrasound. Obstetrics and Gynecology 1987; **70**: 673–6.

Devore GR, Alfi O. The use of color Doppler ultrasound to identify fetuses at increased risk for trisomy 21: an alternative for high risk patients who decline genetic amniocentesis. Obstetrics and Gynecology 1995; **85**: 378–86.

Drugan A, Greb A, Johnson MP, et al. Determinants of parental decisions to abort for chromosome abnormalities. Prenatal Diagnosis 1990; **10**: 483–90.

Duikman R, Goldberg JD. Termination of pregnancy. In: Evans MI, ed. Reproductive risks and prenatal diagnosis. Norwalk (CT): Appleton & Lange, 1992: 299–309.

Evans MI, Johnson MP. Chorionic villus sampling. In: Evans MI, ed. Reproductive risks and prenatal diagnosis. Norwalk (CT): Appleton & Lange, 1992.

Evans MI, Sacks AL, Johnson MP, Robichaux III AG, May M, Moghissi KS. Sequential invasive assessment of fetal renal function, and the in utero treatment of fetal obstructive uropathies. Obstetrics and Gynecology 1991; **77**(4): 545–50.

Ewigman BG, Crane JP, Frigoletto FD, Lefevre ML, Bain RP, McNellis D, and the RADIUS Study Group. A randomized trial of prenatal ultrasound screening in a low risk population: impact on perinatal outcome. New England Journal of Medicine 1993; **329**: 821–7.

Fletcher JC, Evans MI. Maternal bonding in early fetal ultrasound examinations. New England Journal of Medicine 1983; **308**: 392–3.

Freedman AL, Bukowski TP, Smith CA, Evans MI, Johnson MP, Gonzalez R. Fetal therapy for obstructive uropathy: specific outcomes diagnosis. Journal of Urology 1996; **156**: 720–4.

Furlong RM, Black RB. Pregnancy termination for the genetic indications: the impact on families. Social Work in Health Care 1984; **10**: 17–34.

Holmes Seidel M, Ryynanen M, Lindenbaum RH. Parental decisions regarding termination of pregnancy following prenatal detection of sex chromosome anomalies. Prenatal Diagnosis 1987; **7**: 239–44.

Johnson MP, Johnson A, Holzgreve W, et al. First trimester simple hygroma, cause and outcome. American Journal of Obstetrics and Gynecology 1993; **168**: 156–61.

Johnson MP, Bukowski TP, Reitlerman C, Isada NB, Pryde PG, Evans MI. In utero surgical treatment of fetal obstructive uropathy: a new comprehensive approach to identify appropriate candidates for vesicoamniotic shunt therapy. American Journal of Obstetrics and Gynecology 1994; **170**: 1770–9.

Johnson MP, Flake AW, Quintero RA, Evans MI. Shunt procedures. In: Evans MI, Johnson MP, Moghissi KS, eds. Invasive outpatient procedures in reproductive medicine. Philadelphia: Lippencott Raven Publishers, 1997.

Jorgenson C, Uddenberg N, Ursing I. Ultrasound diagnosis of fetal malformations in the second trimester. The psychological reactions of women. Journal of Psychosomatic Obstetrics and Gynæcology 1985: **4**: 31–40.

Kenyon SL, Hackett GA, Campbell S. Termination of pregnancy following diagnosis of fetal malformation: the need for improved follow-up services. Clinical Obstetrics and Gynæcology 1988; **31**: 97–100.

Larsen JW Jr, MacMillin MD. Second and third trimester prenatal diagnosis. In: Evans MI, Fletcher JC, Dixler AO, Schulman JD, eds. Fetal diagnosis and therapy: science, ethics, and the law. Philadelphia: JB Lippincott, 1989: 36–43.

Leon IG. The psychoanalytic conceptualization of perinatal loss: a multidimensional model. American Journal of Psychiatry 1992; **149**: 1464–72.

Lyon MF. X-chromosome inactivations and the location and expression of X-linked genes. American Journal of Human Genetics 1988; **42**: 8–16.

Mathews AL. Known fetal malformations during pregnancy: a human experience of loss. Birth Defects Original Article Series 1990; **26**: 168–75.

Nadler HL. Antenatal detection of hereditary disorders. Pediatrics 1968; **42**: 912.

Nicolaides K, Shawwa L, Brizot M, Snijders R. Ultrasonographically detectable markers of fetal chromosomal defects. Ultrasound in Obstetrics and Gynecology 1993; **3**: 56–69.

Pryde PG, Isada NB, Hallak M, Johnson MP, Odgers AE, Evans MI. Determinants of parental decisions to abort or continue after non-aneuploid ultrasound detected fetal abnormalities. Obstetrics and Gynecology 1992; **80**: 52–6.

Quintero RA, Hume RF, Smith C, Johnson MP, Cotton DB, Romero R, Evans MI. Percutaneous fetal cystoscopy and endoscopic fulguration of posterior urethral valves. American Journal of Obstetrics and Gynecology 1995a; **172**: 206–9.

Quintero RA, Johnson MP, Romero R, et al. In utero percutaneous cystoscopy in the management of fetal lower obstructive uropathy. Lancet 1995b; **346**: 537–40.

Sepulveda W, Romero R, Pryde PG, Wolfe HM, Addis JR, Cotton DB. Prenatal diagnosis of sirenomelus with color Doppler ultrasonography. American Journal of Obstetrics and Gynecology 1994; **170**(5 Part 1): 1377–9.

Verp MS, Bombared AT, Simpson JL, Elias S. Parental decision following prenatal diagnosis of fetal chromosome abnormality. American Journal of Medical Genetics 1988; **29**: 613–22.

Vincent VA, Edwards JG, Young SR, Nachtigal M. Pregnancy termination because of chromsome abnormalities: a study of 26 950 amniocenteses in the Southeast. Southern Medical Journal 1991; **84**: 1210–13.

Warburton D. Outcome of cases of de novo structural rearrangements diagnosed at amniocentesis. Prenatal Diagnosis 1984; **4**: 69–80.

Wertz DC, Fletcher JC. Attitudes of genetic counselors: a multinational survey. American Journal of Human Genetics 1988; **42**: 592–600.

Wertz DC, Fletcher JC. Ethical issues in prenatal diagnosis. Pediatric Annals 1989; **18**: 739–49.

Part V

Prenatal Care as an Integral Component of Women's Health Care

12

Opportunities for improving maternal and infant health through prenatal oral health care

James J. Crall

Introduction

It is not unusual for oral health to be overlooked by those responsible for organizing prenatal care programs, regardless of whether the programs are clinical or educational in nature. After all, until recently, the most commonly cited link between pregnancy and oral health in the clinical literature was a poorly understood and largely inconsequential condition known as "pregnancy gingivitis" (Carranza, 1996). However, applications of modern scientific techniques during the past decade have provided greater insights into the likely etiology of this common phenomenon, and also have demonstrated significant links between conditions in the mouths of mothers and the future oral health of their infants. Other recent epidemiological and laboratory studies have directed attention to a possible link between maternal oral health and the course and outcomes of pregnancy in some women.

For this reason, it seems timely and appropriate to review the available evidence on oral health and pregnancy. This chapter provides an overview of the current state of knowledge about these topics along with suggestions for achieving broader, more integrated involvement among health care professionals and prenatal program administrators in health promotion related to oral health. It begins with a review of common oral health problems, which may be exacerbated during pregnancy, but which may be minimized or prevented through effective prenatal care. Because it may be unfamiliar to many involved with prenatal care, the etiology of conditions affecting oral health is emphasized in this discussion. The second section provides a synopsis of recent scientific reports demonstrating links between maternal oral health and pregnancy outcomes and highlights potential opportunities for improving those outcomes through prenatal care. A summary of recent research findings concerning relationships between maternal oral health and infant oral health follows, along with a discussion of the direct and indirect effects of prenatal oral health care on dental disease in infants. The final section outlines the elements of a new paradigm concerning the importance of maternal oral health within the context of effective prenatal care.

Oral changes during pregnancy

Dental plaque

Dental plaque is a thin film composed of bacteria and salivary components that forms on tooth surfaces. Plaque composition is neither homogeneous nor static. It varies among individuals within populations, as well as within individuals over time and across sites throughout the mouth, depending on a multitude of ecological factors.

Plaque is generally accepted to be a primary etiologic agent for the two most common pathologic dental conditions: dental caries (tooth decay) and periodontal diseases (inflammatory conditions that cause destruction of tooth-supporting structures). However, not all plaque is considered pathogenic or harmful. In the case of periodontal health, certain bacterial species actually are regarded as being protective or beneficial to the host because they prevent more pathogenic bacteria from colonizing susceptible areas (Dzink et al., 1985). Evidence suggests that selective colonization by certain organisms may provide similar protective or moderating effects in the case of dental caries.

It is now widely accepted that certain common oral bacteria (e.g., *Streptococcus mutans* and particular strains of *Lactobaccilli*) produce acids that cause dental caries (Krasse and Newbrun, 1982; van Houte, 1980). Another discrete group of bacteria, including several Gram-negative species, function as periodontal pathogens and are implicated in the etiology of gingivitis (inflammation of the gums, which are the soft tissues surrounding the teeth) and periodontitis (loss of soft tissue attachment and destruction of tooth-supporting bone) (Offenbacher, 1996). This concept has been advanced further in the specific-plaque hypothesis initially described by Loesche (1976), which stipulates that specific forms of periodontal disease have specific bacterial determinants.

Different sites throughout the mouth harbor different mixes of bacteria. Of particular interest is the observation that the disease-producing potential of plaque has been shown to vary by site and to depend on the presence of or an increase in specific microorganisms that produce substances that mediate the destruction of host tissues (Offenbacher, 1996). For example, studies have shown that the odds ratio for future periodontal site breakdown increases sharply from two to seven or eight as the numbers of *Porphyromonas gingivalis* increase from 10^5 to 10^7. This observation also demonstrated that a "threshold" of 10^6 *P. gingivalis* is necessary for progressive attachment loss predictably to occur. Thus, as a general model, increases in pathogenic organisms beyond critical threshold levels lead to site-specific elevations in inflammatory mediators and enhanced pathogenicity or risk of harm to the host (Offenbacher, 1996).

Many physical, environmental, and social variables seem to influence plaque composition and the risk of periodontal attachment loss in individuals (Offenbacher, 1996). Of particular relevance is the finding that if the host is stressed in any manner that leads to increased inflammation, bacterial overgrowth will occur. Changes in hormone levels during pregnancy also have been shown to influence the composition of plaque, with a shift toward a greater percentage of pathogenic anaerobic bacteria, particularly *P. intermedia* (Kornman and Loesche, 1980). These organisms apparently can substitute steroid hormones (e.g., progesterone or estradiol, which increase in gingival crevicular fluid during pregnancy) for vitamin K as a growth factor and thus achieve an ecological advantage. Additional details concerning mechanisms and mediating factors are beyond the scope of this chapter, but can be found elsewhere in the literature (e.g., Offenbacher, 1996).

Periodontal status

Adverse changes in periodontal health are common during pregnancy. Published studies report gingivitis prevalence rates ranging from 50% to as high as 100% in expectant mothers (Löe, 1965). Gingival areas that exhibited only mild levels of gingivitis before pregnancy may become swollen, inflamed, and prone to increased bleeding. The gingival changes are usually painless unless complicated by acute infection and are reversible following the pregnancy, provided that local irritants are eliminated (Carranza, 1996). Fortunately, significant attachment loss or more severe forms of periodontal destruction are uncommon. It is important to note that pregnancy itself does not cause gingivitis or more severe periodontal disease. Rather pregnancy induces changes that exacerbate the typical gingival response to plaque and other local irritants, and results in clinically detectable changes in periodontal tissues (Carranza, 1996).

No notable changes occur in the gingiva during pregnancy in the absence of local irritants. When local irritants such as plaque are present, however, the severity of gingivitis generally increases early on in pregnancy (usually starting in the second or third month), peaks in the seventh or eighth month and diminishes somewhat during the ninth month (Löe, 1965). Expectant mothers with previously unnoticed gingivitis may gradually become aware of the condition when gingival areas become enlarged and edematous, and show a greater propensity to bleed. The aggravation of gingivitis in pregnancy has been attributed principally to increased levels of progesterone, which produce vascular changes and increased susceptibility to mechanical irritation (Mohamed et al., 1974; Nyman, 1971).

Depression of the maternal T-lymphocyte response also has been suggested as a possible explanation for the modified tissue response to plaque observed during pregnancy (O'Neil, 1979).

Occasionally, the gingival tissue displays tumor-like enlargements, commonly referred to as "pregnancy tumors." However the histologic picture of these entities is one of mixed chronic and acute inflammation with an abundance of blood vessels, and is more properly characterized as an angiogranuloma (Maier and Orban, 1949). Studies also report increases in tooth mobility, periodontal pocket depth, and gingival fluid during pregnancy (Lindhe and Attstrom, 1967; Rateit-schak, 1967). Like gingivitis, the severity of these conditions tends to correlate with hormonal levels, primarily levels of progesterone and estrogen. Accordingly, there typically is a partial reduction in severity by two months postpartum and a return to normal within 12 months, provided that local irritants have been eliminated through effective self-care behaviors and professional preventive services (e.g., tooth cleaning).

Dental caries

The literature regarding the incidence of dental caries during pregnancy is both sparse and mixed, with some reports indicating increased caries incidence during pregnancy, while others report no differences compared to women who are not pregnant (Waldman, 1990). In spite of the large number of pregnancies in the U.S., there have been no national clinical studies of oral status in pregnant or recently pregnant women.

Maternal periodontal disease and pregnancy outcomes

Preliminary work by Offenbacher and colleagues at the University of North Carolina suggests that severe periodontitis in pregnant mothers may be a significant risk factor for preterm delivery leading to low birth weight infants (i.e., < 2500 gm). Results of a case-control study on 124 pregnant or postpartum mothers showed a 7.5- to 7.9-fold increased risk for preterm low birth weight infants in mothers with severe periodontal disease (Offenbacher et al., 1996). The investigation controlled for a wide range of possible confounding obstetrical risk factors, including maternal age, tobacco use, drug use, alcohol use, level of prenatal care, nutrition, genitourinary infections, and parity.

Offenbacher et al. (1996) hypothesize that periodontal infections, which serve as reservoirs of Gram-negative organisms, lipopolysaccharide, and inflammatory mediators including prostaglandin E_2 (PGE_2) and tissue necrosis factor (TNF), may pose a potential, unrecognized threat to the fetal–placental unit by triggering a hormonal cascade that results in preterm labor or preterm rupture of membranes. This concept is supported by experiments in the pregnant hamster model (Collins et al., 1994) and a recent case-control study (Offenbacher et al., 1998), which showed a dose–response relationship for maternal gingival crevicular fluid PGE_2 and decreasing birth weight.

Although Offenbacher et al. made an appropriate effort in their research to control for important socioeconomic, behavioral, and other factors that are correlated with poor birth outcome, further studies are needed to confirm the link between periodontal disease in pregnant mothers, preterm delivery, and low birth weight. Larger-scale prospective studies to investigate further the linkages between maternal periodontal disease status and preterm low birth weight, and the impact of possible interventions (e.g., self-care, counseling and treatment to reduce or eliminate periodontal disease during pregnancy) are in progress. Although as yet unsubstantiated, this area of research is a compelling line of inquiry with potentially great impact on the practice and effectiveness of prenatal care.

Relationships between maternal oral health and infant oral health

Fascinating evidence has emerged in recent years, primarily through the work of Scandinavian researchers and Caufield and colleagues at the University of Alabama at Birmingham, concerning the important influence of maternal risk factors and oral health on the future oral health of infants (Alaluusua and Renkonen, 1983; Caufield et al., 1982; Kohler et al., 1988). This new paradigm looks at early infant caries as a common, infectious, transmissible disease with strong maternal determinants (Caufield et al., 1993; Rogers, 1981).

New paradigm for early childhood caries

The results of numerous studies conducted during the 1980s suggested that children acquire *Streptococcus mutans*, the principal etiological bacterial strain associated with dental caries, from their mothers some time after tooth eruption commences (i.e., after 6 months of age) (Rogers, 1981, Caufield et al., 1982). More recent investigations not only have confirmed that vector of transmission, but also have provided additional detail regarding timing and routes of transmission. For example, Caufield and colleagues (1993) discovered that transmission of cariogenic organisms generally occurs within a relatively narrow "window of infectivity" at around two years of age. More recent work using sophisticated DNA "fingerprinting" techniques (Li and Caufield, 1995) has demonstrated a high degree of fidelity between maternal strains of cariogenic organisms and those of their offspring and a lack of commonality of genotypes between fathers and infants. Additional studies have confirmed that transmission of indigenous oral biota occurs vertically (i.e., from mother to infant), not horizontally (i.e., among siblings). On a broader scale, the fidelity of maternal transmission has been shown to differ by race and gender of the offspring, with mother–daughter fidelity being greater than mother–son.

These findings hold considerable promise for identifying high-risk infants and developing targeted therapeutic interventions. Such interventions have only begun to be tested in clinical trials. If successful, these strategies could help to reduce the incidence of early childhood caries, a still-too-common condition that results in extensive dental destruction in infants and frequently requires costly treatment involving hospitalization and general anesthesia.

Improving maternal and infant health through prenatal care

Prenatal programs that seek to deal effectively with the potential risks and consequences of oral diseases during pregnancy should include appropriate assessments of oral health, education, counseling, and necessary professional services. These measures are currently indicated based on the effects of pregnancy on maternal health and the relationship between maternal and infant oral health; additional evidence supporting the link between maternal periodontal disease and pregnancy outcome would make these interventions all the more critical. Ideally, guidelines or recommendations based on sound scientific evidence of the effectiveness and cost-effectiveness of various strategies would be available to outline preferred programs of care. However as with the epidemiology of oral conditions during pregnancy, little scientific information exists concerning the use of dental services by pregnant women in the U.S. or evidence of the effectiveness of different prenatal care programs. Studies of the general population typically report that women are more inclined to engage in self-care behaviors, more likely to visit a dentist, and more likely to report symptoms as compared to men (Radford, 1993). However, the largely anecdotal information available on use of dental services by pregnant women suggests that significant numbers forego needed treatment, even for painful oral conditions (Waldman, 1990).

Dental care during pregnancy: goals and timing

Dental care should be an integral component of prenatal care. Early assessment and counseling are recommended so that expectant mothers can be informed about potential pregnancy-related changes in oral health and can be taught methods that will help them avoid or minimize the need for invasive dental treatment during pregnancy. Personal plaque control behaviors complemented, when necessary, by professional services to remove local irritants are highly effective, non-invasive approaches for preventing undesirable bacterial overgrowth and soft tissue changes, and enhancing oral health throughout pregnancy.

The overall goals of any prenatal oral health care program should be to minimize risks to both mother and developing fetus.

A guiding principle of effective prenatal oral health care is to avoid emergency situations that require surgical treatment if at all possible. Ideally, this means early detection of clinical problems and non-surgical procedures to arrest disease processes or minimize their consequences (e.g., professional teeth cleaning and polishing to remove local irritants and/or procedures to control or eliminate dental caries). If possible, non-emergency treatment needs should be addressed during the second trimester. Regardless of when treatment is performed, appropriate precautions should be taken to avoid or minimize risks associated with radiation exposure, medication administration, and postural complications (Waldman, 1990).

Reducing infant health risks through prenatal care

There is emerging evidence that steps taken to improve mothers' oral health during pregnancy can have direct as well as indirect effects on the health of their offspring. Studies have shown that the initial establishment of *Streptococcus mutans* in infants can be prevented or delayed by caries-preventive measures in mothers who have high levels of this organism (Köhler et al., 1983). The results of further investigations (Köhler et al., 1984) indicate that preventing or delaying transmission of decay-causing organisms reduces the risk of caries in their infants at age three. These findings underscore the importance of taking steps to improve expectant and new mothers' oral health for the sake of their infants as well as for their own well-being. Additional investigations are underway to determine whether reducing the levels of periodontal pathogens that may act as indirect sources of infection and inflammation can reduce the risk of preterm low birth weight and the attendant infant health risks that accompany that condition.

With respect to indirect benefits, considerable research into the linkages between parental health-related attitudes and behaviors and those of their infants has been conducted. Families share health behaviors, including those related to primary prevention (diet and exercise) and tertiary prevention (compliance with health-related regimens) (Baranowski and Nader, 1985). In the case of oral health, the general consensus is that parents play a crucial role in children's health by introducing them to self-care practices (e.g., brushing with fluoride toothpaste and flossing) and shaping their attitudes and behaviors regarding nutrition and use of professional services (Inglehart and Tedesco, 1995).

Conclusion

As pointed out at the onset, oral health has received comparatively little attention in the context of prenatal care. A literature search related to this chapter identified 2500 citations under the heading "dental" and 1850 under the heading "prenatal care." However, the intersection of the two headings produced only two citations. The historical reasons for this void have been identified; so too have the reasons why this situation should not persist.

Pregnancy poses risks to maternal oral health. Beyond that, studies suggest that maternal periodontal conditions may be linked to pregnancy outcomes. Maternal oral health can influence the colonization of infants' mouths by decay-causing bacteria and thus their risk of subsequent dental caries. Equally important is evidence that early attention and relatively simple measures can avoid or minimize the adverse impact of pregnancy on the oral health of expectant mothers and delay or prevent the transmission of cariogenic organisms to their infants, thereby reducing their risk of dental disease. Thus, the case for a new paradigm that emphasizes oral health as part of prenatal care continues to grow.

Much remains to be learned about the links between maternal and infant oral health. Nevertheless, a variety of approaches for improving the health of infants as well as mothers through more effective prenatal care programs are on the horizon. Progressive prenatal care programs will begin now to incorporate and translate existing and emerging knowledge into comprehensive and effective measures that emphasize early assessment, self-care education and counseling, timely professional prevention and treatment, and coordination among various types of health care professionals and programs. Progressive health care professionals will recognize the importance of caring for the overall health of individuals and populations, not merely parts of the body.

REFERENCES

Alaluusua S, Renkonen O-V. *Streptococcus mutans* establishment and dental caries experience in children from 2 to 4 years old. Scandinavian Journal of Dental Research 1983; **91**: 453–7.

Baranowski T, Nader PR. Family health behavior. In: Turk DC, Keans RD, eds. Health, illness and families: a life-span perspective. New York: John Wiley & Sons, 1985: 51–80.

Carranza FA Jr. Influence of systemic diseases on the periodontium. In: Carranza FA Jr, Newman MG, eds. Clinical periodontology. Philadelphia: W.B. Saunders Co, 1996: 193–4.

Caufield PW, Cutler GR, Dasanayake AP. Initial acquisition of mutans streptococci by infants: evidence for a discrete window of infectivity. Journal of Dental Research 1993; **72**: 37–45.

Caufield PW, Wannemuehler Y, Hansen JB. Familial clustering of the *Streptococcus mutans* cryptic plasmid strain in a dental clinic population. Infection and Immunity 1982; **38**: 785–7.

Collins JG, Windley HW III, Arnold RR, et al. Effects of a *Porphyromonas gingivalis* infection on inflammatory mediator response and pregnancy outcome in the hamster. Infection and Immunity 1994; **62**: 4356–61.

Dzink JL, Tanner AC, Haffajee AD, Socransky SS. Gram negative species associated with active destructive periodontal lesions. Journal of Clinical Periodontology 1985; **12**: 648–59.

Inglehart MR, Tedesco LA. The role of the family in preventing oral diseases. In: Cohen LK, Gift HC, eds. Disease prevention and oral health promotion. Copenhagen, Munksgaard; 1995: 271–305.

Köhler B, Andréen I, Jonsson B. The effect of caries-preventive measures in mothers on dental caries and the oral presence of the bacteria *Streptococcus mutans* and *Lactobacilli* in their children. Archives of Oral Biology 1984; **29**: 879–83.

Köhler B, Andréen I, Jonsson B. The earlier the colonization by *mutans* streptococci, the higher the caries prevalence at 4 years of age. Oral Microbiology and Immunology 1988; **3**: 14–17.

Köhler B, Bratthall D, Krasse B. Preventive measures in mothers influence the establishment of the bacterium *Streptococcus mutans* in their infants. Archives of Oral Biology 1983; **28**: 225–31.

Kornman KS, Loesche WJ. The subgingival microbial flora during pregnancy. Journal of Periodontal Research 1980; **15**: 111–22.

Krasse B, Newbrun E. Objective methods for evaluating caries activity and their application. In: Stewart RE, Barber TK, Troutman KC, et al., eds. Pediatric dentistry: scientific foundations and clinical practice. St. Louis: The C.V. Mosby Co., 1982: 610–16.

Li Y, Caufield PW. The fidelity of initial acquisition of *mutans* streptococci by infants from their mothers. Journal of Dental Research 1995; **74**: 681–5.

Lindhe J, Attstrom R. Gingival exudation during the menstrual cycle. Journal of Periodontal Research 1967; **2**: 194–8.

Löe H. Periodontal changes in pregnancy. Journal of Periodontology 1965; **36**: 209–17.

Loesche W. Chemotherapy of dental plaque infections. Oral Sciences Reviews 1976; **9**: 65–107.

Maier AW, Orban B. Gingivitis in pregnancy. Oral Surgery 1949; **2**: 334–73.

Mohamed AH, Waterhouse JP, Friederici HH. The microvasculature of the rabbit gingiva as affected by progesterone: an ultrastructural study. Journal of Periodontology 1974; **45**: 50–60.

Nyman S. Studies on the influence of estradiol and progesterone on granulation tissue. Journal of Periodontology 1971; **7**(Suppl): 1–24.

Offenbacher S. Periodontal diseases: pathogenesis. Annals of Periodontology 1996; **1**: 821–78.

Offenbacher S, Jared HL, O'Reilly PG, et al. Potential pathogenic mechanisms of periodontitis-associated pregnancy complications. Annals of Periodontology 1998; **3**: 233–50.

Offenbacher S, Katz V, Fertik G, et al. Periodontal infection as a possible risk factor for preterm low birth weight. Journal of Periodontology 1996; **67**: 1103–13.

O'Neil TCA. Maternal T-lymphocyte response and gingivitis in pregnancy. Journal of Periodontology 1979; **50**: 178–84.

Radford M. Beyond pregnancy gingivitis: bringing a new focus to women's oral health. Journal of Dental Education 1993; **57**: 742–8.

Rateitschak KH. Tooth mobility changes in pregnancy. Journal of Periodontal Research 1967; **2**: 199–206.

Rogers AH. The source of infection in the intrafamilial transfer of *Streptococcus mutans*. Caries Research 1981; **15**: 26–31.

Romero R, Hobbins JC, Mitchell MD. Endotoxin stimulates prostaglandin E2 production by human amnion. Obstetrics and Gynecology 1988; **71**: 227–8.

Romero R, Mazor M, Wu YK, et al. Bacterial endotoxin and tumor necrosis factor stimulate prostaglandin production by human decidua. Prostaglandins Leukotrienes and Essential Fatty Acids 1989; **37**: 183–5.

van Houte J. Bacterial specificity in the etiology of dental caries. International Dental Journal 1980; **30**: 305–26.

Waldman HB. Oral health status of women and children in the United States. Journal of Public Health Dentistry 1990; **50**(Spec. Issue): 379–89.

13

Family planning: need and opportunities

Lorraine V. Klerman

Introduction

The idea that prenatal care should have objectives beyond the birth of a healthy infant to a healthy mother is not a new one. In recent years, the most forceful expression of an expanded purpose for prenatal care can be found in *Caring for Our Future*, the 1989 report of the Public Health Service's Expert Panel on the Content of Prenatal Care (PHS, 1989). The report stated:

The prenatal period provides an opportunity to look beyond pregnancy and delivery to identify the resources essential for further healthy development of parents and infant. The objectives of prenatal care are concerned with more than the prevention of maternal and neonatal morbidity and mortality; these objectives include other aspects of the woman's health prior to, during, and after pregnancy and include the promotion of healthy child development, positive family relationships, and family planning (p. 2).

The book that followed this report, *New Perspectives on Prenatal Care*, amplified this view, noting that the preconceptional period, the nine months of pregnancy, and the postpartum visit or visits provide a "window of opportunity" to do more than ensure the delivery of a healthy infant (Klerman, 1990). Thus, the Public Health Service panel anticipated the ideas presented in this book, namely that during the prenatal period many women have an intense relationship with one or more providers of care. This interaction should be used not only to ensure a healthy mother and a healthy infant, but also to initiate or continue a program of medical care and health-promoting behavior for the woman herself, aside from her role as mother.

Family planning is a central objective of comprehensive women's health care. One of a woman's most important health-related concerns is her fertility, that is, her ability to have children when she wants them, as well as to not have them when she does not want them; to have healthy infants, and to maintain her health during and after pregnancy. In order to achieve these objectives, the woman and her sexual partner must engage in family planning.

Probably the most important goal of family planning is to reduce the incidence of unintended pregnancies, whether they are actually unwanted or only mistimed. A second goal is to allow an appropriate interval between pregnancies. This chapter will summarize the scope of the problems of unintended pregnancy and of short interpregnancy intervals. The chapter will then present a rationale for including family planning as an integral element of preconceptional care, prenatal care, and well-child supervision, and explore some of the current barriers to realizing this goal.

Unintended pregnancy

The term "unintended pregnancies" usually includes those pregnancies that were mistimed and those that were unwanted at the time of conception.

Definitional and measurement problems

Most studies of unintended pregnancies use the definitions developed by the National Center for Health Statistics for its National Surveys of Family Growth (NSFG). The NSFGs ask a series of questions of a sample of women who have experienced a live birth in the previous five years. The answers to these questions determine whether the birth or births are classified as unwanted (not wanted now or at any time in the future); mistimed (wanted but happened too soon); or intended. Thus, the NSFG reports on unintended *births* not unintended *pregnancies*. In order to estimate the number of unintended pregnancies, researchers add to the calculations a percentage of miscarriages and all abortions, because almost all abortions are the result of pregnancies that are either unwanted or seriously mistimed. Such analyses indicate the number and characteristics of unintended pregnancies, a much larger number than unintended births.

Issues in measuring unintendedness include when to ask the question, because the answer may vary depending on whether it is asked before, during, or after pregnancy; how to word the question, for example to ask directly whether a pregnancy was wanted or to assume this from the answers to other, less direct questions; whether to ask the woman only or also her sexual partner; and problems with recall.

Because questions have been raised about the NSFG intendedness results, the 1995 NSFG added questions that might reduce misunderstanding of the questions and that would validate the responses (Abma et al., 1997). Other researchers are experimenting with new approaches, which are particularly urgent in characterizing adolescent pregnancies. Among adolescents, most unintended pregnancies are mistimed rather than unwanted, and ambivalence and less-than-truthful answers may occur.

Magnitude and risk factors

In its 1995 report, *The Best Intentions* (Brown and Eisenberg, 1995), the Institute of Medicine (IOM) revealed the magnitude of the problem of unintended pregnancy. The IOM found that in 1987, only 43% of pregnancies were intended at conception, 20% were mistimed but resulted in live births, 8% were unwanted but resulted in live births, and 29% were mistimed or unwanted and were terminated. The 1995 NSFG reported a drop from the 1988 survey in the percentage of births that were unwanted by the mother at the time of conception from 12% to 10%. This was due in part to a drop in unwanted births to African American women from 29% to 21% (Abma et al., 1997).

The IOM report found that while women of all economic and social statuses experienced unintended pregnancies, the rates were higher among women at either end of the age span, unmarried women, and poor women (Brown and Eisenberg, 1995). Although there are racial and ethnic differences in the incidence of unintended pregnancies, it is likely that these are a result of economic and educational disparities.

Consequences of unintended pregnancy

There are many reasons to be concerned about the frequency of unintended pregnancies. Obviously an unwanted or even seriously mistimed pregnancy can be life-disrupting for the pregnant woman and often for her male partner and other family members as well. Plans for education, employment, and marriage can be disturbed or even abandoned, often leading to poverty and welfare dependence and even domestic violence. Research also has shown that women with unintended pregnancies, compared with those with intended pregnancies, are less likely to seek prenatal care early and more likely to smoke during pregnancy (Brown and Eisenberg, 1995). Neither of these activities promotes a healthy pregnancy. The data on maternal drinking and other health-compromising behaviors are more controversial, but no research suggests that unintended pregnancy is associated with health-promoting behaviors (Brown and Eisenberg, 1995).

Unintended pregnancies are associated with adverse effects for the infant as well. Several studies find an association between unintended pregnancies and low birth weight, possibly a result of inadequate prenatal care and maternal smoking, and with child abuse and neglect and child behavior problems (Brown and Eisenberg, 1995).

Interpregnancy intervals

Definitional and measurement problems

Again, as in the case of unintended pregnancies, there are problems in defining and measuring interpregnancy intervals. It is possible to measure the number of months using either conception or delivery as the starting point and the ending point. Thus, three measures are possible, an interconception interval (conception 1 to conception 2), an interpregnancy interval (delivery 1 to conception 2), and an interdelivery interval (delivery 1 to delivery 2). The interdelivery interval is the easiest to measure and is the one provided in United States vital statistics reports because the data needed for its calculation are usually provided on birth certificates and have high validity.

Using the interdelivery interval to examine the association between short intervals and pregnancy outcomes may cause a confusion of cause and effect. For example, it is more likely that a short interdelivery interval and an associated low birth weight was caused by a preterm delivery, rather than the preterm delivery and low birth weight being caused by the short interval. This problem can be overcome by adjusting for gestational age, but the information on which gestational age is based is often omitted from birth certificates and, even when present, is frequently of questionable validity (Miller, 1991).

Using the interpregnancy interval rather than the interdelivery interval avoids the cause–effect problem, but not the problem of needing to know the date of the second or higher order conception. Most studies use the date of the last menstrual period as a proxy for the date of conception. This information is requested on all birth certificates in the U.S., but is not as uniformly recorded or as valid as date of last birth. The interconception interval would have the same problem as the interdelivery interval and is not used.

Another problem with the measurement of intervals is that they are usually measured between live births, ignoring spontaneous and induced abortions and fetal deaths. Although the data indicate that elective, early induced abortions do not affect the outcomes of subsequent pregnancies, spontaneous abortions and fetal deaths may be the result of factors that will also cause preterm delivery or intrauterine growth restriction in a subsequent pregnancy. Thus, a subsequent live infant might be preterm or growth-restricted despite a long interval between live births due to an intervening fetal loss caused by an underlying medical problem related both to the fetal loss and the preterm birth or growth restriction. Also, there are indications that women who experience a fetal loss become pregnant again sooner than women who bear a live infant. This would increase the likelihood that short intervals would be associated with a poor pregnancy outcome. Including low weight births that are due to elective early deliveries for medical reasons also may make it difficult to determine the independent effect of the interval.

Magnitude and risk factors

In 1991, the last year for which data from national vital statistics are available, 1.8% of all second and higher order live births occurred between one and 11 months after the prior live births; 12.1%, between 12 and 17 months; 14.4%, between 18 and 23 months; and 71.7%, two years or longer. These percentages exclude what is listed in the federal data as "0 months" (plural deliveries) and "not stated." The modal interval was 24 to 35 months (NCHS, 1993).

As in the case of unintended pregnancies, women of all economic and social statuses experience short interpregnancy intervals. However, a study of birth and fetal death certificates from 1970 to 1977 revealed a direct association between maternal age and mean interval. Also, women bore children sooner after a fetal death than after a live birth. Again, racial and ethnic differences in birth intervals probably reflect economic and educational differences (Spratley and Taffel, 1981).

Consequences

Studies in developing nations have sometimes found an association between short interpregnancy intervals and maternal morbidity (Winikoff, 1983; Winkvist et al., 1992). Little is known about the short- or long-term effects on women in the United States. The consequences for fetus and infant, however, are better known. Short interpregnancy intervals are associated with unintended pregnancies and, therefore, with the consequences of such pregnancies, including late initiation of prenatal care (Klerman et al., 1998). Research suggests that when possible confounding factors are controlled, there is a relationship between short interpregnancy intervals and poor pregnancy outcomes. One study found that intervals of less than six months and possibly less than 12 or 18 months were associated with intrauterine growth restriction. Only intervals as short as less than four months were associated with preterm delivery, raising the question of causation discussed earlier (as reviewed by Klerman et al., 1995).

Opportunities for family planning

Although there is general agreement that family planning is essential for the health of women and their infants and children, there has been insufficient consideration given to when family planning should be discussed with women and their sexual partners. The assumption seems to be that a woman will present herself for family planning assistance at some point after menarche and before her first conception, and then again after each birth until menopause. This is a goal at best. It certainly does not represent reality in the United States in the 1990s.

To make progress toward the goal of providing family planning when it is needed, family planning should be integrated into existing systems of care so that it does not always require an additional appointment or additional trip to a physician or clinic. Family planning should be a standard component of most encounters between a health care provider and a woman between menarche and menopause. During adolescence, family planning counseling could be provided in the course of preventive and treatment visits, including those that occur in school facilities. For other women, family planning could be addressed during preconceptional visits when a pregnancy is being planned; during visits for prenatal care; during the postpartum checkup; in the course of preventive and treatment visits during adulthood; and during visits for well-child supervision.

As a component of preconceptional care

The idea that a woman should have a health assessment conducted before she tries to become pregnant has begun to receive increasing attention. However, most recommendations for preconceptional care are directed at preparing the woman for a pregnancy and improving the outcomes of pregnancy, rather than in preventing or delaying pregnancy or improving women's health.

The Public Health Service Expert Panel on the Content of Prenatal Care was one of the first groups to strongly advocate a preconceptional visit, although it did not list family planning as a component of such care (PHS, 1989, p. 37). A 1993 report sponsored by the March of Dimes stressed the potential benefits of preconceptional care (MOD, 1993), as did an issue of the Alan Guttmacher Institute's *Issues in Brief*, which is addressed to policy makers (Alan Guttmacher Institute, 1993). The latter publication contained this statement:

The nation would be well served by making a commitment to advance preconception services to a similar extent as it has prenatal care. Preconception care, focused on women's overall health and risk assessment and risk reduction prior to pregnancy, will serve as a key component of the next wave of low-birth-weight and infant mortality reduction strategies – and may provide increased savings beyond those experienced from prenatal care alone (p. 1).

Professional organizations now also recommend preconceptional care. The American Academy of Pediatrics (AAP) and the American College of Obstetricians and Gynecologists (ACOG) include several pages on preconceptional care in their 1997 edition of *Guidelines for Perinatal Care* (AAP/ACOG, 1997). ACOG also stresses the importance of preconceptional care and includes family planning as an essential element in its professional publications, technical publications, and patient materials (ACOG, 1993, 1995, 1996).

Guide to Clinical Preventive Services, the report of the U.S. Preventive Services Task Force, lists "unintended pregnancy and contraception" among its counseling interventions for the general population, 11 to 64 years of age, and this could be considered preconception counseling (USPSTF, 1996). Perhaps the most import-ant source of support for preconceptional care has come from the federal govern-ment in its publication *Healthy People 2000: National Health Promotion and Disease Prevention Objectives* (USDHHS, 1991). These objectives included increas-ing to at least 60% the proportion of primary care providers who provide age-appropriate preconception care and counseling.

However, the concept of a preconceptional visit is not yet firmly established. In a March of Dimes survey, 76% of women strongly agreed that it is very important for a woman who is planning to have a child to see her doctor before she becomes pregnant. In contrast, 98% strongly agreed that it is very important for a woman who is pregnant to see her doctor during her pregnancy (MOD, 1995).

Also, women who do not plan their pregnancies are often those at highest risk for poor pregnancy outcomes. A four-state survey of new mothers found that 66.2% of women with unintended pregnancies had an indication for counseling (smoking or drinking in the three months before conception, underweight before pregnancy, or delayed prenatal care after the first trimester) in contrast to 53.6% of mothers with planned pregnancies (Adams et al., 1993).

As a component of prenatal care

Family planning should also be advocated as a component of prenatal care (Klerman et al., 1995). Because the proportion of women who receive prenatal care is very high, a large percentage of women might be influenced if family planning advice were a routine component of this care (Ventura et al., 1997). Although contraception could not be initiated, women could be helped to make preliminary decisions about the timing or avoidance of future pregnancies and about ways to achieve such goals. The prenatal period is an appropriate time to consider whether to request tubal ligation during hospitalization for delivery. Depo-Provera can be safely injected immediately postpartum, Norplant can be inserted at that time as well, and there is no reason why birth control pills should not be prescribed or actually provided at hospital discharge for use later (Hatcher et al., 1994). All of these options require discussion during the prenatal period if a fully informed decision is to be made, because most women are too busy in the day or two in the hospital after delivery to give contraception much thought.

As a component of postpartum care

Most prenatal care providers plan to discuss family planning at a woman's office or clinic visit for a checkup after delivery. Unfortunately, some women do not return for this postpartum visit. In one study of a low income clinic population, 2.7% of women returned within 30 days after their delivery, 62.5% within 60 days, and 68.3% within 90 days (Mulvihill, pers. comm., 1998).

As a component of well-child supervision

Family planning, directed at the mother or both parents, should be a part of visits for well-child supervision (Klerman and Reynolds, 1994). Although it is clear that an unintended pregnancy or bearing another child after a short interval might have an adverse impact on the child already born, pediatricians and family physicians often do not feel comfortable discussing family planning with a mother. They believe that they should focus on the child and that the mother might think that they are asking inappropriate questions if they ask about the mother's family planning practices.

Barriers to family planning

Despite these multiple opportunities for family planning, unintended pregnancies and short interpregnancy intervals continue to be important problems. One reason is that women do not always seek or accept family planning counseling or use contraceptives effectively. A 1994–1995 survey revealed that Americans are skeptical about the effectiveness and safety of contraceptives. Only 64% of the men and women of reproductive age studied thought that oral contraceptives were very effective and only 17% thought they were very safe (Delbanco et al., 1997). Other reasons for unintended pregnancies and short interpregnancy intervals are health systems barriers, including provider reluctance to offer timely family planning counseling.

Before pregnancy

Although several studies have shown the effectiveness of counseling by health care providers in modifying behaviors in areas such as smoking (Dolan-Mullen et al., 1994), drinking (Fleming et al., 1997), and dietary change (Beresford et al., 1997), many clinicians are reluctant to being proactive in areas of health behavior, including family planning. For example, a Commonwealth Fund study found that the majority of women at their last checkups did not receive information or counseling about health-related behaviors. Fifty-four percent were not asked about smoking; 60% received no counseling about diet; 61% were not asked about exercise; 65% were not queried about alcohol use; and 80% were not asked about drug use. Nevertheless, three in five women reported engaging in one or more high-risk behaviors (Brown et al., 1995).

With regard to family planning specifically, a Massachusetts survey of specialists in general practice, family practice, and internal medicine revealed that only 54% considered family planning as "definitely" part of their role (Wechsler at al., 1996). In a study of internal medicine and family practice residents in a large inner-city hospital, 40% failed to indicate that they would provide a healthy woman with information on family planning and rubella immunization or counseling on sexually transmitted diseases (STDs) and safer sex, and 74% would not have discussed congenital anomalies with a diabetic woman seeking pregnancy (Conway et al., 1995). In addition, some states claim to be unable to locate enough funds to meet the need for family planning (Alabama Center for Health Statistics, 1995).

During pregnancy

Despite the logic of providing family planning counseling during prenatal visits, the recommendations of most authoritative bodies are vague and there is scant evidence that it is actually provided. The Public Health Service Expert Panel cited "postpartum activity, including family planning" in its recommended health promotion activities starting in the seventh pregnancy visit (38th week) for nulliparous women and sixth pregnancy visit (39th week) for parous women and continuing in all visits until delivery (PHS, 1989, pp. 66–70). In contrast, the report of the U.S. Preventive Services Task Force does not list family planning among the counseling interventions for pregnant women except under STD prevention, where it suggests "use condoms," but this was not intended to be a family planning recommendation (USPSTF, 1996).

Family planning is mentioned in the context of prenatal care in some manuals prepared for obstetricians. *Guidelines for Perinatal Care* does not mention family planning in its prenatal care section, but includes in Appendix A on the Antepartum Record a check-off box for counseling about "Postpartum Birth Control." (AAP/ACOG, 1997). The Educational Objectives of the Council on Resident Education in Obstetrics and Gynecology mentions postpartum sterilization and postpartum birth control in its section on prenatal care (Council on Resident Education in Obstetrics and Gynecology, 1996). *Guidelines for Outpatient Perinatal Care* recommends at the 28th through 36th week prenatal visits that the clinician review plans for contraception and, if sterilization is requested, obtain written informed consent. The 37th through 40th week visits include instructions to bring the sterilization papers when the woman goes to the hospital for delivery (Chez at al., 1995).

State and local health department manuals are more prescriptive. For example, the manuals for nurses who provide services for pregnant women in one county health department are very clear in this regard (Jefferson County Department of Health, 1994, 1995). Nurses must include family planning covering birth control methods in their third trimester education activities. The accompanying guide notes that the woman should decide during pregnancy whether or not she will want to use birth control after delivery and, if so, which method. The clinician is to stress that she can become pregnant again, even before she has a menstrual cycle, and that a pregnancy so soon would be very difficult on her both physically and emotionally and on the baby. The Comprehensive Health Record Instruction Manual of the Alabama Department of Public Health states that women are to be counseled about tubal sterilization in the first trimester and about postpartum family planning and tubal sterilization in the third trimester (Alabama Department of Health, 1997). Family planning as a possible component of prenatal care also has been mentioned in articles about prenatal care for special populations, such as teenagers (Stevens-Simon and Beach, 1992), and in a special issue of a nursing journal that dealt with pregnancy classes, women with physical disabilities, women in homeless shelters, and women in the workplace (O'Connell, 1993; Podgurski, 1993; Rogers, 1993; Shapiro, 1993).

Little is known about whether family planning is actually discussed during prenatal care. Few studies of the content of prenatal care examine whether family planning is included, probably reflecting the limited recommendations that it should be. For example, the analyses of mothers' reports on the content of prenatal care in the 1988 National Maternal and Infant Health Survey could not include family planning among the seven types of advice or counseling studied, because it was not a recommended service and thus not on the survey instrument (Kogan et al., 1994). A small questionnaire-based survey of pregnant women seen in a public clinic and in private practice found that only 37% of private patients reported receiving information from their prenatal care provider about contraception and family planning as compared to 74% of those in public clinics. In contrast, 89% of private patients and 98% of public patients received information about vitamins (Freda et al., 1993).

In the intrapartum period

The restriction on the number of days in the hospital following delivery makes long counseling sessions on birth control procedures unlikely in that setting. Also, women who deliver in Catholic hospitals face special problems with regard to making plans for birth control during their hospitalization. Moreover, even women who have signed sterilization papers may not have the procedure done while they are still in the hospital because of reimbursement policies. Some policies will not allow a physician and/or a hospital to be paid for two procedures during the same hospitalization, that is, both the delivery and the ligation. Also, obstetricians report that residents are reluctant to do tubal ligations after their first few cases because it is an easily learned and unchallenging procedure. This would cause particular problems for economically disadvantaged women who might experience difficulty making arrangements for outpatient surgery at a later date.

Conclusion

There seems to be little disagreement that family planning is essential to the health of women and their infants. There also is increasing consensus about the need for pre- and interconceptional care. However, these two types of care will need much more encouragement in terms of provider and consumer education, and financial reimbursement before they become accepted standards of care. The public health and obstetric establishments try very hard to educate women about the importance of prenatal care, usually neglecting to state that prenatal care begins with preconceptional care. Moreover, the potential for family planning during the well-child supervision visit has barely been considered.

The high rate of unintended and short-interval pregnancies indicates that women are not effectively using family planning. The United States should continue to devote considerable resources to making family planning services more accessible financially, geographically, culturally, and in other ways. Public health and other agencies should not only increase their outreach efforts to bring women into family planning facilities, they should also consider incorporating family planning into health-related visits that are made for other purposes. Integrating family planning into prenatal care might be another way to reach women, particularly those unlikely to make an extra trip to the doctor specifically to discuss family planning, even if that means risking an unintended pregnancy or one with a short interpregnancy interval.

Acknowledgments

Margaret Snively's assistance with the preparation of this paper is gratefully acknowledged. The work on which this paper is based was supported in part by the Agency for Health Care Policy and Research (Contract #290–92–0055), the Maternal and Child Health Bureau (MCJ 9040), and by the General Endowment Fund, Health Services Foundation, University of Alabama at Birmingham.

REFERENCES

Abma J, Chandra A, Mosher W, Peterson L, Piccinino L. Fertility, family planning, and women's health: new data from the 1995 National Survey of Family Growth. Hyattsville (MD): National Center for Health Statistics; Vital and Health Statistics; 1997 May. Series 23, Number 19. DHHS Publication No. (PHS) 97–1995.

Adams MM, Bruce FC, Shulman HB, Kendrick JC, Brogan DJ, and the PRAMS Working Group. Pregnancy planning and pre-conception counseling. Obstetrics and Gynecology 1993; **82**: 955–9.

Alabama Center for Health Statistics. Unplanned pregnancies in Alabama. Health Statistics Surveillance 1995; **4**: 1–4.

Alabama Department of Public Health. Comprehensive health record instruction manual (update No. 2). Montgomery (AL): Alabama Department of Public Health; September 22, 1997.

Alan Guttmacher Institute. Preconception and prenatal care can improve birth outcomes. New York: Alan Guttmacher Institute. Issues in Brief, March 1993.

American Academy of Pediatrics and the American College of Obstetricians and Gynecologists (AAP/ACOG). Guidelines for Perinatal Care, 4th edition. Elk Grove Village (IL) and Washington (DC): American Academy of Pediatrics and the American College of Obstetricians and Gynecologists, 1997.

American College of Obstetricians and Gynecologists (ACOG). Planning for pregnancy, birth and beyond, 2nd edition. Washington (DC): American College of Obstetricians and Gynecologists, 1993.

American College of Obstetricians and Gynecologists (ACOG). Preconception care. Washington (DC): American College of Obstetricians and Gynecologists. Technical Bulletin No. 205, 1995.

American College of Obstetricians and Gynecologists (ACOG). Guidelines for women's health care. Washington (DC): American College of Obstetricians and Gynecologists, 1996.

Beresford SAA, Curry SJ, Kristal AR, Lazovich D, Feng Z, Wagner EH. A dietary intervention in primary care practice: the eating patterns study. American Journal of Public Health 1997; **87**: 610–16.

Brown ER, Wyn R, Cumberland WG, et al. Women's health-related behaviors and use of clinical preventive services. Los Angeles: UCLA Center for Health Policy Research, 1995. (A Special Report for the Commission on Women's Health of The Commonwealth Fund.)

Brown SS, Eisenberg L, eds. The best intentions. Unintended pregnancy and the well-being of children and families. Washington (DC): National Academy Press, 1995.

Chez RA, Cox SM, Egerman R, et al. Guidelines for outpatient perinatal care. Wayne (NJ): Berlex Laboratories, Inc., 1995.

Conway T, Hu T-C, Mason E, Mueller C. Are primary care residents adequately prepared to care for women of reproductive age? Family Planning Perspectives 1995; **27**: 66–70.

Council on Resident Education in Obstetrics and Gynecology. Educational objectives. Core curriculum in obstetrics and gynecology, 5th edition. Washington (DC): Council on Resident Education in Obstetrics and Gynecology, 1996.

Delbanco S, Lundy J, Hoff T, Parker M, Smith MD. Public knowledge and perceptions about unplanned pregnancy and contraception in three countries. Family Planning Perspectives 1997; **29**: 70–5.

Dolan-Mullen P, Ramirez G, Groff JY. A meta-analysis of randomized trials of prenatal smoking cessation interventions. American Journal of Obstetrics and Gynecology 1994; **171**: 1328–34.

Fleming MF, Barry KL, Manwell LB, Johnson K, London R. Brief physician advice for problem alcohol drinkers. A randomized controlled trial in community-based primary care practices. Journal of the American Medical Association 1997; **277**: 1039–45.

Freda MC, Andersen HF, Damus K, Merkatz IR. Are there differences in information given to private and public prenatal patients? American Journal of Obstetrics and Gynecology 1993; **169**: 155–60.

Hatcher RA, Trussell J, Stewart F, Stewart GK, Kowal D, Guest F, Cates W, Policar MS. Contraceptive technology, 16th revised edition. New York: Irvington Publishers, Inc., 1994.

Jefferson County Department of Health. Policy and procedure manual. Birmingham (AL): Jefferson County Department of Health, 1994 and 1995.

Klerman LV. A public health perspective on *Caring for Our Future*. In: Merkatz IR, Thompson JE, Mullen PD, Goldenberg RL, eds. New perspectives on prenatal care. New York: Elsevier Science Publishing Co., Inc., 1990: 633–42.

Klerman LV, Cliver SP, Goldenberg RL. The impact of short interpregnancy intervals on pregnancy outcomes in a low-income population. American Journal of Public Health 1998; **88**: 1182–5.

Klerman LV, Phelan ST, Poole VL, Goldenberg RL. Family planning: an essential component of prenatal care. Journal of the American Medical Women's Association 1995; **50**: 147–51.

Klerman LV, Reynolds DW. Interconception care: a new role for the pediatrician. Pediatrics 1994; **93**: 327–9.

Kogan MD, Alexander GR, Kotelchuck M, Nagey DA, Jack BW. Comparing mothers' reports on the content of prenatal care received with recommended national guidelines for care. Public Health Reports 1994; **109**: 637–46.

March of Dimes Birth Defects Foundation (MOD). Towards improving the outcome of pregnancy: the 90s and beyond. White Plains (NY): March of Dimes Birth Defects Foundation, 1993.

March of Dimes Birth Defects Foundation (MOD). Preparing for pregnancy. White Plains (NY): March of Dimes Birth Defects Foundation, June 1995.

Miller JE. Birth intervals and perinatal health. An investigation of three hypotheses. Family Planning Perspectives 1991; **23**: 62–70.

National Center for Health Statistics (NCHS). Advance report of final natality statistics, 1991. Monthly Vital Statistics Report, 1993 September. Volume 42, Number 3 (supplement).

O'Connell ML. Childbirth education classes in homeless shelters. AWHONN's Clinical Issues in Perinatal and Women's Health Nursing 1993; **4**: 102–12.

Podgurski MJ. School-based adolescent pregnancy classes. AWHONN's Clinical Issues in Perinatal and Women's Health Nursing 1993; **4**: 80–94.

Public Health Service (PHS) Expert Panel on the Content of Prenatal Care. Caring for our future: the content of prenatal care. Washington (DC): U.S. Department of Health and Human Services, Public Health Service, 1989.

Rogers JG. Perinatal education for women with physical disabilities AWHONN's Clinical Issues in Perinatal and Women's Health Nursing 1993; **4**: 141–6.

Shapiro HR. Prenatal education in the work place. AWHONN's Clinical Issues in Perinatal and Women's Health Nursing 1993; **4**: 113–21.

Spratley E, Taffel S. Interval between births: United States, 1970–77. Vital and Health Statistics, 1981 August. Series 21, Number 39. DHHS Publication No. (PHS) 81–1917.

Stevens-Simon C, Beach RK. School-based prenatal and postpartum care: strategies for meeting the medical and educational needs of pregnant and parenting students. Journal of School Health 1992; **62**: 304–9.

U.S. Department of Health and Human Services (USDHHS). Healthy people 2000: national health promotion and disease prevention objectives. Washington (DC): U.S. Government Printing Office, DHHS Publication No. (PHS) 91–50212, 1991.

U.S. Preventive Services Task Force (USPSTF). Guide to clinical preventive services. 2nd edition. Baltimore (MD): Williams & Wilkins, 1996.

Ventura SJ, Martin JA, Mathews TJ, Clarke SC. Report of final natality statistics, 1995. Monthly Vital Statistics Report. Hyattsville (MD): National Center for Health Statistics, 1997 June. Volume 45, Number 11 (supplement).

Wechsler H, Levine S, Idelson RK, Schor EL, Coakley E. The physician's role in health promotion revisited – a survey of primary care practitioners. New England Journal of Medicine 1996; **334**: 996–8.

Winikoff B. The effects of birth spacing on child and maternal health. Studies in Family Planning 1983; **14**: 231–45.

Winkvist A, Rasmussen KM, Habicht J-P. A new definition of maternal depletion syndrome. American Journal of Public Health 1992; **82**: 691–4.

14

Maternal–fetal conflict is not a useful construct

Wendy Chavkin and Peter Bernstein

Introduction

The notion that maternal and fetal health can conflict derives from a framework that separates the two and, at times, positions them as adversaries. This construction has its roots in the debate over the legalization of abortion and is the approach taken by ethicists and legal scholars when tackling issues such as the management of a woman who refuses a cesarean. Maternal–fetal conflict has been defined as the situation in which "the intent or actions of the pregnant woman do not coincide with the needs, interests, or rights of her fetus as perceived by her obstetric caregivers" (Cohen, 1995). (The term "caregivers" could be broadened to include the state or any other outside authority with an interest in the outcome of the woman's pregnancy.) While the caregivers believe themselves to be objective advocates for the interests of the fetus, the true interests of the fetus are unknowable. Therefore, the caregivers are conferring their values on the fetus, which is necessarily passive and dependent because it cannot express its interests. Following this logic, the conflict really can be redefined as one between the pregnant woman and her caregivers.

This legalistic approach attempts to quantify the risks and benefits to a woman and a fetus of a particular course of action, and thus separates them, rather than seeing them as an inseparable whole whose well-being needs to be fostered before, during, and after the pregnancy. By necessity, this approach examines only a snapshot in time. Little attention is given to the woman's past, her social context, or the prospects of either mother or future child. For example, an uninsured pregnant woman may be viewed as indifferent to fetal welfare if she does not comply with a prescribed medical regime, even though she may lack the financial resources to purchase necessary medications.

This approach, if applied broadly, could construe almost all decisions regarding the management of pregnancy as though the mother and her fetus are in conflict. We will divide such decisions into maternal conditions/therapies that place the fetus at risk and fetal ones that put the mother at risk. Through examination of these apparent conflicts, we hope to arrive at a different paradigm.

Maternal conditions/therapies that place the fetus at risk

Pre-eclampsia

It is generally accepted that the only cure for pre-eclampsia is delivery of the fetus. The "conflict" arises when a woman with severe pre-eclampsia is carrying a fetus so preterm that delivery would probably result in severe compromise or death of the newborn. However, if the mother's condition is deteriorating with worsening hypertension, oliguria, or liver, neurologic, or hematologic dysfunction, she needs to be delivered. This state of maternal decompensation represents poor maternal perfusion secondary to vasospasm and is likely to result in impaired uteroplacental blood flow. Thus, in fact, delivery is indicated for both maternal and fetal well-being. (See Chapter 1 for an additional discussion of this condition.)

Epilepsy

It is widely believed that maternal seizures during pregnancy are detrimental to fetal well-being. Seizures have been associated with increased risk of miscarriage, fetal malformations, preterm labor, and stillbirth, all of which have been attributed to anoxia (Orringer et al., 1977; Yerby et al., 1985). These conclusions are based on observational studies of women with epilepsy. On the other hand, numerous reports have documented the teratogenicity of currently used anticonvulsants. In a prospective case-control study, Waters and colleagues (1994) found that the use of phenobarbital, phenytoin, or carbamazepine during pregnancy increased the risk of fetal death or the occurrence of anomalies. Steegers-Theunissen and colleagues (1994) also performed a prospective case-control study and found that anticonvulsant use in pregnancy doubled the risk of abnormal fetal outcomes or minor malformations and that this risk increased with greater duration of maternal epilepsy and maternal use of anticonvulsants. Holmes and colleagues (1994) reported data from a retrospective case-controlled study that showed the prevalence of fetal malformations to be greater among epileptic women using anticonvulsants than among women with epilepsy not taking anti-seizure medications, or among healthy controls. None of the anti-epilepsy drugs has been shown to be significantly more teratogenic than others, with the possible exception of valproic acid, which is more strongly associated with spina bifida (Yerby, 1993).

What is in the best interest of the fetus? Controlling maternal seizures benefits both the pregnant woman and her fetus. Thus, in reality, no conflict exists between the two. The real problem is that we do not have satisfactory treatments to control seizures, nor do we know enough about the currently available medications. Animal studies suggest that some of the newer drugs, such as felbamate, gabapentin, and others, may be less teratogenic. However, these have not undergone clinical trials in pregnant women (Morrell, 1996).

Psychiatric disorders

Psychiatric disorders in pregnant women do not present immediate medical dangers to the fetus in the same way that the previous examples do. Yet, failure to treat schizophrenia, bipolar disorder, or depression adequately may result in maternal suffering and also in suicide attempts or behavior that places the woman and her fetus at risk. More subtle consequences can include familial dysfunction and loss of familial support for the pregnant woman, which might also have consequences for the infant, such as foster care placement. Depression is one of the more commonly treated psychiatric disorders during pregnancy. It is most typically treated with serotonin uptake inhibitors or tricyclic antidepressants. The tricyclic drugs were once thought to increase the rate of limb reduction defects, although this was not confirmed in a Finnish registry study of 2500 cases of birth defects (Idanpaan-Keikkila and Saxen, 1973). Additionally, a more recent company registry-based study examined 796 cases of first trimester exposure to fluoxetane and found no association with fetal malformations (Goldstein et al., 1997).

Until recently, lithium, which is used for treating bipolar disease, had been considered one of the more teratogenic drugs in the psychiatric armamentarium, as it had been associated with cardiovascular anomalies, specifically Ebstein anomaly. The strength of the association has been called into question by one study of 148 women who used lithium during the first trimester of pregnancy and a review of four case control studies involving more than 200 children with Ebstein anomaly (Cohen et al., 1994; Jacobson et al., 1992). Both found little evidence to support the teratogenicity of the drug, although limitations of the study designs preclude certainty. Similarly inconclusive data exist for other psychiatric medications.

Hazardous jobs

In 1982, the Johnson Controls Company prohibited fertile women from holding jobs that might expose them to lead (International Union, 1991). Lead is a known toxin and harmful to children at lower levels than for adults. Safe levels for fetal exposure are unknown, nor have safe levels for pregnant women been established that acknowledge hemodilution, changed calcium absorption, and other metabolic alterations of pregnancy. Numerous studies have suggested that lead exposure during pregnancy can have detrimental effects on the fetus, including post-natal developmental and cognitive deficits (Wong et al., 1992).

The risk to a woman and fetus of lead exposure is difficult to compare with the risk of lost income and health insurance if she is forced to stop working. Moreover, efforts to restrict women from hazardous jobs have been erratic and inconsistent. They have been applied to women moving into higher-paying jobs traditionally held by men and not to women working at traditionally female jobs (which may well include hazardous exposures), such as nursing and teaching.

The conflict here could be redefined as employer–fetal conflict, as the employer is presumably unwilling to incur the costs of providing a work environment that is safe for pregnant women. The employer's motivation may be based more on other interests, such as avoiding potential legal liability (as asserted in the Johnson Controls case) than in doing what it perceives is best for the fetus. The Supreme Court decision in the Johnson Controls case put it succinctly:

> Concern for a woman's existing or potential offspring historically has been the excuse for denying women equal employment opportunities… It is no more appropriate for the courts than it is for individual employers to decide whether a woman's reproductive role is more important to herself and her family than her economic role. Congress has left this choice to the woman as hers to make (*International Union* v. *Johnson Controls*, 1991).

Substance abuse during pregnancy

As a number of chapters have noted, smoking and alcohol and other drug use have significant and negative effects on the health of pregnant women and their fetuses. Cigarette smoking is associated with a range of adverse pregnancy outcomes and appears, through a variety of mechanisms, also to have a negative impact on reproductive health. Several studies have demonstrated that the risk of ectopic pregnancy in smokers is 2.2 to 4 times greater than for non-smokers (Campbell and Gray, 1987). Placentia previa, abruptio placenta, and premature rupture of the membranes are the leading causes of perinatal loss associated with smoking (U.S. Surgeon General, 1990). More than 100 epidemiologic studies have shown that birth weights of smokers' infants are significantly reduced (by approximately 200 gm) and smokers have 3.5 to 4.0–fold increased risk of delivering small-for-gestational-age babies (Hellerstein and Sachs, 1993). A strong association has been recently documented between smoking and sudden infant death syndrome (SIDS), stronger than the association between SIDS and opiates, cocaine, or alcohol.

Heavy alcohol use is associated with fetal alcohol syndrome, which comprises a constellation of anomalies that includes intrauterine growth restriction (IUGR), central nervous system (CNS) dysfunction, and characteristic facial dysmorphology. Heroin use has been significantly associated with fetal growth restriction. Methadone use has been associated with higher birth weight, although this may be confounded by participation in treatment and associated reductions in the hazards of illicit drug use (Kandall et al., 1976). There is a well-described neonatal abstinence syndrome following in utero exposure to opioids, which includes central and autonomic nervous system signs and gastrointestinal and respiratory abnormalities. This syndrome can be successfully medically managed with non-specific supportive measures, such as substitute opiates (paregoric), or CNS depressants (phenobarbital) (Kandall and Garnter, 1974). There is no true abstinence syndrome among cocaine-exposed newborns. A self-limited mild neurologic dysfunction characterized by irritability, poor interactive behavior, and poor organizational response to stimuli has been described, although not rigorously documented (Doberczak et al., 1988). Preterm delivery, placental abruption, low birth weight, and increased pregnancy loss, all consistent with the known vasoconstrictive action of cocaine, are increased in crack-using mothers and their infants.

Some view drug use as a selfish choice that is not in the interest of the fetus, and have advocated punishing women who use illegal drugs during pregnancy. However, the medical definition of addiction is that it is a compulsive disorder, with destructive consequences for the addict and often for those around her. Once again, it is not that the interests of the mother and fetus are colliding. In fact, they coincide: treating the pregnant woman's addiction may improve both of their conditions.

Unfortunately, we do not offer much assistance to women who want to escape their addictions. Little money has been allocated for substance abuse treatment. Few advances have been made in the treatment of such common conditions as tobacco addiction. It has been estimated that cigarette smoking during pregnancy may contribute up to 10% of perinatal mortality (Kleinman et al., 1988). Very few studies have addressed the risks and benefits of using transdermal nicotine replacement or nicotine gum in helping pregnant women to quit smoking; those that have been performed are only preliminary, such as the study conducted by Wright and colleagues (1997) on six pregnant women to determine the pharmokinetics of transdermal nicotine replacement. This is despite the fact that during pregnancy, women may be more receptive to interventions that aid them in breaking their addiction. The Food and Drug Administration (FDA) has assigned transdermal nicotine delivery systems to Pregnancy Category D ("positive evidence of risk"). Nevertheless, these risks to the fetus may not outweigh the benefits to the pregnant woman and her fetus of helping a woman who has had difficulty in quitting smoking.

Management of pain in labor

Narcotics given either intravenously or intramuscularly during labor cross the placenta and rapidly enter the fetal circulation. They can cause significant neonatal respiratory depression at birth, which must subsequently be managed with supportive care and medications, such as naloxone (Barreir and Sureau, 1982). Epidurals may also present risks for the fetus. Several studies report higher rates of cesarean section among women who receive epidurals for inadequate progress in labor (Lieberman et al., 1996; Thorp et al., 1993). Thorp and colleagues (1993) performed a randomized, controlled trial of epidural versus narcotic analgesia in nulliparous women in labor at term and found that epidurals were associated with a greater rate of cesarean sections due to difficult or abnormal labor (dystocia). Cesarean deliveries, in turn, are associated with neonatal respiratory problems and other morbidities (Bryan et al., 1990). Transient tachypnea of the newborn has been observed more frequently among neonates born by cesarean section (Brice and Walker, 1977). These studies are, of course, observational studies, and it is difficult to draw solid conclusions from them because it is impossible to control completely for complications that occurred during the pregnancy, the labor, or the delivery that may have contributed to the decision to perform a cesarean section.

Even in the absence of cesarean section, epidurals may be associated with risks to the fetus. Lieberman and colleagues (1997) reported on an observational study of 1657 nulliparas at full term in labor; they found that there was a significantly higher rate of intrapartum fever among women receiving epidurals (14.5% vs. 1.0%) even after controlling for length of labor. This translated into greater rates of neonatal evaluations for possible sepsis and neonatal treatment with antibiotics.

The preceding two examples of substance use during pregnancy and pain management in labor illustrate the inconsistency and bias entangled with medical management decisions. Illicit drug use during pregnancy is perceived as maternal–fetal conflict; social response is more mixed and confused when the drugs are legal, such as with tobacco and alcohol. Finally, although many women are concerned about risks to the fetus associated with use of pain medication or anesthesia during labor, few would construe use of these drugs as instances of maternal–fetal conflict.

Clinical trials in pregnant women

Two drugs widely used on pregnant women several decades ago, thalidomide and diethylstilbestrol (DES) were shown to be teratogens. DES was also shown to be a transplacental carcinogen (Christie, 1962; Herbst et al., 1981). The public response was to protect pregnant women from participating in research (although neither case involved research, but rather clinical practice). In 1975, Department of Health and Human Services regulations identified limited conditions under which an institutional review board could approve research on pregnant women and fetuses, and classified pregnant women as a "vulnerable population." In 1977, the FDA recommended that women of "childbearing potential" be excluded from early phases of drug trials except in the case of life-threatening disease (FDA, 1977).

However, in 1985, the U.S. Public Health Service Task Force on Women's Health Issues reported that a lack of research specifically addressing women had compromised both the state of knowledge and the quality of health care (USPHS, 1985). In 1993, the FDA revised its 1977 restriction on the inclusion of fertile women in early phases of clinical trials (FDA, 1993). Pregnant women have been excluded from clinical trials because of fear of exposing a fetus to an agent of unknown teratogenic potential. While this is certainly a grave concern shared by all, it too often leaves clinicians adrift when treating pregnant patients. They end up using medications to treat clinical disease in pregnant women without knowing clearly whether the drug has consequences for fetal development, or even whether different dosages are necessary because of pregnancy-altered pharmacokinetics.

One result is that drugs are commonly used to treat conditions in pregnancy even though they have largely been abandoned in the treatment of non-pregnant patients. The use of methyldopa in treating chronic hypertension during pregnancy is a prime example. Another result is the use of drugs known to be potentially harmful to the fetus because new ones that are possibly safer have not been tested for use during pregnancy. The use of anticonvulsant medications for the treatment of epilepsy in pregnancy is a good example. The list of drugs that have not been adequately studied during pregnancy is long and includes antibiotics, psychotropic drugs, and anti-HIV medications.

Fetal conditions/therapies that place the pregnant woman at risk

Cesarean section for fetal indications

Labor carries with it an implicit risk of cesarean section for fetal indications, such as fetal distress or malpresentation. This in turn presents an increased risk of maternal morbidity and mortality. One study, reporting on approximately 1 000 000 births in 1978, found the rate of maternal deaths to be 9.8 per 100 000 live births for vaginal deliveries and 40.0 for all cesarean deliveries (Rosen, 1982). More recently, Lilford and colleagues (1990) found a five-fold increase in the maternal death rate associated with cesarean section compared to vaginal delivery, even after controlling for pre-existing maternal medical complications. This 1990 study was based on more than 263 000 deliveries in Cape Town, South Africa.

Cesarean section is also associated with greater morbidity for the woman than is vaginal delivery. There tends to be significantly greater blood loss than during a vaginal delivery. In addition, 20–30% of women undergoing cesarean section have been reported to have febrile complications resulting from endomyometritis, pneumonia, atelectasis, urinary tract infections, wound infections, ileus, superficial thrombophlebitis, and thromboembolic disease (Bowes, 1994).

Given the poor predictive value of diagnoses such as fetal distress (a term that has never been rigorously defined), it is noteworthy how often we expect women to undergo a procedure as risky as cesarean section. Fetal distress is typically determined using fetal heart rate monitoring during labor, and yet interpretation of fetal heart rate tracings is subject to a great deal of interobserver variation (van Geijn et al., 1991). Trials of fetal heart rate monitoring have not been able to show improved outcomes among fetuses, especially among those considered to be "low risk" who are continuously monitored during labor, but they have observed significantly higher cesarean section rates in the monitored groups (Cibils, 1996; Prentice and Lind, 1987). One of the largest of the studies to look at intrapartum fetal heart rate monitoring was the Dublin randomized controlled trial of intrapartum fetal heart rate monitoring. It involved 12 964 women and demonstrated a higher rate of operative deliveries in the group receiving continuous electronic fetal monitoring compared to those receiving intermittent auscultation, but no differences were noted in long-term neonatal outcomes (Grant et al., 1989; MacDonald et al., 1985).

Women usually are willing to take on the risk of cesarean section in order to err on the side of protecting their fetus, even though we cannot quantify the risk to the fetus. It has become an unchallenged expectation that pregnant women should accept this risk.

About 24% of births in the United States are by cesarean section (ACOG, 1996); this represents one of the highest rates in the world (CDC, 1993). Much of the rise in cesarean section rates in the United States during the 1970s and early 1980s was due to repeat cesarean deliveries, cesareans for dystocia, and cesareans for fetal distress (Taffel et al., 1987). In recent years there has been an effort to reduce the rate of cesarean deliveries. Part of the motivation stems from a concern that many of these operations are not believed to improve neonatal outcome and subject women to unnecessary risks; part has been to control health care costs because cesareans are much more expensive than vaginal deliveries.

Intrauterine fetal surgery

Some women have been willing to undergo intrauterine correction of fetal anomalies, such as diaphragmatic hernia and posterior urethral valves. These therapies can require hysterotomies, tocolytic therapy, and cesarean delivery for the current pregnancy and any future ones. However, these conditions have poor prognoses despite the surgery (Ford, 1994; Manning et al., 1986). In such cases, pregnant women have exposed themselves to risk on behalf of fetal welfare, despite the limited prospects for success.

Trials are being conducted to develop more effective treatments for fetuses with anomalies such as diaphragmatic hernia. In the recent past, attempts had been made to treat this condition with primary repair of the diaphragm during fetal life since large herniations of bowel and liver into the fetal chest often resulted in failure of the lungs to develop. This, therefore, doomed the fetus to death soon after it was born despite technologies such as extracorporeal membrane oxygenation. Prenatal repair has been attempted and requires maternal laparotomy, hysterotomy, partial exteriorization of the fetus, and then repair of the diaphragmatic defect. This operation sometimes must be performed in two steps, subjecting mother and fetus to risks twice. Complications include the need for tocolytic therapy, preterm delivery, and all other complications of major surgery. Despite these efforts, the fetal/neonatal outcomes have not been good (Harrison et al., 1993).

More recently, some surgeons have attempted to reduce the failure and complication rates by performing in utero occlusion of the fetal trachea. This allows the fluid naturally produced by the fetal lungs to accumulate, forcing the lungs to inflate and thus push the herniated organs out of the chest. After delivery, but before the umbilical cord is cut, the tracheal occlusion is cleared. The neonate subsequently undergoes surgery to repair the diaphragmatic defect. Harrison and colleagues (1996) reported their results from a trial in which they performed this procedure on eight fetuses, only one of whom survived.

Acquired immunodeficiency syndrome

Acquired Immunodeficiency Syndrome (AIDS) Clinical Trials Group 076 established that it was possible to decrease the rate of vertical transmission of human immunodeficiency virus (HIV), that is, transmission from mother to fetus during pregnancy. This study found that the use of zidovudine (AZT) in pregnant women with early stage HIV disease significantly reduced the rate of maternal transmission of the virus to the fetus (Connor et al., 1994).

The use of zidovudine to decrease vertical transmission has become standard and widespread, despite concerns raised by some that its use during pregnancy for this purpose may cause the development of virus that is resistant to the drug and decrease its therapeutic benefit when it is needed later in the course of the woman's illness. Once the virus has become resistant to zidovudine, other drug regimens are often less efficacious. Thus far, resistance has not been a major concern since it has been shown in non-pregnant individuals that zidovudine-resistant viral strains have not emerged in patients with early-stage HIV disease who have received less than 18–24 months of continuous therapy (Richman et al., 1990).

Unfortunately, at the present time, it is not known whether the benefits of zidovudine in preventing vertical transmission remain in pregnant women with later-stage disease, although studies are underway. These women may be at greater risk of developing resistant viral strains.

This appears to be the first real example of maternal–fetal conflict, but in fact, zidovudine may pose fetal risks as well, such as teratogenicity, oncogenicity, or development of viral resistance in the neonate who is infected despite the in utero prophylactic use of the drug. Zidovudine has been shown to be teratogenic when administered in extremely high doses in pregnant rats (Burroughs Wellcome, 1993), and it has been shown to be carcinogenic in mice and rats when they are exposed to high doses for long periods of time (Ayers, 1988). As a result, it has been classified by the FDA as a Pregnancy Category C drug ("either studies in animals have revealed adverse effects on the fetus and there are no controlled studies in women, or studies in women and animals are not available").

Studies are now being undertaken to examine the potential benefits and complications to the fetus and the pregnant woman of other drugs used to treat HIV, such as protease inhibitors. Semba and colleagues (1994) have noted that the risk of HIV transmission from mother to fetus is greater among women with lower levels of serum vitamin A. Their study of HIV-positive women in Malawi has many confounding variables, most notably the poor nutritional status of many of the women involved. Nonetheless, the study has sparked interest that vitamin A supplementation may be able to decrease vertical transmission, and studies are being undertaken to examine this.

Inconsistency/uncertainty in the medical management of pregnant women

The preceding examples illustrate that the true risks and benefits to the pregnant woman and her fetus of any plan of management cannot be precisely quantified, but are instead characterized by uncertainty. As a result of this uncertainty, clinical practice may be affected by many factors besides objective data from medical research. These factors include the values and attitudes of the caregiver, race of the patient, socioeconomic status of the patient, the specific medical condition, and the prevailing local customs regarding care. Kolder and colleagues (1987) illustrated the problematic nature of these aspects of medical practice in their survey of court-ordered cesarean sections, in which they found that the majority of coerced procedures were performed on minority women.

As noted earlier, inconsistency can be seen in the differing attitudes concerning the use of "recreational drugs" during pregnancy as compared to the use of pain medications in labor, despite the fact that each poses risks for the fetus. This inconsistency is also apparent in the readiness of many to conduct research on in utero fetal therapies for conditions with extremely poor prognoses, thereby subjecting women to significant risks, while, on the other hand, being reluctant to study new therapies for maternal conditions out of fear of harming the fetus. This is not to suggest that new fetal therapies should not be investigated, but that we need to acknowledge the discrepancies in our attitudes toward women and their fetuses and recognize that new therapies that effectively treat maternal conditions are likely to benefit the fetus in the long run.

Uncertainty pervades the practice of medicine in general, and obstetrics in particular. The development of modern medicine has been characterized by the pursuit of certainty, and uncertainty has often paralyzed action. It is, for example, much easier to decide to deliver a baby prematurely, knowing the significant morbidities associated with prematurity, if we are certain that this is the only correct course of action. We do not have satisfactory answers for the medical dilemmas posed here and thus can not accurately quantify the risks and benefits for a particular patient.

Even if we could do so, the meaning accorded to those risks and benefits can only be interpreted by the women who experience them. We recognize this to some extent when counseling about prenatal diagnosis of Down's syndrome. Women are provided with an estimated risk of carrying a fetus with Down's syndrome, based on their age and the results of serum screening tests, and told the risk of miscarriage associated with subsequent diagnostic procedures, such as amniocentesis. They then must decide whether they consider it more important to know whether the fetus has the condition or to avoid an increased risk of miscarriage.

Chervenak and colleagues (1993) have discussed the hypothetical example of a woman who presents to the labor floor at 39 weeks of gestation with the clinical diagnosis of placental abruption. A prolonged bradycardia on the fetal heart monitor is considered evidence of fetal distress. The woman is offered a cesarean section for fetal indications, but refuses. The obstetric team decides to perform the surgery without the women's consent on the basis of what the authors term their "beneficence-based obligations" to the fetus.

This is an example of the arrogance that medical certainty can breed. The obstetricians here are willing to perform surgery, despite the likelihood that it may already be too late to save the fetus, who may die despite the intervention. Another likely possibility is that the fetus would be neurologically devastated. The caregivers are certain about the proper course of action, and yet the outcome is unclear. The physicians believe that the best option is to maximize the chance that this baby will survive. Alternatively, the woman may consider the best option to be one that minimizes the risk of a seriously impaired infant. From her perspective, it may be better to allow the fetus to die rather than be forced to care for a child who is neurologically devastated.

We must understand what patients value, especially because we cannot guarantee the outcome. We do not even clearly understand how best to manage some obstetric situations even when woman and doctor agree on the desired outcome.

Nurturing the whole

The pregnant woman and her fetus are not co-equals. The fetus is entirely dependent and silent. All fetal experience is mediated through the mother. Any compromise in maternal health may have consequences for the fetus. This holds true for chronic conditions that precede and those that follow the pregnancy. For example, women with diabetes whose serum glucose is poorly controlled before pregnancy have worse neonatal outcomes. Addicted women may expose the fetus to drugs and infectious diseases during pregnancy and to the risk of a chaotic household or foster care after the birth.

Similarly, the woman with a medical condition who chooses to continue a pregnancy is vulnerable. That medical condition may be complicated by her pregnancy, as is seen among women with hypertension who develop superimposed pre-eclampsia. Rather than considering woman and fetus to be adversaries, they should be seen as fundamentally interdependent. The approach of the caregivers should be to foster the health of both, given their basic interdependence and mutual needs. In fact, caregivers could look at pregnancy as an opportunity to identify maternal conditions and plan for the mother's subsequent health care, both for her sake and her child's, thus broadening their interest in the patient and her future child beyond the time period of the pregnancy.

New directions

By recognizing that when we speak of "maternal–fetal conflict," we are superimposing our own values regarding "fetal interests" and by recognizing our own uncertainty in how best to manage medical conditions during pregnancy, we arrive at the uncomfortable conclusion that the best way to care for a pregnant woman is to involve her completely in the management decisions. After all, she and her child will have to live with the consequences.

Thus, physicians must learn to share authority with their patients, something with which they are traditionally uncomfortable. The typical response of providers is that the patient cannot understand the complexity of the medical situation. The patient can just as easily respond that the doctor does not understand the complexity of her own needs and values. As Jay Katz (1984) writes:

... no single right decision exists for how the life of health and illness should be lived ... both parties [physicians and patients] need to relate to each other as equals and unequals. Their equalities and inequalities complement one another. Physicians know more about disease. Patients know more about their own needs. (p.102)

This holds true as much for the pregnant patient as the non-pregnant patient. The additional factor in the equation, the fetus, does not significantly complicate the issue. The pregnant woman or the physician cannot know the interests of the fetus with certainty. Each comes from a different perspective – the physician from the medical point of view, and the woman from the personal one that understands her and her family's circumstances and values.

By relying on this approach, we may be able to formulate more clinical trials that involve therapies for pregnant women. By involving patients in the discussion and design of the trials and by acknowledging our uncertainty and the conceivable risks involved, we may be able to resolve the inconsistency noted earlier between the well-publicized trials to treat lethal fetal anomalies, which place the pregnant woman at risk, and the dearth of trials for maternal conditions, which are avoided out of fear of harming the fetus. As we have learned, it is generally to the benefit of both when the health of the pregnant woman is maximized.

Using this new approach to the relationship between the pregnant woman and her caregiver, we are attempting to shed the characterization of the pregnant woman in opposition to her fetus and to see them as growing together. Their relationship does not end when the umbilical cord is cut; neither should our efforts to care for them both.

REFERENCES

American College of Obstetricians and Gynecologists (ACOG). Rate of vaginal births after cesarean delivery. Washington (DC): American College of Obstetricians and Gynecologists; ACOG Committee Opinion, November 1996, 179.

Ayers K. Preclinical toxicology of zidovudine: an overview. American Journal of Medicine 1988; **85**: 186–8.

Barrier G, Sureau C. Effects of anæsthetic and analgesic drugs on labour, fetus and neonate. Clinical Obstetrics and Gynæcology 1982; **9**: 351–67.

Bowes W. Normal and abnormal labor. In: Creasy R, Resnik R, eds. Maternal–fetal medicine: principles and practice. Philadelphia: WB Saunders Company, 1994: 527–57.

Brice JE, Walker CH. Changing pattern of respiratory distress in newborn. Lancet 1977; **2**: 752–4.

Bryan H, Hawrylyshyn P, Hogg-Johnson S, et al. Perinatal factors associated with the respiratory distress syndrome. American Journal of Obstetrics and Gynecology 1990; **162**: 476–81.

Burroughs Wellcome. Comprehensive information for investigators: retrovir. Research Triangle Park (NC): Burroughs Wellcome, 1993.

Campbell O, Gray R. Smoking and ectopic pregnancy: a multinational case-control study. In: Rosenberg MJ, ed. Smoking and reproductive health. Littleton (MA): PSG Publishing, 1987: 70–4.

Centers for Disease Control and Prevention (CDC). Rates of cesarean delivery – United States, 1991. MMWR. Morbidity and Mortality Weekly Report 1993; **42**: 285–9.

Chervenak F, McCullough L, Skupski D. An ethical justification for emergency, coerced cesarean delivery. Obstetrics and Gynecology 1993; **82**: 1029–35.

Christie GA. Thalidomide and congenital abnormalities. Lancet 1962; **2**: 249.

Cibils LA. On intrapartum fetal monitoring. American Journal of Obstetrics and Gynecology 1996; **174**: 1382–9.

Cohen L, Friedman J, Jefferson J, Johnson E, Weiner M. A reevaluation of risk of in utero exposure to lithium. Journal of the American Medical Association 1994; **271**: 146–50.

Cohen WR. Maternal–fetal conflict I. In: Goldworth A, Silverman W, Stevenson DK, Young EWD, eds. Ethics and Perinatology. New York: Oxford University Press, 1995: 10–28.

Connor E, Sperling R, Gelber R, et al. Pediatric AIDS Clinical Trials Group Protocol 076 Study Group. Reduction of maternal–infant transmission of human immunodeficiency virus type 1 with zidovudine treatment. New England Journal of Medicine 1994; **331**: 1173–80.

Doberczak TM, Shanzer S, Senie RT, Kandall S. Neonatal neurologic and electroencephalographic effects of intrauterine cocaine exposure. The Journal of Pediatrics 1988; **115**: 770–8.

Food and Drug Administration (FDA). General consideration for the clinical evaluation of drugs. Rockville (MD): Food and Drug Administration, Bureau of Drugs, 1977. Report No. FDA77–3040.

Food and Drug Administration (FDA). Guidelines for the study and evalution of gender differences in the clinical evaluation of drugs. Notice. Federal Register, July 22, 1993; **58**: 39406–16.

Ford WD. Fetal intervention for congenital diaphragmatic hernia. Fetal Diagnosis and Therapy 1994; **9**: 398–408.

Goldstein D, Corbin L, Sundell K. Effects of first-trimester fluoxetine exposure on the newborn. Obstetrics and Gynecology 1997; **89**: 713–18.

Grant A, O'Brien N, Joy M, Hennessy E, MacDonald D. Cerebral palsy among children born during the Dublin randomised trial of intrapartum monitoring. Lancet 1989; **2**: 1233–6.

Harrison MR, Adzick NS, Flake AW, et al. Correction of diaphragmatic hernia in utero VI: hard-earned lessons. Journal of Pediatric Surgery 1993; **28**: 1411–18.

Harrison MR, Adzick NS, Flake AW, et al. Correction of congenital diaphragmatic hernia in utero VIII: response of the hypoplastic lung to tracheal occlusion. Journal of Pediatric Surgery 1996; **31**: 1339–48.

Hellerstein S, Sachs BP. Smoking in pregnancy. ACOG Technical Bulletin 80. Washington (DC): American College of Obstetricians and Gynecologists, 1993.

Herbst AL, Hubby MM, Azizi F, Makii MM. Reproductive and gynecological surgical experience in diethylstilbestrol-exposed daughters. American Journal of Obstetrics and Gynecology 1981; **141**: 1019–28.

Holmes LB, Harvey EA, Brown KS, Hayes AM, Khoshbin S. Anticonvulsant teratogenesis: I. A study design for newborn infants. Teratology 1994; **49**: 202–7.

Idanpaan-Keikkila J, Saxen L. Possible teratogenicity of impramine/chloropyramine. Lancet 1973; **2**: 282–4.

International Union, UAW, v. Johnson Controls. Vol. 113: SC, 1991: 158.

Jacobson S, Jones K, Johnson K, et al. Prospective multicentre study of pregnancy outcome after lithium exposure during the first trimester. Lancet 1992; **339**: 530–3.

Kandall SR, Albin S, Lewison J, Bearle B, Eidelman A, Gartner L. Differential effects of maternal heroin and methadone use on birth weight. Pediatrics 1976; **58**: 681–5.

Kandall S, Garnter LM. Late presentation of drug withdrawal symptoms in newborns. American Journal of Diseases of Children 1974; **127**: 58–61.

Katz J. The silent world of doctor and patient. New York: The Free Press, 1984.

Kleinman J, Peirre M, Madans J, Land G, Schramm W. The effects of maternal smoking on fetal and infant mortality. American Journal of Epidemiology 1988; **127**: 274–83.

Kolder V, Gallagher J, Parsons M. Court-ordered obstetrical interventions. New England Journal of Medicine 1987; **316**: 1192–6.

Lieberman F, Lang JM, Cohen A, D'Agostino R, Jr, Datta S, Frigoletto FD, Jr. Association of epidural analgesia with cesarean delivery in nulliparas. Obstetrics and Gynecology 1996; **88**: 993–1000.

Lieberman E, Lang JM, Frigoletto F, Jr, Richardson DK, Ringer SA, Cohen A. Epidural analgesia, intrapartum fever, and neonatal sepsis evaluation. Pediatrics 1997; **99**: 415–19.

Lilford RJ, van Coeverden de Groot IIA, Moore PJ, Bingham P. The relative risks of cæsarean section (intrapartum and elective) and vaginal delivery: a detailed analysis to exclude the effects of medical disorders and other acute pre-existing physiological disturbances. British Journal of Obstetrics and Gynæcology 1990; **97**: 883–92.

MacDonald D, Grant A, Sheridan-Pereira M, Boylan P, Chalmers I. The Dublin randomized controlled trial of intrapartum fetal heart rate monitoring. American Journal of Obstetrics and Gynecology 1985; **152**: 524–39.

Manning F, Harrison M, Rodeck C. Catheter shunts for fetal hydronephrosis and hydro-cephalus. Report of the International Fetal Surgery Registry. New England Journal of Medicine 1986; **315**: 336–40.

Morrell MJ. The new antiepileptic drugs and women: efficacy, reproductive health, pregnancy, and fetal outcome. Epilepsia 1996; **37**: S34–S44.

Orringer C, Eustace J, Wunsch C, Gardner L. Natural history of lactic acidosis after grand mal seizures. New England Journal of Medicine 1977; **297**: 796–9.

Prentice A, Lind T. Fetal heart rate monitoring during labour – too frequent intervention, too little benefit? Lancet 1987; **2**: 1375–7.

Richman D, Grimes J, Lagakos S. Effect of stage of disease and drug dose on zidovudine susceptibilities of isolates of human immunodeficiency virus. Journal of Acquired Immune Deficiency Syndromes and Human Retrovirology 1990; **3**: 743–6.

Rosen M. Summary of consensus development conference – childbirth by cesarean delivery.

Journal of the Louisiana State Medical Society. 1982; **134**: 94, 98.

Semba RD, Miotti PG, Chiphangwi JD, et al. Maternal vitamin A deficiency and mother-to-child transmission of HIV-1. Lancet 1994; **343**: 1593–7.

Steegers-Theunissen RP, Renier WO, Borm GF, et al. Factors influencing the risk of abnormal pregnancy outcome in epileptic women: a multi-centre prospective study. Epilepsy Research 1994; **18**: 261–9.

Taffel S, Placek P, Liss T. Trends in the United States cesarean section rate and reasons for the 1980–85 rise. American Journal of Public Health 1987; **77**: 955–9.

Thorp J, Hu D, Albin R, et al. The effect of intrapartum epidural analgesia on nulliparous labor: a randomized, controlled, prospective trial. American Journal of Obstetrics and Gynecology 1993; **169**: 851–8.

U.S. Public Health Service (USPHS). Report of the Public Health Service Task Force on women's health issues. Public Health Reports 1985; **100**: 73–106.

U.S. Surgeon General. The health benefits of smoking cessation: a report of the Surgeon General. Publication No. (CDC) 90–8416. Washington, DC: U.S. Department of Health and Human Services, 1990.

van Geijn HP, Copray FJ, Donkers DK, Bos MH. Diagnosis and management of intrapartum fetal distress. European Journal of Obstetrics, Gynecology, and Reproductive Biology 1991; **42**: S63–S72.

Waters CH, Belai Y, Gott PS, Shen P, De Giorgio CM. Outcomes of pregnancy associated with antiepileptic drugs. Archives of Neurology 1994; **51**: 250–3.

Wong G, Ng T, Martin T, Farquharson D. Effects of low-level lead exposure in utero. Obstetrical and Gynecological Survey 1992; **47**: 285–9.

Wright L, Thorp JJ, Kuller J, Shrewsbury R, Ananth C, Hartmann K. Transdermal nicotine replacement in pregnancy: maternal pharmokinetics and fetal effects. American Journal of Obstetrics and Gynecology 1997; **176**: 1090–4.

Yerby M. Epilepsy and pregnancy. Neurologic Clinics 1993; **11**: 777–86.

Yerby M, Koepsell T, Daling J. Pregnancy complications and outcomes in a cohort of women with epilepsy. Epilepsia 1985; **26**: 631–5.

15

Linking prenatal care with women's health care

Paul H. Wise and Marisa Brett

Introduction

In different ways and to differing extents, all the chapters in this book suggest that the effectiveness of prenatal care is dynamic. The changing demography of childbearing in the United States and the remarkable innovation that has occurred in the clinical management of pregnancy and the perinatal period are constantly reshaping the match (and relative mismatch) between needs and capability. Recognition of this dynamic character is important because it inherently condemns static programs and policies. Rather, it invites constant reconsideration of prenatal care's structure and content.

Among the more prominent and recurring insights to emerge recently is the relative isolation of prenatal care from other components of women's health care in the United States. The discussions in a number of chapters in this book provide ample evidence for this insight. In both the clinical and programmatic arenas, current systems of prenatal care could be enhanced if greater coordination across clinical disciplines and preventive programs could be developed. Important recommendations have been made in this regard, including both technical and administrative improvements.

The obstacles to making prenatal care a more integrated part of women's health are not due to technical and administrative considerations alone, however. They are also deeply rooted in questions of justice. Prenatal programs and policies are not derived exclusively from technical knowledge or clinical capability. They are also the product of our deep anxieties over the plight of children in the United States, coupled with a continued ambivalence over the social roles of women in American society. In this context, the effort to link prenatal care to broader systems of women's health care is not only one of technical revision, but also of political commitment. Indeed, greater respect for emerging technical insights as well as a greater willingness to question longstanding political postures will be required to effectively link prenatal care to women's health, and thereby enhance our systemic capability to ensure the health and well-being of newborns and women for years to come.

Maternal deviance and the epidemiology of prenatal risk

One troubling threat to a more comprehensive vision of prenatal care is the tendency to explain poor birth outcomes as being primarily the result of deviant maternal behaviors. All too often, teen pregnancy, a lack of prenatal care, illicit drug use, and marital status are portrayed as the major determinants of our infant mortality problem, or at least of racial and social disparities in infant mortality in the U.S. While the intent of such assertions is often directed at generating ameliorative concern, their impact tends to diminish women's interests and undermine comprehensive approaches to women's health.

To understand these effects, it is useful to recognize that the prominence given to adverse maternal behaviors, while clearly propelled into public discourse by a variety of political agendas, actually has its roots in the scientific community. This is because the source for much of the emphasis on maternal actions has been the enormous proliferation in epidemiologic studies concerned with intrauterine risk. Although this body of work has provided many important insights, much of it is characterized by the identification of individual risk associations, or risk factors, for adverse birth outcomes.

Significantly, the higher the relative risk associated with a specific risk factor, the higher it tends to be elevated in public discourse. The problem with this tight focus on individual risks associated with fetal and newborn outcomes is that it may offer little actual insight into the primary determinants of poor birth outcomes in large populations and can actually distract our attention from the true pathways of causation.

Teen pregnancy is an illustrative case and a helpful example because there are abundant data on this issue and because it is so often invoked as a major cause of the infant mortality problem in the United States. Indeed, there have been a large number of studies that have reported a high relative risk of low birth weight or infant death associated with births to teenage women (Fraser et al., 1995; Jones et al., 1985). There can be little doubt that childbirth to teenagers is a serious problem in the United States. Approximately one in five sexually active teenage women in the United States will become pregnant before reaching her twentieth birthday (Taffel et al., 1995). More than half of these pregnancies will end in a live birth. In 1996, an estimated 505 514 women under 20 years of age gave birth, with two-thirds of these births reported to have been unintended (CDC, 1997). The relationship between teen pregnancy and neonatal mortality also has been well documented. The risk of neonatal mortality increases substantially for births to teens (Ventura et al., 1994). If it is true that teen pregnancy is associated with an increased risk of infant death, why then is a focus on teen pregnancy unhelpful in addressing elevations in infant mortality?

The answer lies in the fact that while the greatest risk for neonatal death lies at the extremes of maternal age, the largest portion of neonatal deaths occurs not on the extremes, but in the middle of the age distribution, among women in their twenties. This distribution, of course, reflects directly the fact that the vast majority of births in the United States occur to women in their twenties and early thirties (NCHS, 1996). Therefore, while the risk of neonatal death is disproportionately high for teens, its actual contribution to the overall neonatal mortality rate is relatively small (Goldenberg and Klerman, 1995). This suggests that as risk rises, its prevalence tends to fall; conditions that convey an extremely high relative risk are likely to be quite rare. If we did away with the risk associated with teen pregnancy tomorrow, our neonatal mortality rate and the racial disparity in neonatal mortality would fall by less than 10%.

Comprehensive women's health is threatened by the misinterpretation and misrepresentation of the epidemiology of relative risk as the epidemiology of contribution. Risk association studies may define what is true, but they may say little about what is relevant. As a result, it is the public perception that our infant mortality problem in the United States is the product of a series of extremely high risk conditions or behaviors. An isolated public focus on factors that convey high relative risk tends to push the public debate over birth outcomes to the margins, to the extremes of risk. This "marginalization" of neonatal and infant mortality causation is not confined to teen pregnancy, but also occurs in the discussion of a number of other adverse maternal behaviors, including heavy cocaine or alcohol use in pregnancy and lack of prenatal care. Clearly, these issues represent major problems and require the provision of greatly expanded services. However, one cannot dismiss national neonatal mortality rates as being due to the high relative risks associated with these maternal behaviors. The data suggest that neonatal mortality in the U.S., as well as social and racial disparities in neonatal mortality, occur not on the margins of risk but in the mainstream of births in this country.

While marginalization raises a series of interesting technical questions, it is more than an abstract or technical concern. Rather, marginalization continues to have a major impact on the public deliberation of infant mortality reduction efforts in the U.S. First, such a heavy focus on the extremes of risk tends to feed destructive stereotypes of women by framing the causes of infant mortality, and particularly racial disparities in infant mortality, as being largely due to deviant maternal behavior (Eberstadt, 1991). This helps generate an undercurrent of resentment toward young women which, in turn, acts to reduce public support for policies directed at meeting their needs.

Second, marginalization has found troubling expression in the development of local initiatives to reduce infant mortality. Operationally, the preoccupation with extremes of risk has helped generate a predisposition of many communities to direct specialized programs toward a relatively small group of women at extremely high risk. Although these efforts can provide important services to women in acute need, these programs are often developed as major infant mortality reduction efforts. The marginalization of infant mortality causation is transformed into the marginalization of intervention. Such programs tend to divert attention and resources from the basic infrastructure of comprehensive health care and social service provision in these very same communities. In community after community, as more and more infant mortality reduction programs are targeted at extremes of risk in pregnancy, funding for entities that provide comprehensive services, community health centers or broad-based neighborhood women's and infant health programs, have deteriorated. It is no coincidence that the initial funding proposal for the federal Healthy Start Initiative, the largest specialized infant mortality reduction effort ever undertaken in this country, involved the transfer of funds to Healthy Start from the migrant and community health center budget.

The impulse to target innovative prenatal care strategies on the extremes of risk, therefore, not only tends to generate counterproductive perceptions of women's contribution to the death of their infants, but can also undermine broad, integrated approaches to improving the health of reproductive-aged women. More comprehensive strategies will require a far more careful representation of empirical research and a fuller appreciation of the harm that can be done by turning the public gaze away from the broad mainstream toward the dramatic margins of risk.

Extreme prematurity and the shrinking window for isolated prenatal care

A substantial portion of neonatal mortality in the U.S. is now concentrated among premature infants. Deaths in premature infants are also responsible for a significant part of the racial disparity in neonatal mortality (Overpeck et al., 1992; Wise et al., 1995). The distribution of neonatal deaths in the U.S. is shown in Figure 15.1. For 1988, for example, some 63.7% of the entire racial disparity in neonatal mortality in the United States was due to deaths occurring to neonates born at less than 26 weeks gestation. Almost 32% of the disparity occurred in newborns of less than 24 weeks gestation – an age that is, in fact, under the legal abortion limit.

The concentration of mortality into the most premature newborns has important implications for the traditional strategy of improving birth outcomes through tightly focused prenatal interventions. By the time a woman knows she is pregnant, presents for prenatal care, has risks identified, is referred to high-risk

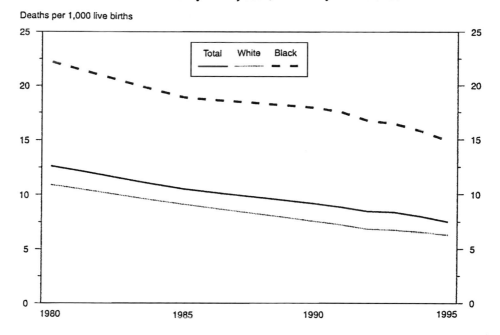

Figure 15.1   Distribution of neonatal deaths in the U.S. (from NCHS, 1990).

programs, and arranges for specialized or home visiting services, the first visit that actually takes place – the initial opportunity for intervention – is likely, in most large-scale programs, to be at about 20–21 weeks gestation. Given the large portion of neonatal deaths occurring to newborns of 25 weeks of gestation or less, this approach does not provide for a large window of opportunity to prevent extreme prematurity.

This ever-decreasing window for traditional prenatal care approaches is a relatively recent trend. The striking concentration of mortality in the most premature groups is largely the result of the major reductions in the mortality of critically ill newborns born at gestations greater than 28 weeks (Paneth et al., 1982; Williams and Chen, 1982). Although survival rates have improved for newborns at all gestations and birth weights over the past two decades, mortality among newborns born at the horizon of viability remains high. Extremely premature newborns, therefore, account for a larger portion of all neonatal deaths than in previous years. These recent trends must be seen as raising important practical challenges to the traditional approach of attempting to enhance services for high-risk women only after they are pregnant.

In addition to the practical difficulties inherent in attempting to intervene early enough in pregnancy to prevent extreme prematurity, the underlying determinants of prematurity and other adverse birth outcomes themselves suggest a need for a broader approach to prenatal care. As described throughout this book, many of the risk factors associated with prematurity not only generally predate pregnancy, but also generally require prolonged and continuous interventions. This is true for chronic medical conditions, prior adverse reproductive outcomes, abusive relationships, inadequate social conditions, inadequate nutrition, and behavioral factors such as smoking, drug or alcohol use. Some important interventions, such as folate supplementation to prevent birth defects (Holmes et al., 1997), act so early in pregnancy that they must be operative before conception. As discussed in Chapter 4 and as shown in other studies, recent evidence suggests that certain low-grade infectious processes may be an important cause of premature labor and that antimicrobial therapy could reduce a significant portion of the expected premature births (Goldenberg et al., 1996; Hauth et al., 1995; Hillier et al., 1995a,b; Meis et al., 1995). However, although the mechanisms of infectious etiologies remain poorly understood, this may be another case in which early intervention is essential. There are indications that the effectiveness of antimicrobial therapy may be enhanced if the treatment of longstanding infections could be initiated before pregnancy begins (Meis et al., 1995). In yet another case, that of HIV, it is clear that although new therapies have proven successful in interrupting transmission to the fetus (Connor et al., 1994), much earlier prevention of HIV transmission among adults is by far the preferable goal.

The confined vision of prenatal care also ignores the importance of other forms of reproductive health services, particularly family planning and abortion, in improving birth outcomes. The beneficial effects of these services include the prevention of unwanted and high-risk pregnancies (Jamieson and Buescher, 1992). The majority of all pregnancies in the United States are unintended, while 12% are unwanted (Forrest and Singh, 1990; NCHS, 1990; Williams and Pratt, 1990). Forty-seven percent of all unintended pregnancies are due to contraceptive failure or imperfect use of a contraceptive method. The remaining 53% occur to the 10% of women at risk for unintended pregnancy, sexually active women who use no contraceptive method at all. An unplanned or unwanted pregnancy can reduce birth intervals and generate a number of social, economic, psychological, and medical challenges to women's health and well-being (Meier and McFarlane, 1994; Miller, 1992; Rawlings et al., 1995). The importance of family planning as a component of prenatal care, and women's health care generally, is discussed at length in Chapter 13.

The isolation of prenatal services has also found programmatic expression, influencing profoundly the way maternal and child health initiatives have been implemented in communities across the country. A recent survey of state maternal and child health directors in 50 states and the District of Columbia found that virtually all had infant mortality initiatives (48), with a large majority providing prenatal care (44) and infant care services (39) (Chavkin et al., 1995). However, only five of these efforts included a women's health component (Chavkin et al., 1998). In most infant mortality reduction programs, women are eligible for services only after they become pregnant, and they are dropped from the program soon after delivery. This lack of concern for women when they are not pregnant not only raises questions of fairness, but also tragically ignores opportunities to enhance the health of reproductive-aged women and their infants.

To move beyond the tight focus on the prenatal period means that the child health community must address the requirements of women's health regardless of pregnancy status. The recent interest in what has been labeled "preconceptional" care generally involves short-term evaluation and treatments focused expressly on preparing for pregnancy (Brown, 1998). Although useful in some situations, preconceptional care does not include the scope of interventions necessary to significantly improve current levels of prematurity and other adverse birth outcomes, given that the majority of pregnancies are unplanned (Forrest and Singh, 1990). In addition, as noted earlier, the problems most likely to result in poor birth outcomes generally require sustained care. Similarly, "interconceptional care," which focuses on improving the health of women once they have a child in order to improve the outcome of subsequent pregnancies, is a useful step forward (Klerman and Reynolds, 1994), but raises some important concerns. Interconceptional care could not address the approximately half of all births that occur to women who have never had a prior birth. Preconceptional and interconceptional care are constructive and needed recommendations. At the same time, our programs and policies ultimately will have to recognize that more comprehensive strategies to provide services to women, regardless of pregnancy status, are warranted.

In some measure, the infant mortality problem in the United States is a legacy of the poor general health status of women of reproductive age. The challenge lies in transforming our current vision of prenatal care from a first step in *child* health care to an important component of *women's* health care over the course of a lifetime. The reduction of infant mortality and the equitable provision of prenatal care services must remain goals. However, approaches limited to pregnancy alone defy the medical and programmatic mechanisms that ultimately root birth outcome in the underlying health experience of women. Equally important, they can also devalue women's general claim to health care.

Confronting antagonisms between women's and infants' interests

The integration of prenatal care into comprehensive women's health care not only requires a reconstruction of policies and programs, it also demands a fundamental reconsideration of how the plight of young children is portrayed in public discourse. Of particular relevance to a broader vision of prenatal care are arguments that elevate fetal well-being above the well-being or autonomy of pregnant women. The identification and, often, the dramatization of the plight of newborns born to women exhibiting a variety of adverse behaviors has led to a host of punitive or coercive public policies directed at pregnant women. The problem with this approach is that policies that hold little regard for the autonomy or health of women can and have generated a series of profoundly counterproductive and, too often, unjust results.

There can be no meaningful dispute that once a woman has chosen to bear a child, society has a legitimate interest in developing policies that will improve the likelihood her baby will be healthy. What is at issue are the specific means employed to reach this objective (Annas, 1987). Many concerned with infant health, including the official policymakers of the American Academy of Pediatrics (AAP, 1995), have embraced what is largely a facilitative model that attempts to improve maternal behaviors through education and improved access to relevant services. However, in many areas of the country, another impulse has emerged as the primary strategy to ensure improved infant health. Rather than supporting facilitative service provision, a highly adversarial posture has developed that advocates the use of governmental action to force women to change behaviors or submit to medical procedures in order to serve the rights or best interests of the fetus.

This approach has been expressed in a variety of forms (Johnsen, 1992; Larson, 1991). State agencies have attempted to impose imprisonment, civil commitment, surgery, or the loss of child custody for a variety of maternal behaviors. These include not following physician advice (*People* v. *Stewart*, 1987), failing to receive adequate health care (*Reyes* v. *Superior Court*, 1977), inadequate nutrition (Des Moines Register, 1980), selecting vaginal delivery instead of cesarean section (Cole, 1990; *Jefferson* v. *Griffin*, 1981), smoking cigarettes (Chavkin et al., 1995), engaging in sexual intercourse against medical advice (Meier and McFarlane, 1994), drinking alcohol (Daly, 1989; Loth, 1989), and taking prescription drugs (*Grodin* v. *Grodin*, 1980). Although many of these cases have had complex legal histories, virtually all have ended in acquittal or have been overturned on appeal.

An adversarial approach is, for some, strongly related to the issue of abortion, though for many in the child health community, it is not. For them, this adversarial position grows from the recognition of prenatal risk and a longstanding tradition of child protection (Osowski, 1992). While child protection remains an essential component of caring and effective child health services, its use as a model for dealing with maternal actions in pregnancy is highly problematic (Meier and McFarlane, 1994). First, the law has proven highly respectful of women's autonomy during pregnancy and what has been called the "bright line of birth" in blocking the extension to the fetus of statutes intended to protect liveborn children. The assumption that the concept of child abuse has a clear parallel in "fetal abuse" has not been borne out. Second, punitive or coercive policies can have the effect of driving women away from the health care delivery system, thereby rendering useless whatever clinical capability exists in prenatal care to ensure a healthy woman and newborn. Third, the invocation of policies that disregard the interests and autonomy of women can only help to generate deep antagonisms between the women's health and infant health communities, a political effect that is counterproductive to the development of an integrated women's health agenda.

Rethinking the elevation of the child: implications for prenatal care policy

Because antagonisms between women's and infants' health stem so directly from a singular focus on children's well-being, it is inevitable that any effort to fundamentally reframe prenatal care will meet resistance from the broad undercurrent of traditional advocacy positions that separate children's interests from those of women in particular and young adults in general. There being no way to avoid these positions, they deserve critical scrutiny.

It is useful to begin by recognizing that the underlying dilemma confronting all those who care for children in the United States is that a child's claim to justice is inherently tied to that of his or her parents. Children's access to societal resources is operationally dependent upon the legitimacy of the parents' claim. This linkage is derived from the longstanding belief in the primacy of familial responsibility for children in the United States.

A clear tension develops, however, when families cannot provide adequately for their children. Then, concern for the well-being of children clashes with traditional attachments to familial autonomy and responsibility (Ellwood, 1988). What emerges is a policy logic by which resources flow to children only when the parental claim to resources is deemed legitimate. Under the recently enacted welfare legislation, the 1996 Personal Responsibility and Work Opportunity Reconciliation Act, for example, children may be considered truly needy, but declared ineligible for state assistance if their parents refuse to seek work. Politically, voters may have real compassion for poor children, but they hesitate to support expanded welfare funding because of their misgivings over the parental actions that allowed these children to become poor in the first place and the fact that these funds are, in effect, used as much to support the parents as the children.

The tension between the needs of children and those of their parents has been at the heart of a number of advocacy efforts to reframe the debate over child welfare concerns. The primary attempt has been to uncouple, rhetorically and politically, children's and parental claims and then elevate the claims of children above those of their parents. This logic emerges from the presumption that the case for allocating resources to children may be far more compelling than a case based on the needs of their parents. Services for homeless young children may enjoy far greater public favor than services for their homeless young fathers.

Advocacy based on the elevation of children's interests have resulted in some important improvements in the state's commitment to children. However, they may, if not carefully amended, ultimately undermine greater linkages between women's and children's interests, and, therefore, a strengthened constituency for comprehensive social reform. Broadly speaking, these approaches can be distilled into three general themes: children as innocents; children as legacy; and children as investment. In many ways, these themes have shaped the mainstream discourse regarding children's interests in the United States.

Children as innocents

For most Americans, childhood is equated with innocence. Virtually by definition, therefore, childhood suffering is perceived as inherently unjust. No infant, regardless of life circumstance, deserves to be impoverished; no newborn deserves to be born with heroin in its blood; no infant deserves to go hungry. Not surprisingly, child innocence serves as a foundation for all child advocacy and is often used to elevate the claims of children above those of their parents. However, innocence as a basis for policy formation can backfire when responsibility for childhood suffering is assigned to "non-innocents" – almost always the parent. If, for example, advocacy to improve services for newborns exposed to cocaine in utero dramatically characterizes these infants as innocent victims, then virtually by definition, their mothers are cast as assailants. This dynamic has helped generate a public rage against drug-addicted women, particularly minority women, that has led to many highly coercive state actions against women, developments that virtually all child advocates recognize as ultimately counterproductive (Johnsen, 1992).

Children as legacy

The elevation of the child's claim has also been expressed through the notion of children as legacy. This refers to the strong current in American sensibilities concerned for the well-being of children as it relates to the future of our society. The phrase "children are our future" can be quite compelling and undoubtedly touches a strong chord in the discussion of the current needs of children. However, this approach as a basis for policy can also be problematic, for it ignores the essential reality that if children are our future, their parents are our present. A reliance on children as legacy to mobilize resources generates a logic that diminishes the current claims of young adults and tends to write them off as a lost cause. Once again, although on its face children as legacy may seem appealing, the policy dynamic it instigates may not serve the best interests of children, who, for the most part, are poor because of the deteriorating economic position of their parents.

Children as investment

The third theme invoked to elevate children's claims is children as investment. Here, arguments for improved services for children are based on the need to produce a vibrant work force in the future to advance our national interests in an increasingly competitive world economy. This has clearly played a large role in the recommendations from the business community for increased services to children. However, like legacy arguments, this approach shifts concern away from the claims of those already in the work force. It calls for state action to remedy what, in some measure, is the product of the inability of current industrial policies and wage scales to keep families with children out of poverty. Moreover, this human investment approach can at times confine the social claims of children to the indifferent requirements of the national economy.

Conclusion

The premise of this discussion is that the full integration of prenatal care into women's health care will require a fundamental search for commonality between women's and children's interests. As long as the health of women is of importance only to the extent that it affects that of the newborn, prenatal care will always remain an isolated, vulnerable policy domain. The central question for all concerned with prenatal care is, ultimately, what is the nature and scope of our commitment to the general health of women? The answer to this question will not come easily. It will require a more critical awareness of the dynamic nature of adverse birth outcomes as well as a recognition of the tortured translation of prenatal risk identification into a highly fractious public discourse. More fundamentally, it will require a new level of self-examination and willingness to amend longstanding approaches to improving birth outcomes and child well-being. Only in this manner can the revision of prenatal care transcend current programmatic and policy antagonisms and link a societal commitment to healthy childbearing to the larger struggle of protecting the health and social claims of women.

REFERENCES

American Academy of Pediatrics (AAP). Drug exposed infants. Pediatrics 1995; **96**: 364–7.

Annas GJ. Protecting the liberty of pregnant patients. New England Journal of Medicine 1987; **316**: 1213–14.

Brown S., ed. Reaching mothers, reaching infants. Washington (DC): Institute of Medicine, 1998.

Centers for Disease Control and Prevention (CDC). State-specific birth rates for teenagers – United States, 1990–1996. Morbidity and Mortality Weekly Report 1997; **46**: 837–42.

Chavkin W, Breitbart V, Wise PH. Efforts to reduce perinatal mortality, HIV, and drug addiction: surveys of the states. Journal of the American Medical Women's Association 1995; **50**: 164–6.

Chavkin W, Breitbart V, Wise PH. National survey of the states: policies and practices regarding drug using women. American Journal of Public Health 1998; **88**: 117–19.

Cole HM. Legal interventions during pregnancy. Journal of the American Medical Association 1990; **264**: 2663–70.

Connor EM, Sperling RS, Gelber R, et al. Reduction of maternal–infant transmission of human immunodeficiency virus type 1 with zidovudine treatment. Pediatric AIDS Clinical Trials Group Protocol 076 Study Group. New England Journal of Medicine 1994; **331**: 1173–80.

Daly CB. Woman charged in death of own fetus in accident. Washington Post, November 25, 1989: A4.

Des Moines Register. Baby placed in foster home: doctor claims prenatal abuse. April 3, 1980.

Eberstadt N. America's infant mortality puzzle. Public Interest 1991; **3**: 30–47.

Ellwood DT. Poor support. New York: Basic Books, 1988.

Forrest JD, Singh S. The sexual and reproductive behavior of American women, 1982–1988. Family Planning Perspectives 1990; **22**: 206–14.

Fraser AM, Brockert JE, Ward RH. Association of young maternal age with adverse reproductive outcomes. New England Journal of Medicine 1995; **332**: 1113–17.

Goldenberg RL, Kelbanoff MA, Nugent R, Krohn MA, Hillier S, Andrews WW. Bacterial colonization of the vagina during pregnancy in four ethnic groups. American Journal of Obstetrics and Gynecology 1996; **174**: 1618–21.

Goldenberg RL, Klerman LV. Adolescent pregnancy – another look. New England Journal of Medicine 1995; **332**: 1161–62.

Grodin v. *Grodin*, 102 Mich. App. 396, 401, 301 N.W.2d 869, 871 (1980).

Hauth JC, Goldenberg RL, Andrews WW, DuBard MB, Copper RL. Mid-trimester treatment with metronidazole plus erythromycin reduces preterm birth only in women with bacterial vaginosis. New England Journal of Medicine 1995; **333**: 1732–6.

Hillier SL, Krohn MA, Cassen E, Easterling TR, Rabe LK, Eschenbach DA. The role of bacterial vaginosis and vaginal bacteria in amniotic fluid infection in women in preterm labor with intact fetal membranes. Clinical Infectious Diseases 1995a; **20**: S276–8.

Hillier SL, Nugent RP, Eschenbach DA, Krohn MA, Gibbs RS, Martin DH. Association between bacterial vaginosis and preterm delivery of a low-birth-weight infant. New England Journal of Medicine 1995b; **333**: 1737–42.

Holmes L, Harris T, Oakley GP Jr, Friedman JM. Teratology Society Consensus Statement on the use of folic acid to reduce risk of birth defects. Teratology 1997; **55**: 381.

Jamieson DJ, Buescher PA. The effect of family planning participation on prenatal care use and low birth weight. Family Planning Perspectives 1992; **24**: 214–18.

Jefferson v. *Griffin*. Ga. 86, 88, 274 S.E.2d 457, 459 (1981).

Johnsen D. Shared interests: promoting healthy births without sacrificing women's liberty. Hastings Law Journal 1992; **43**: 569–614.

Jones EF, Forrest JD, Goldman N, et al. Teenage pregnancy in developed countries: determinants and policy implications. Family Planning Perspectives 1985; **17**: 53–63.

Klerman LV, Reynolds DW. Interconception care: a new role for the pediatrician. Pediatrics 1994; **93**: 327–9.

Larson CS. Overview of state legislative and judicial responses. The Future of Children. 1991; **2**: 72–84.

Loth R. DA sees no politics in fetal death case. Boston Globe. September 16, 1989: 25.

Meier KJ, McFarlane DR. State family planning and abortion expenditures: their effect on public health. American Journal of Public Health 1994; **84**: 1468–72.

Meis PJ, Goldenberg RL, Mercer B, et al. The preterm prediction study: significance of vaginal infections. American Journal of Obstetrics and Gynecology 1995; **173**: 1231–5.

Miller CA. Wanting children. American Journal of Public Health 1992; **82**: 341–3.

National Center for Health Statistics (NCHS). Use of family planning services in the United States: 1982 and 1988. Advance Data, Monthly Vital Statistics Report, 1990; **184**: 1–8.

National Center for Health Statistics (NCHS). Health, United States, 1995. Hyattsville (MD): Public Health Service, National Center for Health Statistics, 1996: 87.

Osowski BD. The need for logic and consistency in fetal rights. North Dakota Law Review 1992; **68**: 171–208.

Overpeck MD, Hoffman HJ, Prager K. The lowest birth-weight infants and the US infant mortality rate: NCHS 1983 linked birth/infant death data. American Journal of Public Health 1992; **82**: 441–3.

Paneth N, Kiely JL, Phil M, et al. Newborn intensive care and neonatal mortality in low-birth-weight infants. New England Journal of Medicine 1982; **307**: 149–55.

People v. *Stewart*, No. M508197 (Cal. Mun. Ct. Feb 26, 1987).

Rawlings JS, Rawlings VB, Read JA. Prevalence of low birth weight and preterm delivery in relation to the interval between pregnancies among white and black women. New England Journal of Medicine 1995; **332**: 69–74.

Reyes v. *Superior Court*, 75 Cal. App. 3d 214, 217, 141 Cal. Rptr. 912, 913 (1977).

Taffel SJ, Mosher WD, Wilson JB, Henshaw SK. Trends in pregnancies and pregnancy rates: estimates for the United States, 1980–92. Monthly Vital Statistics Report. Hyattsville (MD): National Center for Health Statistics, 1995. Volume 43.

Ventura SJ, Martin JA, Taffel SM, Mathews TJ, Clarke SC. Advance report of final natality statistics, 1992. Monthly Vital Statistics Report. Hyattsville (MD): National Center for Health Statistics, 1994. Volume 43, Number 5 (supplement).

Williams LB, Pratt WF. Wanted and unwanted childbearing in the United States: 1973–88. Hyattsville (MD): U.S. Department of Health and Human Services, Public Health Service, 1990; **189**: 1–8.

Williams RL, Chen PM. Identifying the sources of the recent decline in prenatal mortality rates in California. New England Journal of Medicine 1982; **306**: 207–14.

Wise PH, Wampler N, Barfield W. The importance of extreme prematurity and low birthweight to US neonatal mortality patterns: implications for prenatal care and women's health. Journal of the American Medical Womens' Association 1995; **50**: 152–5.

16

A European perspective on perinatal care: an integrated system

Jacques Milliez

Introduction

The ultimate success of a system of care for women and children that is designed to safeguard the health of women during pregnancy, improve birth outcomes, and ensure the healthy development of young children is critically dependent on its comprehensiveness. To meet its goals at a societal level, it must encompass women of childbearing age and their children at all socioeconomic levels, and it must address the full range of their health concerns and determinants.

The preceding chapters of this book have addressed successes and limitations of prenatal care in the United States. This chapter will present an example of a European system of prenatal care, specifically the French system, which strives to meet this goal of comprehensiveness. In France, prenatal care is generally linked to postpartum care and pediatric services for young children, and will therefore be discussed here under the umbrella of "perinatal" rather than "prenatal" care.

Western European countries are inclined to present their public health policies as a model, based on their commitment to the health of pregnant women and infants. It is useful to ask whether the achievements of these policies justify this characterization. This chapter attempts to answer this question by describing the French system, and reviewing its accomplishments as well as its limitations. In doing so, we hope to present a useful comparison to the American system.

The history of perinatal welfare in France

Concern for the welfare of children and pregnant women has a relatively long history in France, beginning in the eighteenth century. At that time, the rate of infant mortality in Europe was around 250 per 1000 live births, which meant that one quarter of each generation was destined to disappear by the end of its first year. In order to preserve the population, basic policies were adopted for the "conservation" of children, namely measures to feed them adequately.

By the end of the nineteenth century, the rate of infant mortality in France was still between 150 and 200 per 1000 live births. In the aftermath of the war against Prussia, the first law in favor of children was enacted in 1874, thanks to the initiative of physician Théophile Roussel. The Parliament voted for this law in order to protect (the word appears for the first time) children, and to control the health conditions of infants fed by wet nurses. In 1889, the law was extended to other categories of children, including battered, ill-treated, and abandoned children.

In 1892, French obstetrician Pierre Budin established the first outpatient clinics for healthy children. Their creation introduced the notion of preventive surveillance of child health and growth. He was followed by Gaston Variot, a pediatrician, and Léon Dufour, a general practitioner, who invented the first welfare centers for children, called "Drop of Milk."

In 1913, Paul Strauss, French Minister of Health, created free medical assistance for childbirth to needy pregnant women and passed a compulsory act granting eight weeks of maternity leave to pregnant workers. Low income pregnant women on leave also received a daily financial allocation during their maternity leave. Later, in 1920, Paul Strauss was the first to advocate the "Carnet de Santé," a health logbook for children.

It was during the early twentieth century that the concept of "protection for mother and infants" – a term actually coined by French obstetrician Adolphe Pinard – became an organizing principle for the management of services. In 1914, the military government of Paris created a Central Office for Maternal and Infant Assistance in order to provide social and medical services to low-income pregnant women and their children under the age of three. In 1927, this agency became the Office for Protection of Mothers and Children and assumed the mission of coordinating all services for mothers and children, most of which were provided at the time by private charity organizations subsidized by the government. In 1931 Camille Blaisot, Minister of Health, urged all of the country's Department Councils (the local governing bodies that manage France's Departments, which are intermediate in size between a U.S. county and a state) to create Centers for the Protection of Mothers and Children (Protection Maternelle et Infantile, or PMI). At the same time, he created a corps of nurses, known as "home visitors," who were dedicated to home supervision of at-risk pregnant women and children.

The real breakthrough in the promotion of perinatal welfare in France occurred after World War II with a 1945 Act that established the protection of mothers and children as a national principle. This crucial PMI legislation, which was part of a post-war policy to encourage births, prescribed universal social and medical protection of pregnant women and their children up to the age of six years and included all classes of society without discrimination. Free consultations were provided for pregnant women, for infants under the age of two, and for children between two and six. The government funded all services. Pregnant women complying with prenatal surveillance recommendations received monthly allocations. Those who worked were granted 90% of their salary during their maternity leave, several weeks before, and several weeks after delivery. The 1945 legislation extended Blaisot's 1931 recommendations by expanding PMI centers nationwide, providing government support to ensure continued funding, and linking them to national maternity insurance through compulsory prenatal visits.

Since its inception, the PMI legislation has been periodically revisited and improved. For example, a category of pediatric nurses for neonates called "puéricultrices," requiring an extra year of training, was created in 1947. In the 1960s, the country's Departments were requested to organize one outpatient neonatal clinic for every 8000 residents and one outpatient prenatal clinic for every 20 000 residents, and family planning and contraception were included under PMI services. In the early 1970s, a perinatal program was launched to reduce prematurity and births risks; the number of compulsory prenatal visits increased from two to four. (In 1992, the number of compulsory visits increased again, to seven.) In 1975, abortion was legalized and provided by PMI centers. A December 1989 law introduced a compulsory maternity logbook for the follow up of pregnancy and changed the focus of mothers' and children's health initiatives from *protection* to *health promotion*. During this time period, perinatal mortality decreased from 70 per 1000 live births in 1945, to 8 per 1000 live births in the early 1980s. It must be noted, however, that a causal link between decreases in perinatal mortality rates and the medico-social PMI network has not been documented.

Currently, the National Health Division of Social Security funds up to 20% of the budget of PMI centers, with the remaining 80% subsidized by Department Councils' budgets. PMI centers are scattered within urban communities, and are often located in public hospitals' maternity clinics. Their number depends on the public health policy passed by each Department. Some Departments have more than a hundred PMI centers, others have none at all.

The health insurance structure

France's perinatal care system depends on the health care financing system that supports it. The health insurance system in France is part of a Social Security system, the basis of which was established in the aftermath of World War II. The Social Security system currently covers more than 99% of France's 60 million citizens. It is a compulsory universal program covering health insurance, pensions, family support, and maternal and child support. Any legal resident, either French or non-French, is entitled to Social Security, provided that he or she works 120 hours per month or 200 hours per trimester, receives unemployment or welfare subsidies, is a single parent, or benefits from a spouse's enrollment in a private insurance plan. All health expenditures, to private as well as public providers of care, are funded almost totally by the Health Division of Social Security.

The Social Security budget in France is $200 billion. It is a separate fund of money that is equal to the national state budget. Half of this budget, $100 billion, is dedicated to health insurance. Though large, the sum amounts to only one-tenth of the U.S. expenditure on health costs, which are currently $1 trillion. Per capita expenditures in France are also much lower than in the U.S. In France, health expenditures represent 9.4% of the gross domestic product (GDP), whereas they are 14% of the GDP in the U.S. (Bok, 1996) and expected to reach 17% of the GDP by the end of the decade (Frigoletto, 1997). It is useful to note that despite the relatively greater expenditure on health care in the U.S., more than 40 million citizens in the U.S., or 15% of the population, including 10 million children, do not have health insurance (Bok, 1996).

Unlike the British National Health Service, which is supported by taxes, only 20% (and this proportion has recently been increased) of the funds for the French Social Security system is provided by taxes on company profits and by a universal income tax called Generalized Social Contribution (Contribution Sociale Général-isée, or CSG). The remaining 80% originates from a wage and salary levy, requested partly from the employer and partly from the employee (Bertrand, 1989). This levy is raised by an independent board called Union de Recouvrement des Cotisations de la Securité Sociale et des Allocations Familiales (URSSAF). These funds, plus the 20% raised through taxes, are then managed and spent by the National Office for Health Insurance (the Caisse Nationale d'Assurance Maladie, or CNAM), a board consisting of elected representatives of the Workers Trade Unions and Patrons Unions. In fact, however, due to frequent conflicts between Workers and Patrons Unions, the government has assumed an arbitration role and drives the budgetary allocations through the use of financial experts appointed by the Ministry of Health.

Both health care providers and patients are considered to be the consumers in the national health insurance system. All practicing physicians are linked to the Health Division of Social Security by a collective agreement that is periodically negotiated between the CNAM and the Medical Unions. The agreement states that all patients are to be reimbursed for health costs, up to roughly 70% of their expenses, according to the type of care they receive. The remaining costs for patients are generally covered by a publicly or privately funded Mutual Complementary Insurance policy. Among the population registered with Social Security in France, 25% cannot afford complementary insurance and must pay their remaining costs out of pocket.

The provision of perinatal care

Care settings

Perinatal care in France is currently provided in three different settings: (1) private offices and clinics, (2) PMI centers, and (3) public hospitals. Approximately half of the 750 000 annual births in France occur in private clinics. The remainder take place in maternity clinics located in public hospitals. PMI centers do not provide birthing services; rather, they focus on providing prenatal and pediatric care. Home delivery is a marginal practice, although home supervision of high-risk pregnancy is an increasing trend.

France's private clinics are funded by Social Security on a fee-for-service payment basis. Payments to the clinic are made directly by Social Security or by the patient, who is later reimbursed. Since 1984, all public hospitals in France have been allocated an overall annual budget that varies little from year to year. This form of financing is aimed at containing health costs. The funding of public maternity clinics in public hospitals is part of this budget. More than 70% of the budget is represented by the salaries for physicians, paramedical staff members, and administrators.

One specific drawback to France's hospital system is the lack of effective networks of primary, secondary, and tertiary care birthing centers within each region of the country. Regionalization of perinatal care in France is far behind what it could be and behind most other European countries, especially Scandinavian countries. Aside from a few scattered experiences initiated in the mid-1980s – for example a program in the western city of Nantes (Sagot et al., 1990) – maternal transfers to tertiary centers equipped with neonatal intensive care units (NICU) are scarce. The regionalization of care and the implementation of appropriate referral policies have been recently proposed, but these are far from being fully implemented. During 1991, the estimated number of maternal transfers nationwide among an overall cohort of 750 000 live births was 242 for pregnancies at 26–28 weeks, and 850 for pregnancies at 29–32 weeks (CNAMTS, 1994). Assuming that the population of pregnant women eligible for transfer to a tertiary center represents at least 1% of all births, the figure should be around 7500 transfers each year.

The reason that France's situation departs from the policies developed in other countries is that after 1980, France elected to focus on neonatal emergency transports rather than maternal transfers, mostly as a result of pressure from pediatricians. Reorganization of regional neonatal transfers in the early 1980s did lead to clear improvements in neonatal outcome. In a large survey of the Paris region conducted in 1985, the perinatal mortality rate of outborns (those transferred to tertiary centers equipped with NICUs) and inborns (those not transferred) did not differ significantly (Dehan et al., 1990). During the period 1989–1992, 67 819 births occurred in Seine Saint Denis. Of these, 46.4% of the premature births at less than 33 weeks gestation occurred in a Level 1 maternity center (a center with no full-time pediatrician), 41.5% occurred in a Level 2 maternity center (a center with a pediatric unit, but no NICU), and 11.3% occurred in a Level 3 maternity center (a center with a NICU) (Node et al., 1992). Outborns represented 75% of the population of very premature babies with a birth weight below 1500 gm and/or a gestational age below 32 weeks. Perinatal mortality for these outborns was found to be different, 15.7%, 14.9%, and 8.8%, respectively, depending on the type of maternity center at which they were born. However, the benefits of maternal rather than neonatal transfers appear to be more obvious in preventing neonatal morbidity and brain injury than in preventing neonatal mortality. Indeed, a different series of data recorded in France between 1985 and 1992 (Truffert et al., 1992), showed that for very premature babies with birth weights between 500 gm and 1500 gm, the relative risk of major neurologic handicap was 7.51 for outborns compared to inborns. This suggests a greater advantage of neonatal transfers for the prevention of handicaps than for reducing the risk of perinatal mortality.

These findings have had some impact on the practice of prenatal care in France. Along with improvements in neonatal transports and a slow but steady increase in maternal transfers, a result has been that more and more high-risk pregnancies are initially checked in to tertiary centers, thus saving the need for transfer after the delivery. By 1989, in regions outside Paris where neonatal transports had been less extensively supported, nearly 60% of premature babies less than 1500 gm were born in tertiary referral centers and the trend has been reinforced since (Chale et al., 1997).

Even though much remains to be done to further improve perinatal transports, the overall national results regarding perinatal indicators, perinatal deaths, and prematurity show that striking progress has been achieved during the past 25 years.

Maternity benefits

Social Security in France provides incentives and benefits to pregnant women to encourage their compliance with prenatal care, ensure they are well supported during their pregnancy, and ensure that their babies get off to a good start. Provided she has been living in France legally for at least three months, any woman, either French or non-French, may benefit from Social Security Maternity Insurance, so long as she declares and registers her pregnancy with Social Security before the 15th week of pregnancy.

During pregnancy, any woman who benefits from maternity insurance must complete seven prenatal visits, which are free of charge. Screening tests are mandatory, including blood group and anti-Rh antibody determination, and serology for syphilis, toxoplasmosis, rubella and hepatitis B, red blood cell and platelet count, and hemoglobin concentration. One sonogram per trimester is reimbursed. For patients with high-risk pregnancies, inpatient hospital care is free after the sixth month of pregnancy. Postpartum hospital care in the maternity ward is free of charge for mother and newborn for seven days after an uncomplicated vaginal delivery and 10 days after a cesarean section. It can be legally extended to 12 days in the case of necessity.

Before 1996, all pregnant woman received a monthly prenatal allocation of about $180. Since then, in an effort to contain costs, these incentives have been reserved for lower income couples below a baseline threshold of income. Any pregnant woman is given six weeks maternity leave before delivery (eight weeks if she is multipara or expecting twins) and 10 weeks postpartum. During the course of her maternity leave, she receives 85% of her salary. Patients on sick leave before the regular maternity leave receive 50% of their salary.

An essential element of prenatal care in France is the two maternity logbooks provided to all pregnant women. Women receive the first one from Social Security when their pregnancy has been registered. Each sheet corresponds to a mandatory prenatal visit and must be completed and signed by the obstetrician or the midwife and sent to Social Security in order for the woman to receive maternity insurance benefits. There is an additional sheet for the postpartum visit, which occurs four to six weeks after delivery.

A second maternity logbook registers all medical records concerning the ongoing pregnancy, including vital signs at each visit, sonogram results, and prescriptions. This logbook serves to link all the health care providers involved in the surveillance of pregnancy, including the midwife from a PMI center, the home care medical team, and the family practitioner.

Perinatal care practitioners

Perinatal care in France is provided by midwives, obstetricians and, for less than 4% of pregnancies, by general practitioners. The hallmarks of this care are the active involvement of midwives in most pregnancies and deliveries and the delivery of care by multidisciplinary perinatal teams.

Midwives

Midwifery is an ancient and widely accepted tradition in France. Called matrons in the old times and midwives since the middle of the last century, these professionals are the traditional caregivers for pregnant women. They are considered to be invaluable contributors to the quality and the efficiency of perinatal care.

There are 12 000 practicing midwives in France. The vast majority belong to private or public maternity clinics. Very few midwives practice in private offices of their own. Midwives receive four years of training in one of 40 schools of midwifery and receive a national diploma, as opposed to a university degree. In France, midwives practice within specified limits. For example, in contrast to the practice of Swedish midwives, French midwives are not entitled to perform instrumental deliveries. However, they can conduct certain other procedures and prescribe specific drugs, as well as assist in providing perinatal medicine, infertility treatment, and family planning services. In addition to supervising pregnancies and delivering babies, they care for postpartum and breastfeeding patients, participate in the psychological preparation for delivery, and occasionally assist with neonatal resuscitation in the delivery room. They are part of the neonatal care team in the pediatric unit, and participate in recording computer data and providing sonograms, genetic counseling, and postpartum perineal rehabilitation. Although most midwives are women, a few men have successfully entered the profession.

Perinatal care teams

Since the National Perinatal Policy Implementation Program was instituted in 1994, all birthing centers in France must have a multidisciplinary perinatal care team on call around the clock. The core of this team consists of a pediatrician, an anesthesiologist, a midwife, and an obstetrician.

In large maternity centers, full-time physicians collaborate with private practitioners who are part-time staff associates. For their hospital attendance, these private physicians are paid by salary, not on a fee-for-service basis. They work primarily in outpatient consultations: sonograms, colposcopy, infertility, high-risk pregnancies. Pediatricians, including pediatric cardiologists, generally work in the neonatal unit. In addition to private practitioners, full-time physicians, and midwives, the perinatal team on the maternity ward includes puéricultrices (the pediatric nurses who are specially trained for neonatal care), psychologists, pedopsychiatrists, nutritionists, HIV specialists, pain relief specialists, interpreters, and social workers. Small birthing centers that perform fewer than 500 deliveries a year are steadily closing down because of the financial and other difficulties of complying with the multidisciplinary staffing requirements of the 1994 Perinatal Policy Implementation Program.

Socioceconomic and demographic issues in the provision of perinatal care in France

The vast majority of pregnant women in France (98%) are registered with Social Security. Of the remaining 2%, half have no health insurance at all (Wcilso et al.,

1996), and the remaining half depend on a health insurance program for low-income individuals (Free Medical Assistance), which is the equivalent of Medicaid. Pregnant women not covered by Social Security have pregnancy outcomes that are equivalent to those achieved by the population registered with Social Security, with no significant differences in the rates of maternal or neonatal morbidity, low birth weight, or prematurity (Milliez et al., 1997). This is likely because of the system's provisions for low-income and uninsured pregnant women.

Any French or non-French legal resident not registered with Social Security and with an annual income below $7,200 is eligible for Free Medical Assistance (Wcilso et al., 1996). The program also covers the portion of health expenses not covered by Social Security for those who are enrolled but cannot afford the cost-sharing component. This includes women who are living on unemployment subsidies (4% of pregnant women), or who are being supported by welfare subsidies (2.8% of pregnant women). These social welfare programs are funded not by Social Security, but by the Department Council budgets. Trained social workers in the PMI centers are generally able to enroll from 60 to 80% of women with no previous health insurance in Social Security during the course of pregnancy (Milliez et al., 1997).

Although only 1% of pregnant women nationwide do not have any kind of health insurance, in inner city or suburban hospitals in certain areas, between 13% and 15% of pregnant women do not have Social Security and cannot apply for Free Medical Assistance. This is generally because they are illegal immigrants. They still gain full access to medical assistance, including pregnancy surveillance and delivery, however, because medical care is mandatory for any individual in an emergency medical condition, and pregnancy is considered to be such a condition.

The 1995 National Birth Registry showed that 12% of pregnant women in France are foreigners, and 99% of them are registered with Social Security (Wcilso et al., 1996). Indeed, patients of more than 40 different nationalities attend French maternity centers. They come from all over the world, including North Africa, Africa, Southeast Asia, Sri Lanka, and Eastern Europe. There also has been a recent influx from mainland China. This diversity is not evenly distributed among all hospitals and some inner city and suburban hospitals are particularly affected. To better distribute this uneven financial burden, these patients are now granted free medical support in PMI centers and public hospitals, provided that they attend the health care center of their district of residence.

This extreme diversity among nationalities explains why full-time interpreters are part of the perinatal team. The multiethnic situation also requires a special effort from maternity staff members toward women who may not be accustomed to a Western European health care system or to the medical techniques, common practices during pregnancy or delivery (e.g., prenatal screening for fetal anomalies or cesarean section for fetal distress during labor), and ethical considerations that are part of modern medicine. However, a recent study conducted by student midwives showed that women from West Africa, even those recently immigrated, were aware of the full array of prenatal procedures and complied well during prenatal visits. Their knowledge of prenatal care generally came from neighbors and companions from the same ethnic group, but even more knowledge came from the social workers of their district of residence and the schoolteachers of their older children. This demonstrates the potential for the social network and schools to enhance the successful integration of immigrants into the country's social system (Aladière, 1994).

The results of comprehensive perinatal care

In 1968, the rate of perinatal mortality in France was 2.5%, with 22 000 stillbirths and 40 000 handicapped infants. The financial burden resulting from these accidents amounted to 2.5% of the GDP. Since then, perinatal indicators have dramatically improved (Milliez, 1993). The perinatal mortality rate was 23.4 per 1000 live births in 1970, fell to 12.3 per 1000 in 1981, and is currently less than 10 per 1000 (Milliez, 1993). The rate of prematurity has fallen from 9% in 1972 to around 5% currently.

The national perinatal program that was launched in the 1970s has been thoroughly implemented. The number of effective prenatal visits has steadily increased: 22.2% of pregnant women had six or more visits in 1972, 33.9% in 1976, 38.3% in 1981, and 50.6% in 1989. The number of sonograms per pregnancy has similarly increased: 32.7% of pregnant women had more than two in 1981, and 74% in 1989. Rates of teenage pregnancy also have fallen from 6.2% to 2.9% between 1981 and 1989.

It is difficult to single out one major factor that accounts for France's favorable evolution in perinatal outcomes. A general improvement in social conditions and higher standards of living is one likely explanation for this trend. This is in keeping with an increasing life expectancy for adults. Technical breakthroughs, such as sonography or fetal heart rate monitoring, which were developed during the same period, have also played a role, though their impact has never been evaluated. It is also very likely that legal and social measures that encourage pregnant women to comply with prenatal care recommendations, along with the progressive infrastructure of multidisciplinary perinatal teams, has effectively contributed to the performances achieved in perinatal medicine during the past three decades.

Despite the wide array of social protection programs, however, 1.1% of pregnant French women still receive prenatal care that is substandard by French norms (i.e., less than four prenatal visits) or no prenatal care at all (Blondel and Marshall, 1996). The reasons for this are numerous – undesired or concealed pregnancy, teenage pregnancy, grand multiparity (i.e., a woman who has had six or more previous pregnancies may feel she has a decreased need for medical supervision), illegal residency, absence of health insurance coverage, and extreme poverty among a disadvantaged population that is unable to seek proper social relief. This population of women experience a rate of intrauterine fetal death, low birth weight, and prematurity that is four times higher than the national average (Blondel and Marshall, 1996). These statistics are exemplified by the findings of a study among a population at high social risk, consisting of women under a judicial sentence of child–mother separation and temporary parental disqualification. Despite being registered with Social Security, these women had lower than average compliance with prenatal surveillance, and this was correlated with a higher rate of maternal morbidity (drug addiction, HIV, and hepatitis C infection) and poorer perinatal outcomes (Milliez and Chaplet, 1997). These findings support the view that comprehensive care is linked to favorable outcomes. They also emphasize the fact that welfare policies may affect one dimension of outcome-related socioeconomic health disparities, such as differences in income levels, while leaving others, such as unequal social conditions, untouched.

Conclusion

The French experience demonstrates that lack of prenatal care and poor social conditions combine to increase the risk of significant adverse neonatal outcomes. These two factors cannot be disassociated. Their interdependence reinforces the merits of a strong medical and global social welfare approach and underlines the contribution of multidisciplinary teams to the alleviation of birth risks.

Although the French model has grown out of France's unique history and culture, most European models are generally similar. The ways and means may be different in each country, but Europe's common policy is to offer comprehensive care to pregnant women and their infants. The underlying philosophy is solidarity within the society, in the form of a universal health insurance coverage for all pregnant women and children.

Such a system may not be cost-effective in many aspects, and it is clear that cost-savings efforts are necessary in order to preserve its future. Nevertheless, the concept of universal health insurance coverage is not conceived as a for-profit system, and in no European country is it managed by the equivalent of a managed care organization. Universal maternal insurance is regarded as an investment for the sake of infants that will reduce the burden of disabilities and the costs of birth-related diseases or conditions. Its higher ambition is to provide every infant the best possible start in life and to contribute to alleviating inequalities in access to health care that are linked to social conditions. These inequalities bear heavily upon the poorest populations and perpetuate their disadvantaged circumstances.

REFERENCES

Aladière MC, Clairet J, Perotte F. Le vécu de la grossesse chez les femmes originaires d'Afrique de l'Ouest. Mémoire de fin d'études de sage femme. Paris: Ecole de Sages Femmes de Saint Antoine, 1994.

Bertrand D. La sécurité sociale. In: Brücker G, Fassin D, eds. Santé publique. Paris: Ellipses, 1989.

Blondel B, Marshall B. Les femmes peu ou pas suivies pendant la grossesse. Journal de Gynécologie, Obstétrique et Biologie de la Reproduction 1996; **25**: 729–36.

Bok D. Health care. In: The state of the nation. Cambridge (MA): Harvard University Press, 1996.

Caisse Nationale d'Assurance Maladie des Travailleurs Salariés (CNAMTS). Enquête sur l'activité ostétricale en 1991. Vol. 2. Paris: Caisse Nationale d'Assurance Maladie des Travailleurs Salariés, 1994.

Chale JJ, Papiernik E, Colladon B, et al. Analyse des lieux et des conditions d'accouchement en 1991 des mères d'enfants dont le poids de naissance était inférieur à 1500 g et/ou l'âge gestationnel inférieur strictement à 33 semaines. Journal de Gynécologie, Obstétrique et Biologie de la Reproduction 1997; **26**: 137–47.

Dehan M, Vodovar M, Gougard J, et al. Devenir des prématurés de moins de 33 semaines d'âge gestationnel: résultats d'une enquête menée en 1985 dans la région parisienne. Journal de Gynécologie, Obstétrique et Biologie de la Reproduction 1990; **19**: 25–35.

Frigoletto FD. CPR: can we be resuscitated? Obstetrics and Gynecology 1997; **89**: 1–4.

Milliez J. Antenatal care in industrialized countries. In: Baum JD, ed. Birth risks. New York: Raven Press, 1993.

Milliez J, Chaplet V. Precarity in pregnancy. Paper presented at: 25é Assises Nationales des Sages Femmes, 1997 May, Besançon (France).

Node N, Barbier ML, Dumas C, Chabernaud JL, Lavaud L. Transfers of newborn from maternity: a prospective study in Paris and Seine Saint Denis. Paper presented at: 13th European Congress of Perinatal Medicine, 1992 May 12–15, Amsterdam.

Sagot P, Roze C, Dantal F, et al. Naissance avant 33 semaines d'aménorrhée. Intérêt du transfert in utero au sein d'un Département de Périnatologie. Revue Francais de Gynécologie et d'Obstétrique 1990; **85**: 293–8.

Truffert P, Goujard J, Crost M, et al. Perinatal management of premature newborns and survival without handicaps. Journal of Perinatal Medicine 1992; **20** Suppl 1: 277.

Wcilso M, Blondel B. 1995 French National Birth Registry: National perinatal survey. Paris: Ministère du Travail et des Affaires Sociales. Service des statistiques des études et des systèmes d'information, 1996.

Epilogue

A commentary on the effectiveness and cost-effectiveness of prenatal care

Joanna E. Siegel and Marie C. McCormick

Introduction

The conference that formed the basis for this book was motivated in large part by recurrent questions in the literature regarding the value of prenatal care. Research has examined whether efforts to improve the access of pregnant women to timely prenatal care have been a successful means of improving birth outcomes. Although some reports have enthusiastically supported the accomplishments of prenatal care (IOM, 1985); others have stressed the equivocal nature of the empirical evidence, and their conclusions have been more guarded (Alexander and Korenbrot, 1995; Kogan et al., 1998; Fiscella, 1995).

Some of the more pointed commentaries on the value of prenatal care have occurred in the context of articles addressing cost-effectiveness. Several influential reports and studies have concluded that prenatal care is a cost-effective intervention based on its impact on specific adverse outcomes of pregnancy, namely low birth weight and prematurity. These studies have calculated the monetary savings resulting from the use of prenatal care (IOM, 1985; Gorsky and Colby, 1989; Korenbrot, 1984; Schramm, 1992), figures readily cited in policy debates. However, other authors have sharply contested these conclusions regarding cost-effectiveness (Huntington and Connell, 1994).

Here, we examine some of the issues relevant to assessing the value of prenatal care that have been highlighted in this book. The premise of this book, as described in the Introduction, is that the arguments for and the critiques of the effectiveness and cost-effectiveness of prenatal care are based on a very narrow conceptualization of both prenatal care and the relevant outcomes. This conceptualization reflects the power and limitations of the vital statistics data, which has been the cornerstone of much research on effectiveness. We summarize some of the themes our authors have raised concerning the past and current contributions of prenatal care construed more broadly, and equally important, its potential.

Effectiveness

A critical component of policy discussions regarding the value of an intervention and its cost-effectiveness is the assumptions that are made and the evidence cited about the ability of the intervention to achieve desired outcomes. For an assessment to reflect an intervention's true worth, it is important to consider the full range of its effects. All types of effects should be considered, as should the impact on all affected individuals (Gold et al., 1996). In this latter aspect, the literature on prenatal care has been noticeably deficient. Although prenatal care influences outcomes for two individuals, the mother and her child, the literature on the outcomes of prenatal care is heavily skewed toward a narrow set of fetal outcomes, with only limited recent information on maternal outcomes.

The authors in this book have sought to provide a realistic assessment of the current body of evidence concerning the effectiveness of prenatal care. At the same time, they address contributions and potential contributions of prenatal care that have not been as well recognized and highlight areas where further research is needed to substantiate the true value of prenatal interventions.

The effect of prenatal care on women's health
Complications of pregnancy and chronic illness

As Stubblefield describes in Chapter 1, interventions in the prenatal period have been extremely successful in reducing the risk of child-bearing for all women by reducing morbidity and mortality from such complications of pregnancy as pre-eclampsia. Modern pregnancy management has also permitted women with chronic illnesses, such as diabetes, to have safe pregnancies. These effects are an important part of the impact of prenatal care. However, as Stubblefield notes, because therapies currently exist for most of the life-threatening conditions affecting pregnant women, there are no formal studies (i.e., experimental trials) seeking to demonstrate the value of prenatal care for these conditions. Although he encourages such research, it is with the aim of improving therapies, not in order to substantiate or quantify the impact of current medical interventions for pregnant women.

Although the current low rates of maternal mortality are well documented, there are few studies that address the impact of prenatal care on the comprehensive health of women throughout and following pregnancy. For example, few studies use the more generic health status measurement instruments to assess the impact of interventions on functional status or quality of life of pregnant women. Furthermore, comparatively little research effort has been devoted to assessing different types of prenatal care packages or settings on the health outcomes for women. An important agenda for research is thus to establish the effect of prenatal care on maternal morbidity parallel to work in other health areas, to measure what is clearly an intended outcome of prenatal care.

Health behaviors

Behavioral choices are responsible for a tremendous proportion of the preventable morbidity and mortality affecting the U.S. population generally, but have been the focus of little attention with regard to the allocation of health care resources (McGinnis and Foege, 1993). This pattern holds true in prenatal care. Prenatal care offers an opportunity for providers to institute preventive strategies by focusing on health habits of women during a time when women are particularly receptive to such information. However, as Paine and Garceau's review in Chapter 2 reveals, the literature examining the effectiveness of behavioral interventions in pregnancy is quite limited. Although smoking and alcohol and other drug use cause clear decrements in health outcome, Paine and Garceau found scant research on all but smoking, and some important areas of behavioral change are virtually unresearched. Interventions addressing health behaviors hold promising potential for addressing preventable adverse fetal outcomes, as Rasmussen highlights in Chapter 6 with respect to intrauterine growth restriction. Research to document the impact of behavioral interventions during pregnancy for different groups of women and to assess their long-term preventive worth is a clear priority for future research.

The effectiveness of prenatal care for the child

Prematurity and low birth weight

Perhaps both the most discouraging, and at the same time, heartening, themes in this volume relate to the evidence of the effect of prenatal care on the traditional fetal outcomes of low birth weight and prematurity. The evidence presented by Goldenberg and Rouse, Heffner, and Stoler (Chapters 4, 7, and 9) indicate that, although post-delivery and neonatal interventions have sharply improved survival, current prenatal care interventions have very limited ability to prevent prematurity and low birth weight. Given that many cost-effectiveness studies addressing the value of prenatal care have focused on these outcomes alone, it is not surprising that they have been subject to criticism (Huntington and Connell, 1994).

What is encouraging are descriptions of the advancements in research regarding the pathogenesis of these problems. Savitz and Pastore (Chapter 3) and Goldenberg and Rouse (Chapter 4) cite recent research pointing to a link between bacterial vaginosis and preterm labor. In Chapter 12, Crall notes that new research on the association between severe periodontitis in pregnancy and prematurity may also offer a lead in determining the pathogenesis of adverse outcomes. Thus, it is the hope of several of our authors that current research will provide the foundation for interventions that have a direct effect on prematurity and low birth weight.

Beyond the traditional outcomes

A major point emerging from this volume is that the traditional outcomes of prematurity and low birth weight are not the only important adverse child health outcomes that prenatal care may, now or in the future, strive to prevent. As Stoler describes in Chapter 9, congenital malformations still persist at historic rates with limited information on the etiology and prevention of most. Parad (Chapter 10) and Evans and colleagues (Chapter 11) describe emerging approaches to the diagnosis and treatment of these problems that may become accepted components of prenatal care in the not-so-distant future. Congenital malformations should not be overlooked as part of the burden of adverse fetal outcomes, as failure to account for them will understate the real and potential value of prenatal interventions. This is particularly true because, to the extent that prenatal interventions ultimately are able to prevent premature births, they will probably have an impact on associated congenital malformations.

Researchers and policy makers must look well beyond the divide of delivery to fully appreciate the impact of adverse fetal outcomes on health and the potential value of prenatal care. As McCormick and Nelson describe in their chapters on the long-term outcomes of prematurity and intrauterine growth restriction (Chapters 5 and 8), adverse fetal outcomes increase the risk of a broad range of child health problems. Even if prenatal care is unable to alter birth weight or the distribution of gestational age, prenatal interventions may improve or worsen infant or child morbidity. For example, as Heffner describes in Chapter 7, assessment and timely delivery can improve health outcomes for growth-restricted fetuses, and appropriate care can improve outcomes for small infants who are not growth restricted (and their mothers) by preventing unnecessary intervention. The impact of prenatal care on improving the outcomes for these groups has not been well quantified, and it has not been reflected in cost-effectiveness analyses. Dr. Nelson's discussion of a body of research investigating the potential impact of intrauterine growth restriction on adult-onset chronic illness raises further intriguing questions about the extent to which current research and policies reflect the full importance of interventions to prevent adverse fetal outcomes.

Prenatal care as part of a health care continuum

Assessments of the value of prenatal care may soon need to consider a broader role for this form of health care. Several authors emphasize the importance of placing prenatal care in the context of a continuum of care for women and families. One reason for this is that women have been found to neglect their own health care; prenatal care is one form of care they seek more consistently, and as a result, it is an opportunity to bring women into care more generally.

This argument has a deeper basis, however. The broader goals of prenatal care for women and for children articulated by many of the authors in this book cannot be accomplished during the nine-month span of a pregnancy. Many concerns are much more effectively dealt with before pregnancy. A prime example is reproductive health. The optimal timing of pregnancy is during adulthood, not during adolescence, and should allow for appropriate spacing between pregnancies. Family planning that addresses these issues of timing with respect to a subsequent pregnancy may be an appropriate component of prenatal and postpartum care. However, as argued by Klerman in Chapter 13, if family planning is to successfully address the many ill-timed births and births to adolescents, it clearly needs to begin long before pregnancy, and needs to be a regular component of women's health care between menarche and menopause. Similarly, healthy behaviors related to nutrition, exercise, and substance use, if addressed before pregnancy, could have a significant impact on both the health of mothers and their infants.

Gains in health accomplished during prenatal care can also be expanded and extended if efforts initiated during prenatal care are maintained and linked to ongoing health promotion efforts. As noted above, pregnant women often reduce their use of tobacco, alcohol, and other drugs during pregnancy. They may also improve their diet and address existing medical concerns (e.g., receiving recommended breast and cervical cancer screening) as a result of their prenatal care. These behaviors, if maintained after pregnancy, would enhance the health of women over the longer term as well as that of the family. Similarly, recent studies have demonstrated that carefully targeted home visitation and parenting-support programs that extend substantially beyond what is received during the prenatal and immediate postpartum period can have positive effects on the well-being of children and families (Kitzman et al., 1997; Olds et al., 1997).

The reorientation and reconceptualization of prenatal care as part of a continuum of care faces important obstacles. In Chapter 14, Chavkin and Bernstein discuss the significance of prevalent societal attitudes that frame mother and child as adversaries, in impeding the development of approaches that support the interdependent dyad. As Wise and Brett emphasize in Chapter 15, the success of efforts to link prenatal care to women's health care will depend critically on our ability to develop coordinated systems that span clinical and preventive programs, despite the historical barriers to this type of coordination.

Conclusion

Prenatal care has been regarded using a medical model as a set of interventions designed to cure specific ills that occur during pregnancy, including an initial emphasis on threats to pregnant women's health and a subsequent focus on protection of the fetus. Although health promotion activities have gained ground, most have a limited place in current prenatal care. The authors in this book have argued for greater attention to the causes of decrements to fetal health and to the longer-term health of children and families. They argue for increased attention to research in areas that address these causes, such as investigation of effective strategies to reduce smoking. At the same time, prenatal care delivery must remain cognizant of technological advances in diagnosis, screening, and treatment, including the opportunities they represent as well as the opportunity costs inherent in adopting new interventions.

As Milliez argues in Chapter 16, prenatal care is not an "optional" service, just as pediatrics is not an optional service. Prenatal care is a unique opportunity for delivering care to the infant, mother, and young family. It is important to keep in mind, therefore, that although there are valid questions about the effectiveness and cost-effectiveness of prenatal care as it has been delivered in the past and currently, the relevant question is not the traditional cost-effectiveness one of the value of prenatal care relative to other means of using resources. Instead, the question is how the opportunity of prenatal care can be used to best advantage.

REFERENCES

Alexander GR, Korenbrot CC. The role of prenatal care in preventing low birthweight. The Future of Children 1995; **5**: 103–20.

Fiscella K. Does prenatal care improve birth outcomes? A critical review. Obstetrics and Gynecology 1995; **85**: 468–79.

Gold MR, Siegel JE, Russell L, Weinstein MC, eds. Cost-effectiveness in health and medicine. New York: Oxford University Press, 1996.

Gorsky RD, Colby JP Jr. The cost effectiveness of prenatal care in reducing low birth weight in New Hampshire. Health Services Research 1989; **24**: 583–98.

Huntington J, Connell FA. For every dollar spent—the cost-savings argument for prenatal care. New England Journal of Medicine 1994; **331**: 1303–7.

Institute of Medicine (IOM), Committee to Study the Prevention of Low Birth Weight.

Preventing low birthweight. Washington (DC): National Academy Press, 1985.

Kitzman H, Olds DL, Henderson CR, et al. Effect of prenatal and infancy home visitation by nurses on pregnancy outcomes, childhood injuries, and repeated childbearing. Journal of the American Medical Association 1997; **278**: 644–52.

Kogan MD, Martin JA, Alexander GR, et al. The changing pattern of prenatal care utilization in the United States, 1981–1995, using different prenatal care indices. Journal of the American Medical Association 1998; **279**: 1623–28.

Korenbrot CC. Risk reduction in pregnancies of low-income women: comprehensive prenatal care through the OB Access Project. Mobius 1984; **4**: 34–43.

McGinnis JM, Foege WH. Actual causes of death in the United States. Journal of the American Medical Association 1993; **270**: 2207–12.

Olds DL, Eckenrode J, Henderson CR, et al. Long-term effects of home visitation on maternal life course and child abuse and neglect: fifteen-year follow-up of a randomized trial. Journal of the American Medical Association 1997; **278**: 637–43.

Schramm WF. Weighing costs and benefits of adequate prenatal care for 12 023 births in Missouri's Medicaid program, 1988. Public Health Reports 1992; **107**: 647–52.

Index

Page numbers in *italics* refer to figures and tables